OXFORD MEDICAL PUBLICATIONS

PATHOLOGY IN DENTISTRY

Pathology in Dentistry

•

EDWARD SHEFFIELD

Consultant Senior Lecturer,
Department of Pathology, University of Bristol and
Bristol Royal Infirmary

Oxford New York Melbourne
OXFORD UNIVERSITY PRESS
1996

Oxford University Press, Walton Street, Oxford OX2 6DP

Oxford New York
Athens Auckland Bangkok Bombay
Calcutta Cape Town Dar es Salaam Delhi
Florence Hong Kong Istanbul Karachi
Kuala Lumpur Madras Madrid Melbourne
Mexico City Nairobi Paris Singapore
Taipei Tokyo Toronto
and associated companies in
Berlin Ibadan

Oxford is a trade mark of Oxford University Press

Published in the United States
by Oxford University Press Inc., New York

A catalogue record for this book is available from the British Library

Library of Congress Cataloging in Publication Data
Sheffield, Edward
Pathology in dentistry/Edward Sheffield.—1st ed.
p. cm.—(Oxford medical publications)
Includes bibliographical references and index.
1. Pathology. 2. Dentistry. I. Title. II. Series.
[DNLM: 1. Dentistry. 2. Pathology. WU 140 1995]
RB111.S444 1995 617.6'07—dc20 95–1213
DNLM/DLC for Library of Congress
ISBN 0 19 262422 9 (Hbk)
ISBN 0 19 262421 0 (Pbk)

Typeset by Cotswold Typesetting Ltd, Gloucester
Printed in Hong Kong

PREFACE

This book is written primarily for undergraduate dental students and aims to present pathology in a way relevant to dentistry. Many pathological processes are the same wherever they occur in the body, and pathology is a subject that underpins a great deal of medicine. A grounding in pathology is therefore an essential part of dental training.

The book follows the traditional structure of many textbooks in that there is a section on general pathology followed by systemic pathology. The section on general pathology covers all important aspects of the subject whilst the systemic section tends to have a bias towards areas that are particularly important to dentists. I have also produced a compact book; many demands are made on students' time and if further reading is required in more depth, a list of useful sources is provided. Pathology is a particularly visual subject and therefore much use is made of illustrations and diagrams.

The book generally follows the undergraduates' preclinical course in pathology and the clinical course in human disease given to Bristol dental students, and I appreciate the help that the opportunity to teach these students has given me in the preparation of this book. I wish to acknowledge the advice and help given to me by my colleagues in Bristol. I also acknowledge the help of Dr J. Eveson and Dr C. Kennedy in supplying clinical photographs. Finally, I acknowledge the patience of my family for the time that I have taken from them during the preparation of this book.

Bristol
August 1995

E.S.

CONTENTS

FURTHER READING

Underwood, J. C. E. (1992). *General and systemic pathology*. Churchill Livingstone, Edinburgh.

Cotran, R. S., Kumar, V., and Robbins, S. L. (1994). *Pathologic basis of disease*, (5th edn). W. B. Saunders, Philadelphia.

McGee, J. O'D., Isaacson, P. G., and Wright, N. A. (1992). *Oxford textbook of pathology*. Oxford University Press.

Roitt, I. M., Brostoff, J., and Male, D. K. (1993). *Immunology*, (3rd edn). Mosby, London.

Austyn, J. M. and Wood, K. J. (1993). *Principles of cellular and molecular immunology*. Oxford University Press.

Walter, J. B. and Grundy, M. C. (1993). *Walter, Hamilton and Israel's principles of pathology for dental students*, (5th edn). Churchill Livingstone, Edinburgh.

1 Cellular pathology

1 Cellular pathology

PATHOLOGY is the study of biological processes that underlie disease. There are processes, such as inflammation and immunological reactions, which are similar whatever site or organ system is involved. These processes are covered in the sections on general pathology. Different organ systems have specific disease processes which are covered in the sections on systemic pathology.

CLASSIFICATION OF DISEASE

Disease processes can be classified into a number of different groups. There are different ways this can be done; one such system is given in Table 1.1.

Table 1.1 Classification of disease

Congenital
Acquired
Infective
Nutritional
Environmental
Neoplastic
Inflammatory
Immunological
Vascular
Metabolic
Degenerative

Congenital abnormalities

Human cells contain 46 chromosomes (22 pairs of autosomes, and a pair of sex chromosomes, XX in females and XY in males). Some disorders have both an environmental and genetic origin. However, there are many disorders in which genetic abnormalities involve either large portions of chromosomes, or involve abnormalities of individual genes. These genetic abnormalities are known as mutations. In the case of gene abnormalities, the mutation may only involve one base pair. The term aneuploid is used when the number of chromosomes is not an exact number of a half set (the haploid number, 23). Extra chromosomes may occur, or there may be loss of complete chromosomes. There may be actual structural abnormalities of the chromosomes, with duplication, inversion, deletion, or translocation (movement of one part of a chromosome to another) of chromosome fragments.

The chromosome that carries an abnormal gene may be a sex chromosome (X or Y) or any of the remaining 22 pairs of chromosomes (autosomes). *Alleles* are two genes at an identical place on a pair of chromosomes. If clinical expression of a gene defect requires both alleles to be abnormal, the condition is said to be *recessive*. If only one gene is required to be abnormal, the condition is said to be *dominant*.

A '*carrier*' state can therefore occur in recessive conditions, for example in cystic fibrosis. If both parents are carriers, there is a 1 in 4 chance of a child developing the disease. Genetic abnormalities, as in the case of cystic fibrosis, do not, however, always fully express themselves. Some important conditions associated with genetic abnormalities are described below.

Congenital metabolic abnormalities

These are conditions in which there is a genetic defect that interferes with a particular metabolic pathway. There is usually an abnormality of a gene that is responsible for coding for a particular enzyme or protein. This results in either a structural defect in the enzyme or reduced synthesis of the protein. The genetic defect runs in families, rather than being due to an acquired mutation during early development.

The abnormal function of an enzyme may result in either a reduced production of a metabolite, or an accumulation of an intermediate metabolite, which cannot be metabolized further. Examples of such conditions are:

Phenylketonuria

This is one of the common serious defects in which there is a deficiency of an enzyme called phenylalanine hydroxylase, which converts phenylalanine to tyrosine. Phenylalanine is an amino acid which is derived from the breakdown of proteins in the diet. There is therefore an accumulation of phenylalanine and its metabolite, phenylpyruvic acid, in the body. Children with this defect present at an early age with cerebral damage resulting in mental retardation, loss of skin and hair pigmentation, and fits. The disease occurs in about 1 in 10 000 births, and is now screened for in the population. Treatment is to avoid phenylalanine in the diet until the child is about 8 years old when other metabolic pathways take over the metabolism of this amino acid.

Gaucher's disease

This is a disease where there is accumulation of large amounts of a substance called sphingomyelin, a specialized type of lipid. This occurs because of a defect in an enzyme called glucocerebrosidase. This enzyme is normally found in lysosomes, which are spherical spaces surrounded by membrane present in the cytoplasm of all cells. Lysosomes are generally involved in the breakdown or digestion of molecules or material that the cell has ingested. They contain specialized enzymes such as hydrolases. The material that cannot be metabolized in Gaucher's disease causes defects in cellular function. Lysosomal storage diseases occur when there is a congenital abnormality of an enzyme found in lysosomes. They usually manifest as an accumulation of a metabolic product which cannot be cleared due to a deficiency of a specific enzyme.

Cystic fibrosis

This is the commonest, potentially lethal, congenital defect, which involves an abnormality of a gene found on chromosome 7 coding for a protein which forms chloride channels in cell membranes. The defect is autosomal recessive in type and is found in about 1 in 20 of the population which means the abnormality should occur in about 1 in 400 births. In fact it occurs in 1 in 2000 births due to incomplete expression.

The chloride channel abnormality causes excessively thick secretions in exocrine (ducted) glands. This causes chronic obstruction in organs, such as the liver and pancreas, together with chronic infection in the lung. Liver cirrhosis, chronic pancreatitis, and bronchiectasis in the lung may result. Infants with cystic fibrosis usually present with poor growth and persistent respiratory infection.

The underlying biochemical defect is a reduced reabsorption of chloride from exocrine secretory ducts. The secretion of sodium and chloride is normal, but the impaired chloride absorption causes retention of sodium in the duct. One feature of patients with cystic fibrosis is an increased sodium chloride secretion in the sweat. In the lung there is reduced chloride secretion and therefore reduced sodium secretion onto the mucosal surface. The net effect of these abnormalities is to increase the viscosity of many secretions.

Congenital abnormalities of development

These are defined as abnormalities present at birth, and up to 5 per cent of births show some degree of chromosomal abnormality. It is frequently possible to predict the nature of the underlying chromosomal abnormality by documenting all the apparent anatomical abnormalities and referring to a reference source.

There are many congenital developmental syndromes that are associated with abnormalities of tooth development. These are listed in Table 1.2.

The most common example of a chromosomal abnormality causing severe abnormality is Down's syndrome.

Table 1.2 Abnormalities of tooth development

Cleft lip/palate
Down's syndrome
Ectodermal hypoplasia
Cleidocranial dysplasia
Gardner syndrome

Down's syndrome

This occurs in approximately 1 in 1000 births and is associated with a chromosomal abnormality in which there is an extra chromosome 21 (trisomy 21). Clinical features include retarded mental development, a flat facial appearance, oblique eyelids, and abnormalities of the hands and ears. There is an increased incidence (up to 40 per cent) of congenital heart disease, most commonly septal defects. The risk of Down's syndrome increases with maternal age.

Sex-linked disorders

There is a group of congenital disorders in which the genetic abnormality is found on the X chromosome. Most are recessive, and a well-known X-linked condition is haemophilia. Females with a haemophilia gene do not express the disease, but are *carriers* of the condition in that male children of a female carrier develop the condition.

Developmental abnormalities of organs

Agenesis

This is when an organ fails to fully develop. For example, there may be renal agenesis, the person having only one kidney. Congenital absence of teeth occurs in about 5 per cent of the population (anodontia or hypodontia), and may involve some or all of the teeth. There may be supernumerary teeth (hyperdontia).

Atresia

This is the failure to develop an opening or lumen during fetal development. There may be atresia of a heart valve or of part of the gastrointestinal tract.

Hypoplasia

This is when an organ fails to develop to its full size, for example, the lung in some cases of congenital heart disease. Microdontia is an abnormally small tooth.

Dysgenesis

This term is applied to an organ when it fails to mature fully in embryonic life. Tissue remains that is normally only present in fetal life. There may be marked distortion of development (Fig. 1.1).

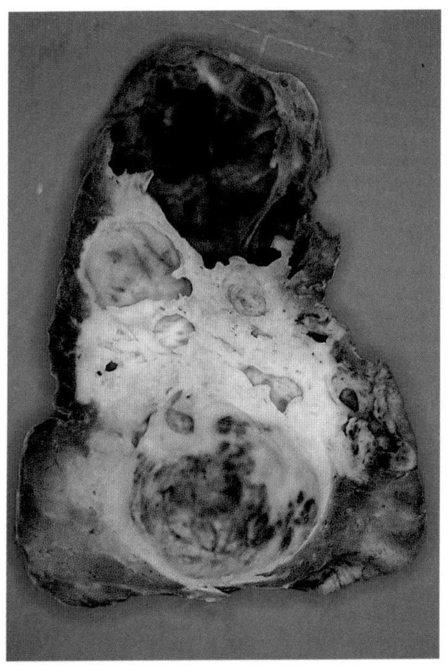

Fig. 1.1 A lung showing a congenital adenomatoid malformation, which is a developmental abnormality which has distorted the lung architecture.

Ectopia

If an organ or part of an organ is found in the wrong place in the body the terms *ectopia* or *heterotopia* are applied. A kidney may be found in the pelvis instead of in its normal position. If there is an additional part of a gland in an abnormal part of the body, the word *accessory* is applied, for example in the case of some adrenal cortex being found in the testis.

Dysplasia

This term is sometimes applied when an organ is abnormally formed in development. For example a kidney may show disordered development, or a tooth

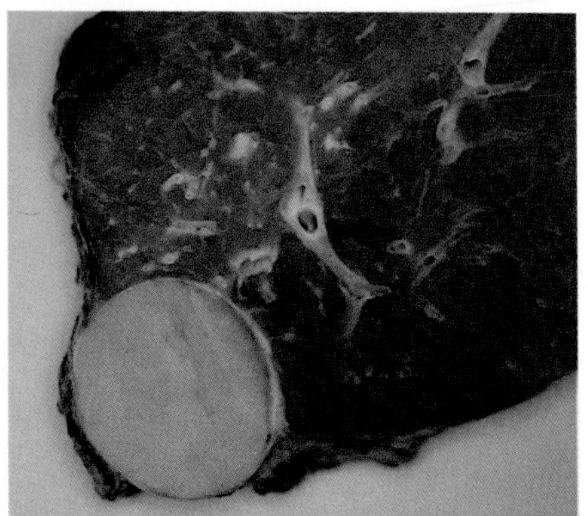

Fig. 1.2 An enteric cyst in the lung filled with mucus.

may show deformity (for example, dilaceration, in which the crown is out of alignment). However, the term *dysplasia* is now usually applied to a lesion which is on the path to cancer development

Cysts

Cysts arising from developmental abnormalities or remnants can be included here. Relevant cysts are *dermoid* cysts, arising from inclusions of skin at embryonic fusion lines in the face, and *branchial* (lymphoepithelial) cysts arising from branchial cleft remnants or salivary gland ducts. Cysts lined by gastric and other intestinal epithelium occasionally occur in the floor of the mouth; these may also be seen in the lung (Fig. 1.2).

Carcinogenesis

The underlying cause of cancer is genetic and many genes are now known to be associated with an increased risk of developing cancer. The association between genetic abnormalities and cancer is covered in the section on carcinogenesis in Chapter 4.

Congenital dental abnormalities

Congenital absence of the teeth is relatively common, occurring in up to 7 per cent of the population. The third molars, permanent maxillary lateral incisors, and second premolars are the teeth most frequently absent. Supernumerary teeth are well described. Many abnormalities of tooth development are associated with congenital syndromes. These include cleft lip or palate, Down's syndrome, and disorders of bone development. Abnormalities of tooth development are described where teeth may be fused or otherwise abnormally united. Congenital syphilis is classically described as producing characteristic hypoplastic changes in the enamel due to damage of the tooth germ by infection by spirochaetes. This gives a characteristic central notch (Hutchinson's incisors). The developmental condition of amelogenesis imperfecta is an inherited abnormality of enamel. Teeth are ectodermal in origin, and this condition involves an abnormality of this layer. It is an autosomal dominant or X-linked condition. There may be abnormal calcification of the teeth, or an abnormal development of the enamel. The teeth may be immature and malformed.

Acquired abnormalities

Infective disorders

Infective causes can be classified into: viruses, bacteria, yeasts, fungi, and parasites. Generally, infections are either due to inherently virulent organisms or they are due to organisms that take advantage of reduced host immunity, termed opportunistic infections.

Viral infections

Viruses and related clinical disease are summarized in Table 1.3.

Respiratory tract infection

Most upper respiratory tract infections are due to rhinoviruses, adenoviruses, and echoviruses. Both echovirus and rhinovirus are single-stranded RNA viruses, adenoviruses being double-stranded DNA viruses. Parainfluenza virus causes upper respiratory tract infection and croup in young children. Rhinoviruses are the main

Table 1.3 Viruses and clinical disease

Virus	Clinical disease
Adenovirus	Common cold, viral pneumonia
Hepatitis	
Hepatitis A	Viral hepatitis
Hepatitis B	
Hepatitis C	
Herpesviruses	
Herpesvirus 1, 2	Vesicular eruptions on mucous membranes and skin, encephalitis
Varicella zoster	Chickenpox, shingles
Cytomegalovirus	Opportunistic viral infection
Epstein–Barr	Glandular fever (infectious mononucleosis)
Myxovirus	
Influenza	Respiratory infection
Respiratory syncytial virus	
Parainfluenza	
Measles	Measles
Mumps	Mumps
Papilloma virus	Many types, with association with epithelial tumours
Picornavirus	
Poliovirus	Poliomyelitis
Coxsackieviruses A, B	Encephalitis, myocarditis, respiratory infection, pancreatitis
Echovirus	Central nervous system disease
Rhinovirus	Common cold
Retrovirus	
Human T cell leukaemia virus (HTLV)	Leukaemia
Human immunodeficiency virus (HIV)	Acquired immunodeficiency syndrome (AIDS)
Togavirus	Rubella (German measles)

cause of the common cold. Lower respiratory tract infections can be due to influenza virus and respiratory syncytial virus, and parainfluenza virus in children.

Mumps

This is a childhood condition caused by a paramyxovirus which presents as acute painful swelling and inflammation of the parotid glands and sometimes other salivary glands. It can involve other organs such as the testes, ovaries, pancreas, and the brain. In children, it is usually a mild self-limiting disease, but in adults may be more severe, causing organ atrophy.

Enteritis

Rotaviruses are a common cause of diarrhoea in children, being responsible from one-third to one-half of all cases of childhood enteritis. There is a group of self-limiting diarrhoeal viral infections which appear to be due to viruses known as Norwalk agents.

Herpes viruses

There are two main types of herpes viruses which are important in human infection, herpes simplex type 1 and herpes simplex type 2. Infection usually presents as bullous eruptions on the skin or mucous membranes. Generally, herpes simplex type 1 infections occur in the upper part of the body and herpes simplex type 2 infections occur in the lower part of the body, particularly the genital tract. Herpes simplex virus is a cause of so-called cold sores that occur around the lips and nose. Herpes simplex may also involve the brain and cause a very serious form of encephalitis which generally involves the temporal lobes. Genital herpes, due to the type 2 virus, is characterized by large numbers of vesicles on the mucous membranes and the external genital skin. In immunosuppression, the virus may cause opportunistic infection with extensive damage to organs.

Varicella-zoster virus

This virus causes two conditions, chicken pox and herpes zoster. Chicken pox is a highly contagious disease of childhood which is characterized by a vesicular skin eruption. It is usually a very mild self-limiting disease and only creates problems in patients with immunodeficiency where it may cause overwhelming infection with pneumonia or encephalitis. After infection and resolution of chicken pox, the varicella-zoster virus lies latent within sensory dorsal root ganglia in the spinal cord. If the patient subsequently becomes immunosuppressed, herpes zoster may result, which is also known as shingles. This effectively is re-activation of the latent varicella-zoster virus and the symptoms relate to the nerve distribution of the sensory nerve involved.

Cytomegalovirus

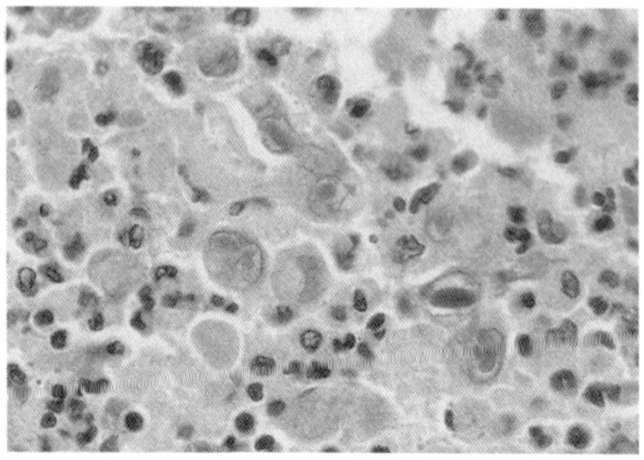

Fig. 1.3 Large purple cytomegalovirus inclusions are seen in nuclei in these lung epithelial cells (bottom right).

This is a very common infection which has many variable presentations depending on the clinical situation and the age of the patient. It may be acquired in the uterus following infection of the mother. It may be acquired during birth, via respiratory transmission in children and adults, by blood transfusion, and organ transplantation. Infection of a fetus may cause serious cerebral damage. Cytomegalovirus infections are very common in the population, most people having acquired the infection with very mild or no clinical symptoms. As with varicella-zoster virus, the infection lies latent and only causes clinical problems if the patient becomes immunocompromised due to, for instance, chemotherapy or AIDS. Cytomegalovirus is a well-recognized cause of viral pneumonia in immunocompromised patients. Cytomegalovirus infection can be recognized by characteristic viral inclusions on histology (Fig. 1.3).

Infectious mononucleosis (glandular fever)

In the West, infectious mononucleosis is primarily a disease of young adulthood. In the rest of the world, however, infectious mononucleosis occurs at a much younger age group. Infectious mononucleosis is caused by the Epstein–Barr virus (EBV), which belongs to the herpes virus group. The name glandular fever comes from the characteristic clinical symptoms of enlarged lymph nodes, fever, and sore throat. Large activated T lymphocytes are seen in the peripheral blood which are reacting against infected B lymphocytes. EBV is frequently secreted in the saliva and is transmitted by kissing and other methods of transmission of saliva. The virus selectively infects B lymphocytes and induces a B lymphocyte proliferation which is then limited by a T cell response. EBV becomes incorporated into the genome of infected cells, and becomes latent. In general, it is a self-limiting disease, although vague symptoms may persist for many months. EBV infection is associated with Burkitt's lymphoma and nasopharyngeal carcinoma.

Human immunodeficiency virus (HIV)

It is now clear that human immunodeficiency virus (HIV) is closely associated with acquired immunodeficiency syndrome (AIDS). HIV is transmitted primarily by body fluids, particularly blood. High-risk groups include homosexuals, intravenous drug abusers, haemophiliacs receiving contaminated factor VIII concentrates, any sort of recipients of blood components, and heterosexual contacts with high-risk groups. HIV is a human retrovirus which primarily infects T cells. There are many different types of HIV, HIV-1 being the most common type. The CD4 molecule on T helper lymphocytes has an affinity for the HIV virus, and therefore T helper cells are primarily infected. There is a glycoprotein expressed on the surface of the virus called gp120 which has an affinity for the CD4 molecule. There is evidence that T cell activation is required for viral infection. HIV is closely related to the human T cell leukaemia virus type 1 (HTLV-1). HIV is an RNA virus with a reverse transcriptase that produces DNA from the RNA genome. Two strands of RNA are present in the viral core. HIV is a lentivirus in that there is a long period between infection and clinical disease.

The initial infection is followed by a mild infleunza-like illness during which an antibody response is mounted and the immune system destroys infected cells. However, the virus is not completely eliminated, and virus replication continues for many years. There is a gradual decrease in the number of circulating T helper cells which mirrors the decrease in cell-mediated immunity. Only a small proportion of these helper T cells are infected; it is possible that non-infected T cells also become the target for the immune system. HIV may also be causing apoptosis, a form of self-induced death. AIDS is almost always a fatal disease. There appears to be little risk of infection of HIV from normal contact in the community, infection requiring blood-to-blood transmission. The risk from infection by occupational exposure to patients is also very small. There is a small risk of infection from accidental needlestick injuries, which has been estimated at 0.5 per cent. There is a very high level of HIV-infected cells in lymph nodes, particularly in early infection. This correlates with the frequent widespread lymph node enlargement seen early in HIV infection. It appears that the first cells to be infected are the antigen-presenting cells which are members of the mononuclear–phagocyte system, which also carry the CD4 molecule. AIDS does not occur in patients who do not have HIV. Although there is a long delay between infection and clinical disease, which can be as much as 15 years, practically all HIV-positive cases eventually become immunosuppressed. The striking feature in AIDS is reduction in the number of CD4 positive helper T cells in the circulation. HIV binds to the CD4 molecule, and then it is transported to the cytoplasm. Reverse transcriptase then acts forming a proviral DNA which then is integrated into the genome of the infected cell. The DNA is then transcribed into RNA which then codes for proteins of the HIV virus. Eventually intact complete virus particles bud from the surface of the infected cell. HIV infection eventually causes death of infected T cells. The cause of this is not clear but death may be due to accumulation of products of the HIV virus or destruction of cells may be due to the host immune system. Other cells express HIV virus, including cells of the monocyte–macrophage system. However, these cells seem resistant to the cytotoxic effects of the virus. Another important site of infection by HIV is the brain. Damage to nerve cells is a striking feature of AIDS. There is evidence that damage to the neurones is due to high levels of the gp120 protein which causes changes in calcium levels within neurones and damage due to

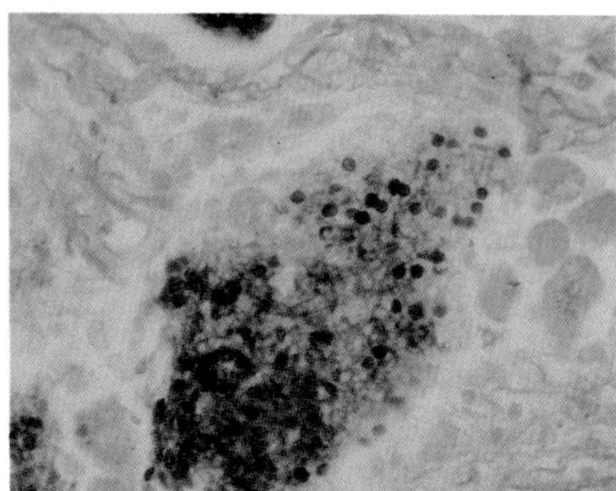

Fig. 1.4 Silver stained pneumocystis organisms in lung exudate are seen as small black spheres.

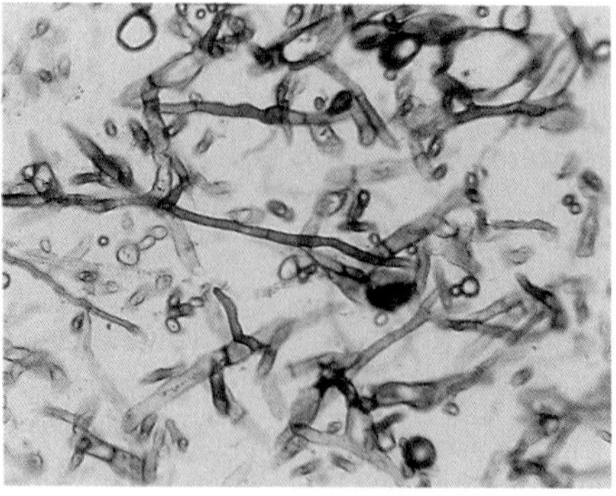

Fig. 1.5 Silver stain showing *Aspergillus* hyphae, seen as branching filaments.

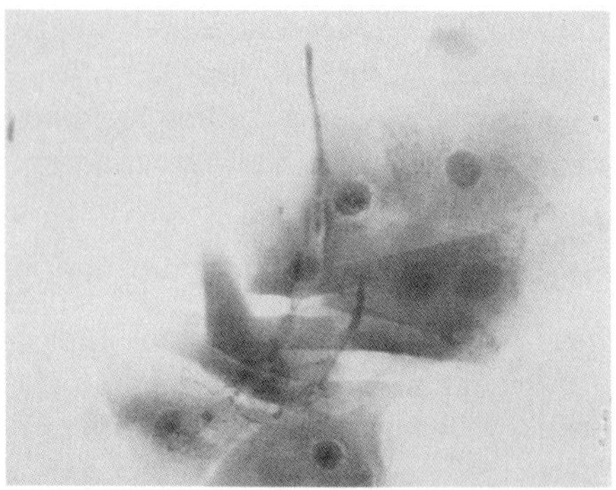

Fig. 1.6 *Candida albicans* pseudohyphae in a throat smear.

over-excitation. The virus appears to infect the connective tissue cells of the brain (the glial cells) and these cells produce a neurotoxic agent.

The main effects of HIV infection are the reduction in CD4-positive helper cells in the circulation, reduction in T cell function, and general stimulation of B cells in a polyclonal fashion. There is also alteration in function of the cells of the monocyte–macrophage system. The generalized reduction in cell-mediated immunity increases the susceptibility of the person to opportunistic infections, particularly intracellular organisms. These include tuberculosis, including typical and atypical forms, pneumocystis (Fig. 1.4) and similar protozoa, fungal infections including *Aspergillus* (Fig. 1.5), *Candida* (Fig. 1.6), *Nocardia*, and overwhelming viral infections. Frequent viral infections seen in AIDS include the activation of cytomegalovirus, varicella-zoster virus, and Epstein–Barr virus. AIDS patients are also prone to developing an unusual vascular proliferation of the skin which may be a tumour or may be a viral-driven process called Kaposi's sarcoma. There is an increased incidence of lymphoma with AIDS, also linked to Epstein–Barr virus.

The virus very rapidly changes its characteristics over time. The reverse transcriptase enzyme has a high error rate, inducing mutations, allowing selection of advantageous forms of the virus. It is therefore difficult for the immune system to mount an effective response; it also makes the production of an effective vaccine very difficult. Drugs that interfere with the viral replication cycle, for instance azidothymidine (AZT) which blocks the action of reverse transcriptase, have been tried with limited success. Prevention still remains the best way of dealing with the disease. Oral diseases caused by infection associated with AIDS are summarized in Table 1.4.

Table 1.4 Oral diseases associated with AIDS

Candida
Necrotizing gingivitis
Herpes simplex
Varicella-zoster
Epstein–Barr virus (hairy leukoplakia)
Cytomegalovirus
Kaposi's sarcoma

The next two microorganisms are not viruses, but are also intracellular organisms and so are included here.

Chlamydia

Chlamydial diseases are caused by intracellular organisms, which are slightly larger than viruses, but are similar to bacteria in that they have a cell wall. They can be recognized histologically by the characteristic vacuolation that they cause in the cell cytoplasm of infected cells. They need to be within cells to multiply. There are three main species, *Chlamydia trachomatis*, *C. psittaci*, and *C. pneumoniae*. Types A, B, and C of *C. trachomatis* are the cause of the disease trachoma, a leading cause of blindness in the developing world. Types D to K are sexually transmitted and are a common cause of acute non-gonococcal urethritis in men and a common cause of acute epididymitis. In females, chlamydial infection causes acute or chronic follicular cervicitis and is a frequent cause of pelvic inflammatory disease. *Chlamydia trachomatis* infection can also cause reactive arthritis, previously known as Reiter's disease. In babies, infection can cause conjunctivitis and pneumonia.

Chlamydia psittaci is a cause of psittacosis, a pneumonia caused by aspiration of infected particles from birds. *Chlamydia trachomatis* is also a cause of lymphogranuloma venereum.

Mycoplasma

These are organisms that resemble bacteria which have a deficient cell wall, so-called L-forms. They are very small free-living organisms, and in humans are a frequent cause of primary atypical pneumonia. Clinical features are very similar to viral pneumonia. There is marked epithelial damage, but it is usually self-limiting.

Bacterial infections

The main groups of pyogenic ('pus-forming') bacteria are summarized in Table 1.5. Staphylococci are a frequent cause of acute pyogenic infection, particularly in surgical wound infection, skin infection, respiratory infections, and impetigo. Staphylococci can also cause infective endocarditis, toxic shock syndrome, and may also produce a toxin which is a cause of food poisoning. *Staphylococcus aureus* is a prime cause of abscesses, and particularly in the case of the lung can cause destructive multiple abscesses. The beta-haemolytic streptococci are best known for causing non-infective complications such as scarlet fever, rheumatic fever, and glomerulonephritis. Pneumococcus is a well-known cause of lobar pneumonia and meningitis. Meningococcus is a frequent cause of acute purulent meningitis. Gonococcus is the cause of the sexually transmitted disease gonorrhoea.

Dental caries is associated with *Streptococcus mutans*, among other oral bacteria. The primary cause of dental caries appears to be the action of acid on the enamel causing decalcification. The acid is derived from the action of bacteria on carbohydrates in the diet. Bacteria present in dental plaque convert sugars in the diet to acid, particularly lactic acid. A very acid microenvironment is then formed against the surface of the enamel, giving rise to leaching out of calcium.

Other normal oral bacteria are:

- *Actinomyces*.
- *Veillonella*.
- Gram-negative rods.

Gram-negative bacteria are summarized in Table 1.6. These are all a frequent cause of opportunistic pneumonia, septicaemia, endocarditis, wound infection, and urinary tract infection. Many Gram-negative bacteria also produce endotoxins which are capable of inducing shock. Bacteroides species, which are frequent in the gut, are a cause of anaerobic infection. *Legionella* species are also Gram-negative bacteria and cause legionnaire's disease. Bacteria causing enteric infections are summarized in Table 1.7—These are all recognized causes of gastroenteritis.

Table 1.5 Pyogenic organisms

Staphylococcus aureus
Staphylococcus epidermidis
Streptococcus pyogenes
Beta-haemolytic streptococci
Streptococcus pneumoniae (Pneumococcus)
Neisseria meningitidis (meningococcus)
Neisseria gonorrhoea (gonococcus)

Table 1.6 Gram-negative bacteria

Escherichia coli
Klebsiella
Proteus species
Pseudomonas
Bacteroides
Enterobacter

Table 1.7 Bacteria causing enteric infections

Pathogenic *E. coli* (e.g. subtype 0127)
Shigella
Vibrio cholerae
Campylobacter
Yersinia
Salmonella

Clostridia

Clostridium tetani—This is a cause of tetanus.

Clostridium botulinum—This is capable of producing a very potent toxin and is a cause of food poisoning. The toxin acts as a neurotransmitter inhibitor and causes paralysis.

Clostridium perfringens—This is a cause of gas gangrene.

Clostridium difficile—This is a cause of pseudomembranous colitis. It frequently colonizes the bowel, particularly in antibiotic treatment, and the bacterium produces a toxin which causes extensive epithelial damage to the colonic epithelium.

Actinomyces

Nocardia and *Actinomyces* are filamentous organisms which share some characteristics of bacteria and fungi. *Nocardia* is an important opportunistic infection in immunosuppressed patients.

Actinomyces can invade soft tissue and colonize wounds following surgery, for example following removal of an appendix, or following dental surgery.

Treponemal infection

Historically, the most important treponemal infection is *Treponema pallidum*, the cause of syphilis. *Treponema pallidum* is a spiral-shaped spirochaete which is approximately 12 micrometres long. It is extremely motile and is primarily a sexually transmitted systemic disease. It can also be transmitted across the placenta from the mother to fetus resulting in congenital syphilis.

Primary syphilis

After initial infection, there is a latent incubation period of approximately three weeks, but this may extend to three months. This is characterized by the development of a chancre, an ulcer with a raised edge and a red centre which occurs at the site of infection. There is a heavy chronic inflammatory infiltrate associated with the chancre with obliteration of small blood vessels. Numerous treponemes are seen in the exudate over the chancre. Regional lymph nodes are also enlarged. At the same time there is a dissemination of spirochaetes throughout the body. The chancre heals within several weeks and then there are no further clinical symptoms.

Secondary syphilis

This follows the primary infection after a time period of several weeks up to six months. The most striking feature is a generalized skin rash. This skin rash is self-limiting and resolves within one to two months. There may also be mucosal involvement, particularly the mucosa of the oral cavity. Red mucosal patches appear in the mouth which shows a chronic inflammatory infiltrate. Linear 'snail-track' oral mucosal lesions also develop. There may also be fever and generalized lymphadenopathy. Syphilis then again enters a long latent period which may last 10 or 20 years.

Tertiary syphilis

The underlying pathology of syphilis, particularly in the tertiary phase, is that of an obliterative inflammation of small blood vessels, known as obliterative endarteritis, and periarteritis. There is also very typically a heavy plasma cell infiltrate which suggests the diagnosis on histology. Small vessels show a concentric proliferation of the intima which slowly occludes the lumen. Common manifestations of tertiary syphilis are in the cardiovascular system, with inflammation of the aorta and aneurysm formation, particularly of the ascending aorta. There is also involvement of the central nervous system with meningo-vascular involvement and involvement of the posterior columns of the spinal cord called tabes dorsalis. This is also the cause of general paralysis of the insane, so-called general paresis. Another manifestation of syphilis is the gumma, which is an area of well-circumscribed necrosis, frequently found in the liver, testis, and bones. Gumma may also be seen in the skin or in the mucosa of the mouth. About a third of infected patients develop tertiary syphilis which may occur many years after the primary infection.

Congenital syphilis

This is infection of the fetus from the mother. Congenital syphilis is characterized by multiple congenital abnormalities, particularly involving the liver, lungs, and central nervous system. A very characteristic dental abnormality is defective formation of enamel which results in notching of the occlusive margins of the incisors. These are called Hutchinson's teeth.

It is fortunate that syphilis has maintained sensitivity to penicillin despite widespread treatment by this antibiotic.

Infections of the mouth

Viral infections

Common viral infections of the mouth include herpes simplex virus types 1 and 2 which causes herpetic stomatitis. Varicella-zoster virus causes chicken pox and shingles. Coxsackie A viruses cause herpangina, and hand, foot, and mouth disease. Epstein–Barr virus causes infectious mononucleosis and is also associated with development of Burkitt's lymphoma and nasopharyngeal carcinoma.

Bacterial infections

It has been claimed that gingivitis is the most common infection in the world. However, the most common bacterial infection to involve the teeth is dental caries. This is loss of enamel due to the action of organisms found in the mouth. As mentioned previously, the primary cause of dental caries appears to be the action of acid on the enamel giving rise to decalcification.

Opportunistic infections are frequently seen in the mouth. Many clinical bacterial infections of the mouth are due to a disturbance in the normal relationships between bacterial normally found in the mouth. One example of this is acute ulcerative gingivitis. There appears to be an over-growth of bacteria in this condition due to a disturbance of the normal symbiotic relationship between organisms. Actionomycosis is a recognized complication of infection of the mouth, particularly of tooth sockets. *Actinomyces* are filamentous organisms which can colonize and invade soft tissues surrounding a tooth extraction. Secondary syphilis may present as mucosal lesions in the mouth; this is now less common.

Fungi

The most frequent fungal infection of the mouth is *Candida*. It is most frequently an opportunistic infection occurring when there is disturbance in normal immune function, for example in AIDS. Immunosuppression due to chemotherapy may also be complicated with oral candidiasis.

Human immunodeficiency virus infection (HIV) and acquired immunodeficiency syndrome (AIDS)

HIV has been dealt with in more detail on p. 00, but the evidence is now very strong that HIV is associated with AIDS. Oral infective manifestations of AIDS include chronic candidosis and chronic gingivitis including necrotizing gingivitis. Opportunistic viral infections occur including Epstein–Barr virus, cytomegalovirus, herpes

Table 1.8 Organisms causing disease in the mouth

Bacteria	
Streptococci	Dental caries
Staphylococci, anaerobes	Periapical abscess
Fusobacteria, spirochaetes	Necrotizing ulcerative gingivitis
Actinomycosis	Chronic suppurative inflammation
Mycobacteria	Tuberculosis, leprosy
Gonorrhoea	Acute inflammatory lesions
Syphilis	Chancre, oral plaques, gumma
Fungi	
Candida	Oral candidiasis
Mucor species	Deep invasive infection (diabetics)
Viruses	
Human papilloma virus	Papillomata
Herpes simplex	Stomatitis
Varicella-zoster	Shingles
Epstein–Barr	Glandular fever
Coxsackie A	Hand, foot, and mouth disease
	Herpangina
Echovirus, rhinovirus	Pharyngitis

simplex virus, human papilloma virus, and varicella-zoster virus. Unusual organisms seen in AIDS include cryptococcus, histoplasmosis, and in certain areas of the world, blastomycosis, coccidioidomycosis, and parcoccidioidomycosis. It is probable that the development of some tumours in the mouth, particular Kaposi's sarcoma, lymphoma, and squamous cell carcinoma are also caused by viral infection.

A summary of organisms that cause disease in the mouth is given in Table 1.8.

Nutritional disorders

Vitamin deficiency

Vitamin deficiencies and malnutrition due to an imbalance between dietary protein, fat, and carbohydrate will be covered. Serious nutritional deficiency, as well as having general effects, may interfere with tooth development.

A deficiency of a vitamin leads to a specific group of clinical features. This is because vitamins are involved at key points in particular metabolic pathways. Vitamins A, D, E, and K are fat-soluble vitamins; the others are water-soluble. The major vitamins (and trace elements) and the effects of deficiency are described in Table 1.9. Vitamins are necessary dietary factors that are required for specific metabolic pathways that cannot be synthesized. Some common vitamins and conditions of deficiency are described below.

Vitamin C (ascorbic acid) An important function of vitamin C is in collagen synthesis, where it acts as a cofactor for an enzyme important for allowing procollagen fibrils to cross-link. A deficiency causes scurvy. Clinical consequences of deficiency include haemorrhages, particularly into soft tissues and the gums, and bone abnormalities. There is softening of bones, with distortion; this can involve the jaw and can result in the loss of teeth. Swelling of the gingiva, haemorrhages from the gums and persistent periodontal infection occur.

Thiamine (vitamin B_1) A common cause for thiamine deficiency in the West is alcoholism; in other parts of the world dietary lack of the vitamin is associated with

Table 1.9 Vitamin and trace element deficiencies

Vitamin	Clinical effects of vitamin deficiency
A	Hyperkeratosis of epithelium; xerophthalmia; increased susceptibility to mucosal infections; reduced night vision
Thiamine (B_1)	Cardiac failure; neuropathy; beri-beri; central nervous system disease
Riboflavin (B_2)	Mucosal inflammation; particularly of the tongue (glossitis) and of corner of lips (cheilitis); dermatitis
Niacin (nicotinamide)	Dermatitis, cheilitis, and glossitis; gastrointestinal mucosal changes; pellagra; central nervous system changes
Folate	Megaloblastic anaemia and glossitis
B_{12}	Megaloblastic anaemia and glossitis; pernicious anaemia; spinal cord degeneration
C	Scurvy; increased bleeding tendency; dermatitis; poor healing
D	Rickets in children; osteomalacia in adults
K	Clotting factors II, VII, IX, and X; reduced production
E	Neuropathy and anaemia
Iron	Microcytic, hypochromic anaemia
Iodine	Hypothyroidism; goitre
Fluoride	Dental caries
Zinc	Poor healing

refined foods. The clinical consequences affect the heart (wet beri-beri due to heart failure causing oedema), the peripheral nerves (dry beri-beri), and the central nervous system (Wernicke–Korsakoff syndrome).

Riboflavin (vitamin B_2) This is described because a deficiency of this vitamin is associated with atrophy of the tongue, and keratotic inflammatory lesions at the corners of the mouth (called cheilosis). Inflammatory lesions of the skin and eyes also occur.

Niacin (nicotinamide) A deficiency of this vitamin results in a condition called pellagra, which includes dermatitis, mucosal inflammation of the intestine with diarrhoea, and dementia associated with spinal cord abnormalities.

Vitamin B_{12} and folate These are grouped together because a reduced intake produces similar results, with anaemia showing enlarged red cells (megaloblastic anaemia). Vitamin B_{12} deficiency also results in neurological deficits. This is discussed in more detail in the chapter on haematology (p. 000). Vitamin B_{12} and folate are both coenzymes in the DNA synthetic pathway. In the production of red cells there is continued cell enlargement without corresponding mitosis.

Vitamin A Retinol is the main form of vitamin A, and is required for normal visual function. It is also involved in epithelial differentiation. The main effects of deficiency are corneal damage with keratinization, and suppression of the immune system. Squamous metaplasia of glandular epithelium also occurs.

Deficiency of vitamin A has been linked to an increased incidence of epithelial dysplasia and carcinoma. For example, leukoplakia of the oral cavity with dysplasia and oral carcinoma have been linked to oral cancer.

Vitamin D Vitamin D helps maintain normal blood calcium levels by increasing the absorption of calcium from the intestine, and with parathyroid hormone increasing calcium resorption from the bone and the distal tubules of the kidneys. One effect of vitamin D deficiency is a low blood calcium. Vitamin D is also needed for normal bone calcification.

The skeletal effect of vitamin D deficiency is a abnormal bone formation, with excessive amounts of non-mineralized collagenous matrix (osteoid). This can be demonstrated in a bone biopsy. In adults this results in bone weakness, but in children the abnormal bone forms in growth areas, particularly where cartilage is transforming to bone. There is deformation of load-bearing areas, particularly the legs, pelvis, and ribs. This condition in children is known as *rickets*.

Vitamin D_3 is mainly synthesized in the skin by the action of sunlight (ultraviolet light) on 7-dehydrocholesterol (an endogenous source). Vitamin D_2 comes from the diet (an exogenous source). Both these vitamins are metabolized to 25-hydroxy-vitamin D in the liver, and then to active 1,25-dihydroxy-vitamin D (calcitriol) in the kidneys. Renal disease can therefore interfere with calcium metabolism.

Vitamin E This is involved in protection from highly reactive and unstable radicals. Deficiency results in nerve damage.

Vitamin K The synthesis of the blood clotting factors II (thrombin), VII, IX, and X are dependent on the presence of vitamin K. In newborn infants, deficiency results in a risk of haemorrhage, particularly into the brain, known as haemorrhagic disease of the newborn. A bleeding tendency can also result in the adult with malabsorption, giving rise to gingival bleeding, for example.

The anticoagulant, warfarin, acts by blocking the recirculation of vitamin K.

Malnutrition

Chronic malnutrition with deficient energy intake leads to loss of body fat stores, muscle wasting, and reduced growth in childhood. The term 'marasmus' is used for this condition, particularly in areas of the world where nutritional deficiency is endemic.

If there is sufficient energy intake, but insufficient high quality protein intake, there is associated oedema, liver enlargement due to fatty change, electrolyte abnormalities, and reduced albumin in the serum. The name 'kwashiorkor' has been applied to this, and it occurs when there is a very high proportion of carbohydrate in the diet.

States of malnutrition occur between the spectrum described above. All malnutrition is associated with an increased risk of infection. Malnutrition is not only associated with poverty; it is seen in association with chronic disease, alcoholism, psychiatric illness, old age, and malabsorption syndromes such as coeliac disease.

Iron deficiency A deficiency of iron may result from chronic blood loss, malabsorption, or reduced dietary intake. Gastrointestinal bleeding is a very common cause of chronic blood loss. Increased demands for iron, as in pregnancy, may also result in a deficiency. Iron deficiency results in anaemia, with small pale red cells (a hypochromic, microcytic anaemia).

Environmental disorders

Under this heading can be placed mechanical, heat, extreme cold, and radiation injury. Also, the effects of environmental toxins will be described.

Physical causes

Certain physical agents, such as a high acid diet, can cause decalcification of teeth. Chronic abrasion of teeth can cause attrition which is loss of tooth substance. Increased attrition of teeth may be due to a diet with a high content of abrasive material. In addition, certain habits, such as chronic chewing of tobacco and pipe smoking, may result in excessive erosion of teeth.

Neoplastic disorders

This can be summarized as an imbalance between cell production and cell loss. A neoplasm ('new growth') is a loss of normal growth control within a tissue.

Inflammatory disorders

This is essentially the reaction of a tissue to injury. Inflammatory reactions are generally a non-specific stereotyped response.

Inflammatory conditions of the teeth, particularly gingivitis and periapical periodontitis, are common reasons for tooth loss apart from caries. The inflammatory reactions in the mouth and teeth are identical to inflammatory reactions anywhere else in the body. In view of the high vascularity of the periapical tissue, there is also marked capability of healing if the underlying cause of the inflammation is treated. Chronic gingivitis associated with dental plaque can progress from the marginal gingiva, down the tissue surrounding the teeth, and initiate periapical inflammation. Dental plaque appears to be the underlying initiating cause of periodontal inflammation. All the typical features of acute inflammation are seen in early gingivitis, including vasodilatation, exudation of fluid, and acute inflammatory cell infiltrate, predominantly of polymorphonuclear neutrophils. Repeated episodes of acute inflammation then progress to chronic inflammation, and there is infiltration by lymphocytes and fibrosis, with laying down of collagen from gingival fibroblasts. The adjacent squamous epithelium shows typically marked hyperplasia. Loss of epithelium—ulceration of the gingival epithelium against the tooth (the gingival pocket) occurs. Lymphocytes and plasma cells increase in number and there is continued destruction of gingival tissue with fibrosis. In advanced gingivitis there will be healing responses, including development of granulation tissue and increased fibrous tissue. Immunological mechanisms then come into play, with evidence of cell-mediated immunological reactions. There is also evidence of humoral immune mechanisms in periodontal disease. With extension of periodontal inflammation down to the apex of the tooth, a frequent complication is the development of a periapical granuloma. The word granuloma in this sense is inappropriate in that a true macrophage granuloma is not seen. It really describes the abundant granulation tissue and organizing blood clot that is seen in this condition. An abscess develops with this organization. There is also resorption of adjacent bone which is replaced by chronic inflammatory tissue. There is frequently a marked foreign body giant cell reaction to cholesterol material derived from the chronic haemorrhage. There is also frequently hyperplasia of epithelial rests of Malassez. These epithelial rests are small embryonic remnants of squamous epithelium commonly seen near the root of the tooth derived from the epithelial root sheath. This squamous epithelium may eventually line the cyst and form a well-circumscribed radicular cyst (Fig. 1.7). Periapical disease may progress to form a

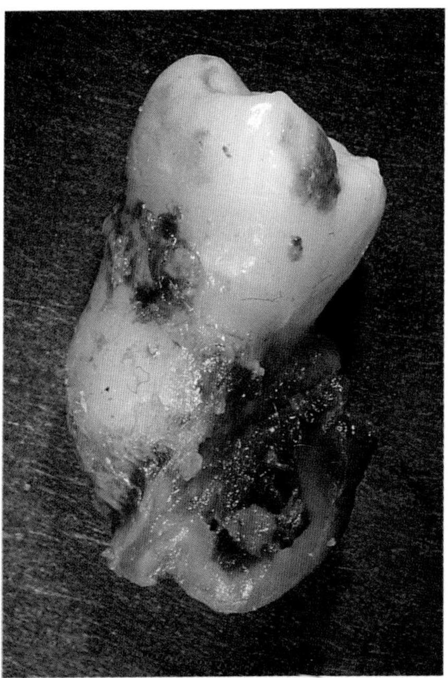

Fig. 1.7 A radicular cyst associated with an extracted tooth.

very large abscess with possible erosion into underlying bone and pointing of the abscess externally. Also, inflammation may spread into the underlying and surrounding connective tissue forming a cellulitis.

Immunological disorders

An immunological reaction is specific and has memory, in contrast to an inflammatory reaction. Immunological reactions are protective, but in some situations, such as in hypersensitivity or allergy, they may be harmful. Some diseases are caused by an inappropriate attack by the immune system on the host's own tissues, known as autoimmune disease.

Vascular disorders

Most frequently, vascular disorders arise from a reduced blood supply to an organ. This gives rise either to compromised nutrition and oxygenation (ischaemia), or necrosis (infarction). Vascular disorders also include thrombosis, embolism, and inflammatory diseases of vessels known as vasculitis.

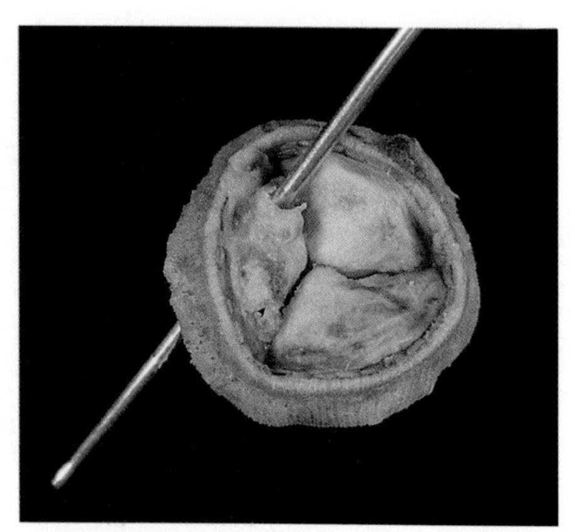

Fig. 1.8 A pig valve used in a patient for 15 years shows 'degenerative' perforation of a cusp (probe).

Metabolic disorders

These involve abnormalities of certain metabolic pathways. Diabetes mellitis, a disorder of carbohydrate metabolism, is an example of such a condition (see p. 000).

Degenerative disorders

This is a less well-defined group of conditions. The word degenerative is applied to conditions where tissue breakdown or loss is the main feature. Examples include tissue calcification or osteoarthritis, although it can be argued that osteoarthritis is a metabolic or even an immunological disorder. The term is also applied to processes of 'wear and tear' (Fig. 1.8).

CELLULAR PATHOLOGY

A concept which is very helpful to an understanding of pathological processes is that the processes occurring at a cellular level manifest themselves at a clinical level in the individual concerned. In other words, just because something is small it does not mean it is insignificant.

Cells can be regarded to some degree as free-living, independent, and sometimes expendable biological factories. They are, however, extremely reliant on each other. Cells have varying functions and varying degrees of specialization. This characteristic of specialization is known as *differentiation*.

Although all cells contain all the genetic material which has the theoretical ability to create a whole organism (the genotype), in the process of differentiation only selected genes are expressed. Therefore, cells show a specialization in structure and function (the phenotype). There is close cellular control of gene expression, which is regulated at all levels from transcription of DNA, processing of RNA, and modification of proteins after translation.

Factors in the extracellular environment, such as the extracellular matrix, basement membrane components, and growth factors, influence cellular differentiation. Examples are given below:

Epithelial differentiation is characterized by cells forming confluent sheets, with cell cohesion and the development of intercellular junctions. The cells produce basement membrane material and associate with basement membranes.

Examples of epithelial differentiation are:

- Squamous: the cells show intercellular bridges (desmosomes, representing 'rivet-like' structures holding the cells together) and produce keratin.
- Glandular: the cells form tubes and/or produce mucin (mucin consists of a polypeptide chain with carbohydrate side-chains).

Connective tissue is characterized by cells lying within extracellular material or 'matrix'. The cells show little or no cohesion and intercellular junctions are infrequent.

- Fibrous tissue: spindle cells (fibroblasts) produce collagen, forming an extracellular matrix. Collagen is a common structural protein in the body.
- Cartilage: chondrocytes produce a specialized proteoglycan matrix.
- Bone: osteoblasts produce osteoid which goes on to calcify (ossify), making bone.
- Muscle: cells produce abundant contractile proteins, either of striated (voluntary) or smooth (involuntary) type.
- Fat: the cells store large amounts of fat, termed lipocytes.

The terms below usually come under the subject of 'cellular pathology' and will be discussed in turn.

Cellular injury

This can be due to a wide variety of causes, some of which are listed below.

Trauma

Trauma involves physical forces that directly disrupt tissues to cause cell death. There will be physical disruption of cell membranes and other structures, and damage to blood vessels which introduces ischaemia. Any form of surgery inevitably induces some degree of cell death at the site of incision and tissue manipulation.

Extremes of temperature

Mild heat damages enzyme function and metabolic pathways, but the effects may be reversible. Severe heat denatures proteins and causes cell death directly. It is important to note also that excessive cold can damage tissue. Slow freezing in particular damages tissue because of the formation of large ice crystals that disrupt cell structures. The faster that tissue can be frozen the smaller the resultant crystals. If ice crystal formation can be inhibited completely by solvents that have an 'anti-freeze' function, then cells in culture can survive freezing and thawing.

Drugs and chemicals

Many drugs are therapeutic within only a certain range of concentrations. Above this therapeutic range, many drugs become toxic, either to specific organs or to more general metabolic pathways.

Immunological reactions, particularly hypersensitivity

Damage to cells can occur as a secondary event in some immunological reactions, particularly in hypersensitivity reactions, where an excessive immune reaction can

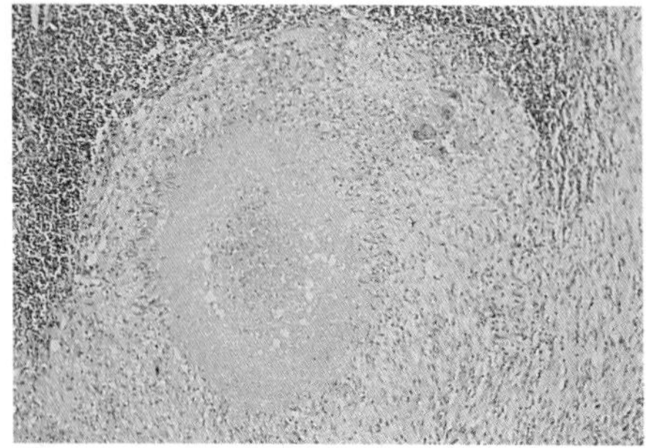

Fig. 1.9 Necrosis in a tuberculosis granuloma is seen as a granular amorphous change. Necrotic tissue usually looks like this in most situations.

result in areas of cell damage and death. In many cases, thc necrosis that occurs, in particular in necrotizing tuberculosis, is due to high concentrations of highly active cytokines (Fig. 1.9).

Agents that cause cellular injury or death may interfere with any number of cell processes. However, major cell processes that are frequently damaged are the production of the cellular energy source adenosine triphosphate (ATP) which requires oxygen, and the stability of normal osmotic and ion concentration in cells. A low ATP level in a cell is a marker of cellular injury. The concentration of sodium outside cells is much higher than in inside cells; with potassium the reverse is the case with high levels of intracellular potassium. Ion 'pumps' in the cell membrane driven by ATP maintain these ionic concentrations. A change in these ion levels is also a marker of cell injury. There may be damage to the cell nucleus and interference to specific metabolic pathways in the cell.

Other mechanisms of cell injury include damage and disruption to cell membranes, and the toxic effect of radicals, which are highly reactive unstable molecules with an unpaired electron. Radicals are frequently produced from oxygen. These molecules cause cell injury by reacting with lipids in cell membranes, proteins, and DNA. An insoluble brown pigment called *lipofuschin* is frequently formed when lipids have reacted with radicals. The heart and liver are frequent sites of deposition of lipofuschin, particularly in older people.

An important point is that cells have a capability to resist and repair injury. The degree of injury is dependent not only on the type of damaging agent, ut on the length of time and the severity of the exposure.

Genetic disorders

Inborn errors of metabolism may result, for example, of an accumulation of a metabolic byproduct which may reach toxic levels.

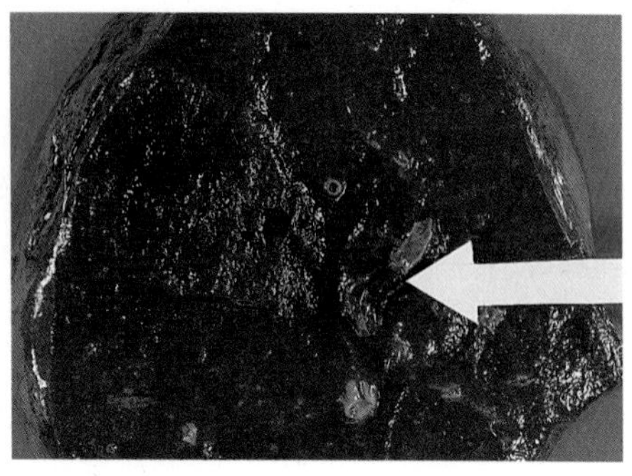

Fig. 1.10 A lung infarct due to a pulmonary embolus (arrow). It is typically seen as a wedge-shaped red area.

Infective agents, particularly viruses

Many bacteria, particularly those of Gram-negative type, produce toxic metabolites such as endotoxins or exotoxins. These may have a local toxic effect or have a more generalized systemic effect. Endotoxins can induce circulatory shock or generalized microvascular damage resulting in, for example, adult respiratory distress syndrome. Some exotoxins are toxic for a specific organ; for example, diphtheria bacilli produce a metabolite that is toxic for the myocardium.

Some of the byproducts of the inflammatory response to the infection may cause cell necrosis. For example, in an abscess, a great deal of cell death is due to the excessive realease of toxic lysosomal products such as lysozyme from neutrophil polymorphonuclear cells.

Table 1.10 Common sites of infarction

Myocardium
Spleen
Brain
Intestine (particularly small bowel)

Reduced blood supply (ischaemia)

Cell injury and death can be caused by the accumulation of toxic waste products due to insufficient circulation. Also, there will be an insufficient delivery of nutrients and oxygen to the tissue. Essential metabolites include glucose and vitamins. Necrosis due to ischaemia is termed *infarction* (Fig. 1.10). Tissues prone to infarction are listed in Table 1.10.

Lack of oxygen (hypoxia)

The cell damage that occurs with reduced or absent blood supply, termed ischaemia, is primarily due to hypoxia. Some tissues, such as muscle, can adapt to ischaemia and build up an oxygen 'debt'. The myocardium of the heart can also do this, and reduce its metabolic activity as a protective response, termed 'hibernation'. The oxygen requirements of a tissue are reduced by cooling.

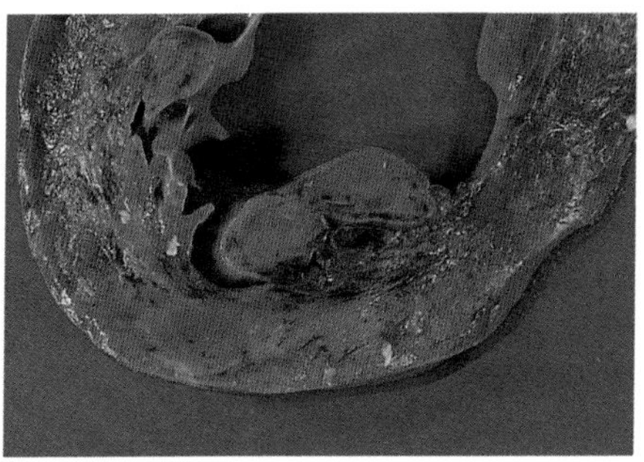

Fig. 1.11 Greenish discoloration in an acute myocardial infarct, aged 3–5 days.

Morphology

In cell necrosis, although biochemical changes are rapid, microscopic changes take several hours to develop. For example, irreversible injury to myocardial cells in the heart occurs after loss of blood supply for longer than 40 minutes. Necrosis due to loss of blood supply is termed *infarction*. However, microscopic changes are not seen for about six hours, and naked eye (macroscopic) changes do not appear for 24 hours. Microscopic changes include swelling of the cell cytoplasm, damage to organelles, such as mitochondria, lysosomal disruption, and nuclear breakdown. Macroscopic changes include pallor with adjacent congestion, followed by yellow/green discoloration after a few days due to an inflammatory infiltrate (Fig. 1.11). If the tissue has little in the way of connective tissue in it the infarct may become soft or liquify; the brain is a good example of this so-called *liquifactive* necrosis. Infarcts in different tissues are dealt with in the chapters on organ systems.

Different tissue have varying susceptibility to injury, particularly due to ischaemia and hypoxia. Muscle cells in a limb can survive several hours without blood, whilst, as mentioned above, myocardial cells can only survive 40 minutes. This is because of the high reserve of energy-providing glycogen within skeletal muscle cells and the ability of this tissue to obtain energy from anaerobic metabolism. Neurones in the brain can only survive four minutes of ischaemia.

The term *gangrene* is applied to areas of necrotic tissue involving multiple regions of tissues and there is frequently infection by microorganisms. This often occurs in necrotic intestine in view of the high bacterial load in the lumen. Some organisms that infect wounds, such as *Clostridium perfringens*, by the production of toxins, can cause further tissue necrosis. *Clostridium perfringens* is an anaerobic gas-forming organism commonly found in the gut and soil.

Gangrenous tissue turns a dark green or black colour due to the reaction of haemoglobin with hydrogen sulphide from bacteria.

Ionizing radiation

Much of the cellular damage that occurs in radiation exposure is due to the production of small, highly reactive molecules called *radicals*. These are short-lived molecules with an unpaired electron which avidly form chemical bonds with other molecules. In biological processes they are produced to aid intracellular killing of bacteria by phagocytic cells such as neutrophils and macrophages. If the injury is severe enough it may become irreversible and lead to cell death, termed necrosis.

Apoptosis

This is a term which literally means 'leaves falling off a tree' and refers to an interesting phenomenon of programmed cell death. It is a process that is genetically controlled and requires energy. It is characterized by a break up of the nucleus into typical clumps on electron microscopy, and a cutting up of the DNA into short fragments by enzymes. It is really a form of cell suicide and is important in the control of tissue mass and in embryogenesis.

Apoptosis is induced in target cells by lymphocytes in cells infected with virus, in transplant rejection, and in autoimmune disease. It is a normal phenomenon within germinal centres in reactive lymph nodes. Apoptosis frequently occurs in tumours. It is the process by which many tumour cells are killed with chemotherapy or radiotherapy.

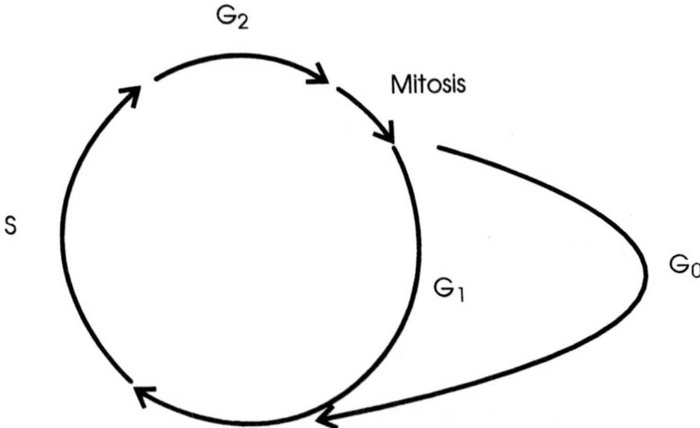

Fig. 1.12 A summary of the cell cycle.

A gene called *bcl*-2 is part of a family of genes involved in apoptosis. This gene is expressed when a cell is 'rescued' from apoptosis, for example, in developing lymphoid follicles in lymph nodes. The gene is activated when a cell is selected for survival and maturation. The *bcl*-2 gene product appears to act as an inhibitor of the process of apoptosis induced by either cytokines or a protein called p53 (see p. 000).

Cellular proliferation

The different stages that a cell goes through when it divides are grouped together and referred as the 'cell cycle' (Fig. 1.12). Cells that are not within the cell cycle and 'resting' are described as being in the G_0 phase. Cells that are fully differentiated and incapable of further division, such as neurones, are in this state permanently. Most cells only spend a limited time in G_0 phase. Cells enter the cell cycle at a stage termed G_1 (gap 1). It is this stage that varies with slowly or rapidly dividing cells. After the G_1 phase, the cell then starts synthesizing DNA (the S phase). At the end of this phase the cell has twice the amount of DNA it had before the S phase. The cell then enters a G_2 phase, and then undergoes mitosis (M phase), the phase of nuclear division. Cytoplasmic division then occurs, and the resultant cells then enter G_1 again.

Control of cell proliferation

Normal cell proliferation is under the influence of growth factors. These factors bind to specific receptors on the cell surface membrane and initiate a chain of biochemical events that result in cell division. Growth factor receptors are specialized proteins that are embedded in the cell membrane, and have three parts: an extracellular part that binds the growth factor, a part within the cell membrane, and a part that projects into the cell cytoplasm. This intracellular portion has tyrosine kinase activity, or relates to a specialized protein called a G-protein; the name is derived from its ability to bind guanosine 5′-triphosphate (GTP).

After a growth factor has bound to its respective growth receptor, the activity of the associated tyrosine kinase or G-protein is altered and this influences the phosphorylation of a series of specialized proteins and molecules in the cytoplasm.

G-proteins exert their effect through an intermediate metabolic pathway that involves phospholipases acting on the cell membrane (in particular phosphatidylinositol). Metabolic products of these phospholipases (inositol 1,4,5-triphosphate, IP_3, and diacyloglycerol, DAG) influence cytoplasmic calcium. This then alters the activity of protein kinase C.

The two pathways above are brought together in that both tyrosine kinase and

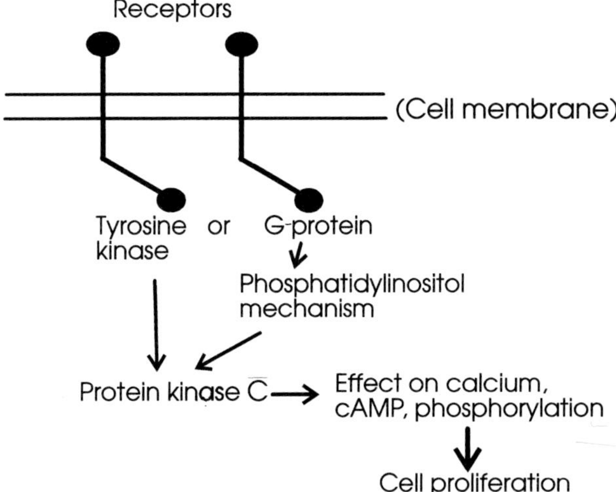

Fig. 1.13 A summary of processes involved in growth factor receptor binding.

protein kinase C phosphorylate a series of proteins involved in ion transport and membranes, influencing genes involved in cell proliferation. This process is summarized in Fig. 1.13.

Oncogenes code for many of the proteins and enzymes involved in the processes described above. As will be seen later, in the process of carcinogenesis, abnormalities are acquired in these pathways (see p. 000).

Cellular differentiation

The process of cellular specialization is called differentiation. It is primarily under genetic control, although the local environment of a cell can cause a change in differentiation. For example, basement membrane components and the extracellular matrix have an influence on cell differentiation. Cytokines and hormones also influence cell growth and differentiation. All cells have a complete complement of genetic information and the process of differentiation involves the selective expression of certain genes, with suppression of others.

Cellular adaptation

This is a response of cells to an external stimulus. This stimulus is usually directly or indirectly environmental in nature.

Atrophy

This is a reduction in cell size accompanied by a reduced number and function of cell organelles. It may be seen in association with reduced nutrition, work, blood supply, hormonal stimulus, and nerve supply, and as an age change. If atrophy occurs in cells throughout an organ, then the organ will reduce in size. There may also be a reduction in the number of cells, which may occur due to apoptosis. It may be physiological or pathological.

Physiological atrophy

- Thymic atrophy in adult life.
- Ovarian atrophy following the menopause.
- Atrophy of structures during fetal development.

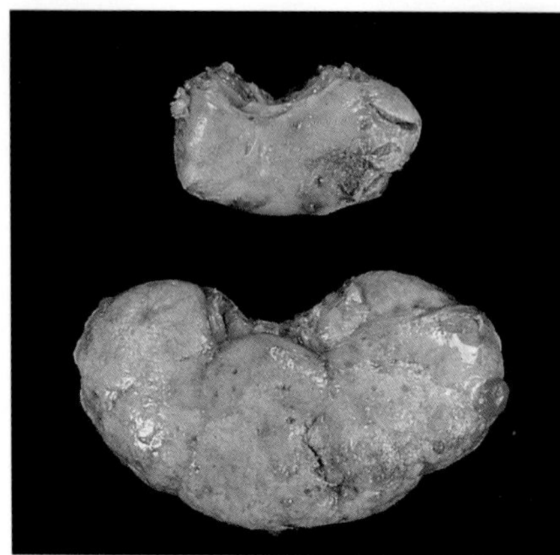

Fig. 1.14 A small atrophic kidney compared to a normal kidney (below).

Pathological atrophy

- Muscle wasting due to disuse.
- Renal atrophy due to renal artery stenosis causing reduced blood supply (Fig. 1.14).
- Muscle atrophy due to loss of innervation due to trauma.
- Loss of hormonal influences.

Hypertrophy

This is characterized by an increase in cell size, without an increase in cell number. There is, therefore, no proliferative activity and no DNA synthesis. It may be physiological as a normal response to increased work demanded of a tissue, or pathological.

Physiological hypertrophy

- Muscle hypertrophy due to exercise.
- Uterine hypertrophy due to pregnancy.
- Enlargement of a kidney when the opposite kidney is lost.

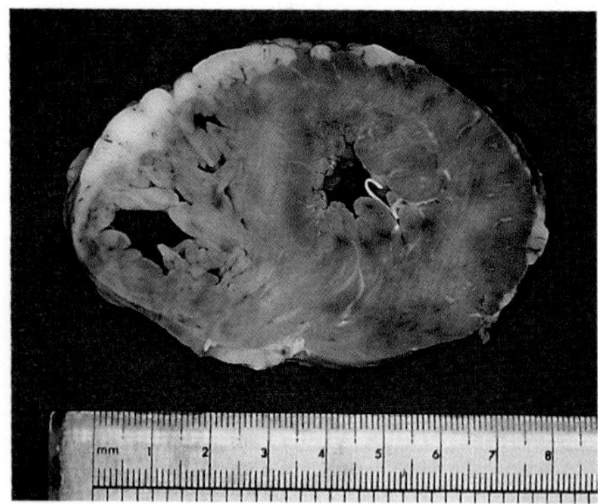

Fig. 1.15 Thickening of the right ventricle (on the left transversely) in pulmonary hypertension. It normally should only be about 4 mm thick.

Pathological hypertrophy

- Hypertrophy of the left ventricle of the heart in hypertension and aortic stenosis.
- Hypertrophy of the right ventricle of the heart with increased blood pressure in the pulmonary artery (Fig. 1.15).
- Gum hypertrophy associated with the anti-epileptic drug phenytoin.

Hypoplasia

This term is usually applied to developmental abnormalities when an organ has not been normally formed.

- Lung hypoplasia due to diaphragm abnormalities.
- Abnormalities in the development of teeth—enamel hypoplasia.

Hyperplasia

This is defined as an increase in cell number without an increase in cell size. There is proliferative activity with DNA synthesis; mitotic activity is seen in hyperplastic tissue. As above, this process may be physiological or pathological.

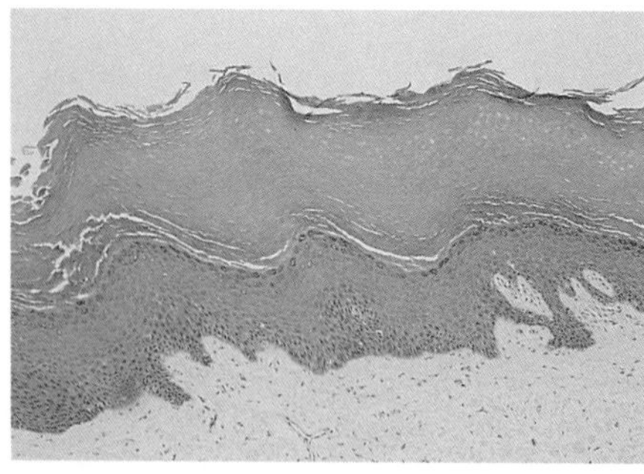

Fig. 1.16 This skin shows marked thickening of the keratinized corneal layer, the red amorphous layer above the epidermis. This is due to chronic trauma.

Physiological hyperplasia

- Increase in size of a lymph node as a response to infection.
- Skin as a response to increase wear and tear (Fig. 1.16). In an endocrine organ, such as the adrenal or thyroid, where increased function is required.
- The breast in pregnancy.
- The increase in cementum with mechanical stress to a tooth.
- Hyperplasia of the oral mucosa as a response to chronic trauma from a denture or tooth.

Pathological hyperplasia

- Prostatic hyperplasia in elderly men.
- Increase in size of the thyroid due to iodine deficiency.

- Adrenal nodular hyperplasia giving rise to Cushing's syndrome.
- Inflammatory oral mucosal papillary hyperplasia associated with ill-fitting dentures.
- Bone marrow following blood loss.

Hyperplastic lesions of the oral mucosa

Hyperplastic lesions of the oral mucosa, presenting as small nodules are relatively common. They are frequently removed in view of anxiety of neoplasia. Hyperplastic lesions frequently involve the connective tissue underlying the mucosa, but similar lesions may also involve the vascular tissue and present as a so-called pyogenic granuloma. There may be marked hyperplasia of the mucosa due to chronic irritation from dentures or malpositioned teeth. Fibroepithelial polyps appear to be associated with chronic trauma.

Metaplasia

This is the change of one type of differentiated tissue into another type of differentiated tissue. It is potentially reversible.

- Respiratory epithelium to squamous epithelium due to chronic irritation from smoking.
- Bladder transitional epithelium to squamous epithelium due to bladder stones.
- Intestinal metaplasia in chronic gastritis; the stomach mucosa begins to resemble small intestinal mucosa.
- Mucous columnar metaplasia of the oesophagus due to reflux of gastric acid.
- Ossification of soft tissue due to trauma.
- Squamous metaplasia of the ducts in minor salivary glands, particularly in a condition called necrotizing sialometaplasia, which can be mistaken for invasive squamous cell carcinoma on histology.

Dysplasia

This is a term that is applied to a process of disordered growth with a high risk of malignant change. It is best observed in epithelium where it is characterized by loss of normal differentiation of cells towards the surface, cytological atypia with enlarged and variably sized nuclei, and mitoses away from the normal proliferative basal area. Dysplasia is covered further in the chapter on neoplasia. The processes described above are summarized in Fig. 1.17 and Table 1.11.

IONIZING RADIATION

Types of radiation

The greater the degree of ionization induced by the radiation, the greater the biological effect. Ions form when a high energy photon removes an electron from an atom or molecule. Radiation that has the greatest ionizing effect is *electromagnetic radiation*.

Particulate radiation

Alpha particles (positively charged particles with the structure of a helium nucleus), beta particles (high-energy electrons from isotopes), and neutrons. Particulate radiation may be produced from radioactive decay or artificially from accelerators.

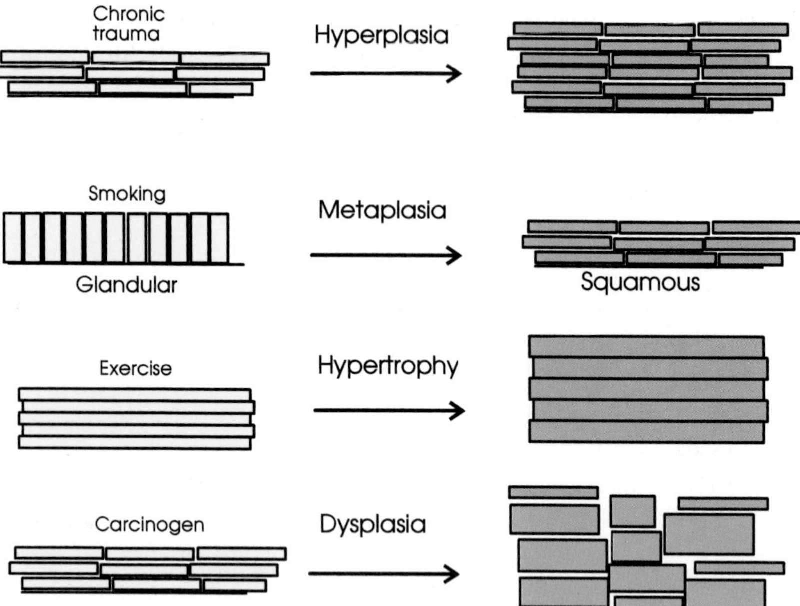

Fig. 1.17 A summary of cellular responses.

Table 1.11. Tissue characteristics and growth abnormalities

Feature	Description
Hypoplasia	Reduction in number of cells (aplasia is acquired, agenesis is congenital)
Hyperplasia	Increase in number of cells in a tissue
Metaplasia	A change in type of one differentiated tissue into another differentiated tissue
Dysplasia	Abnormal cell proliferation which has malignant potential
Neoplasia	A tumour produced by an imbalance between cell production and cell loss. The tumour is autonomous, persists after the initiating stimulus has been removed, frequently shows increased proliferative rate, and has a detrimental effect

In general, ionizing radiation that has significant biological effect is of very short wavelength, shorter than ultraviolet light, with high energy. If this radiation is produced artificially by collisions of electrons with a target, for instance, it is called X-ray radiation. If it is produced by natural decay of unstable isotopes it is called gamma radiation. The term *photon* applies when any electromagnetic radiation is being considered as being composed of small packets of energy.

Ultraviolet light has less of an ionizing effect than higher-frequency radiation, but is capable of causing genetic damage. Lower-frequency radiation, such as microwave and other radio frequency radiation, has a heating effect at high power, but appears not to have any specific biological effect other than cataract development in the eye in the case of microwaves.

Sources of radiation

The whole population is exposed to background radiation, 90 per cent of which comes from the decay of naturally occurring isotopes in rocks. Granite is a common source of such radiation, in the form of radon, a radioactive gas.

Only 10 per cent of background radiation is derived from artificial sources, and the majority of this in most people (up to 90 per cent or more) is from medical investigations or treatment with, for example, X-rays. Only a very small amount of background radiation comes from industrial or military sources.

Units of measurement

The effects on biological tissues vary depending on the type of radiation the tissue is exposed to. Particulate radiation, such as alpha radiation, has more of an ionizing effect than electromagnetic radiation such as X-rays. Also, different tissues have variable sensitivity to radiation, as described below.

The current units of radiation measurement are:

- *Becquerel* (Bq). 1 Bq = 1 atomic decay per second. This reflects the actual rate of decays occurring.
- *Gray* (Gy). 1 Gy = 1 joule of energy absorbed per kilogram. This is a measure of energy transferred by the radiation. (1 gray = 100 rad in alternative units.)
- *Sievert* (Sv). 1 Sv = 1 joule of energy absorbed per kilogram. However, before the unit is calculated, corrections are made for the type of radiation and the sensitivity of the exposed tissue to this radiation. The sievert is therefore a *dose-equivalent* unit of radiation measurement.

Biological effects

Radiation can cause direct molecular damage, but the biological effect of radiation is mediated predominantly by the formation of *radicals*, such as hydroxyl groups (—OH), by the interaction of the radiation and water molecules. These radicals are highly reactive, short-lived molecules, and if oxygen is present, oxygen radicals, such as superoxide, then form.

These radicals react very rapidly with surrounding molecules, including proteins and DNA. Radicals cause *breaks* in DNA molecules, requiring repair. Patients with a defect in the DNA repair mechanism, such as the congenital *xeroderma pigmentosum*, are very sensitive to radiation exposure, particularly ultraviolet light. These patients have a high incidence of permanent genetic mutation after background ultraviolet exposure to the skin, and frequently develop basal cell and squamous cell carcinomas.

Radicals also cause permanent, strong cross-linking of DNA strands. Pyrimidine dimers and actual breaks in the DNA are caused. Also, mutations in the base pair sequence can be induced.

Different types of radiation have a variable effect, depending on the production of the highly reactive molecules mentioned above.

The effect of radiation is enhanced in well-oxygenated tissues, demonstrating the role of oxygen in the generation of radicals. Particulate radiation, such as alpha particles, beta particles, and neutrons, produce more radicals in their path than electromagnetic radiation. This ability to produce ions and radicals relates to the so-called linear energy transfer (LET) of the radiation.

Effects in tissue

Early or *acute* effects of radiation are seen predominantly in cells that are rapidly dividing. Cells are most susceptible to injury at the time of mitosis. They are most resistant to radiation during DNA synthesis. Rapidly dividing cells include the *bone marrow*, epithelium of the *gastrointestinal tract*, *skin*, and the *testis*. There is suppression of stem cell proliferation and subsequent production of differentiated cells. Tumours in which the cells are rapidly dividing are also more susceptible to damage by radiation than are more slowly growing tumours. Slowly growing or non-dividing cells, such as muscle cells or neurones, are relatively resistant to radiation.

Hypoplasia of tooth enamel is associated with radiation exposure.

Late or *chronic* effects of radiation exposure are mainly *vascular* in origin. Irradiated tissue shows intimal hyperplasia and lipid-laden cells within subendothelial tissues. These changes gradually occlude the lumen and cause ischaemia to the tissue supplied by that vessel. This results in fibrosis and associated atrophy. Frequently, changes in the appearance of nuclei are seen, particularly in connective tissue cells such as fibroblasts. Nuclei appear enlarged and irregular and cells may be multinucleate. This feature may persist for many years and be a marker for previous radiation exposure. These nuclear changes are a pointer to underlying genetic damage that has been induced by the previous radiation.

The genetic damage referred to above is manifested as a late effect by the increased incidence of tumours in tissues that have been irradiated. Radiation has a *carcinogenic* effect, which has a delay or latent period before being expressed. This latent period may be up to 20 years or more. There is generally a linear relationship between the dose of radiation and the risk of tumour development in a particular tissue. Examples of radiation-induced tumours include leukaemias and thyroid cancer after exposure to radiation from nuclear fission bombs, and thyroid tumours and other tumours after radiation therapy. Even dental radiography, particularly tomograms, give a significant radiation dose. Radiation can induce chromosomal abnormalities, such as translocations and deletions, and damage proteins.

Exposure to ultraviolet light is well known to be responsible for an increased incidence or skin tumours, particularly squamous and basal cell carcinomas, and malignant melanoma.

The genetic damage that is induced by radiation is also manifest by its *mutagenic* effect in the developing fetus resulting in congenital malformations. Clinical effects are listed in Table 1.12.

Radiation as a treatment

The susceptibility of rapidly dividing malignant cells to damage by radiation is used as a method of treatment for tumours. Therefore, poorly differentiated, 'high-grade' tumours with a high mitotic rate are the most amenable to therapy. Examples of tumours frequently treated this way are lymphomas, small cell lung carcinoma, breast carcinoma, cervical carcinoma, and testicular cancer.

Radiotherapy also relies on the reduced ability that malignant cells have for repair after radiation damage as compared to normal tissue. If the radiation dose is given at

Table 1.12 Effects of radiation

Dose (grays)	Clinical effects
0.5–1	No overt clinical effects
1–3.5	Mild reduction in leucocyte count and gastrointestinal effects
3.5–7.5	Severe gastrointestinal effects, 20–50% mortality rate within 6 months Severe reduction in all types of blood cell
10	Rapidly fatal

time intervals with a period allowing the normal tissues to recover faster than the tumour cells, there will be a net reduction in the tumour size. This technique of giving small multiple doses rather than less frequent large doses is called *fractionation*.

Complications of radiation, as described above, apply to the treatment of tumours, and these have to be taken into account in the planning of radiotherapy.

Total body irradiation is used to eradicate host haemopoetic and neoplastic cells in preparation for a bone marrow transplant.

VASCULAR PATHOLOGY

Thrombosis

A thrombus is defined as a solid mass formed from *all* blood constituents within a *living* blood vessel. It therefore differs from a clot in that it does not just involve the fibrin-producing clotting cascade; platelets are also involved. Also, clotting can occur in the extracellular tissues as a bruise and *in vitro* within a glass jar, both situations forming a mass which is not defined as thrombus.

In general, for thrombus to form there are abnormalities of the blood, abnormalities of the blood flow, or abnormalities of the blood vessel intimal lining. These three factors are known as Virchow's triad. Clinical examples of thrombus are as follows.

Venous thrombosis

This commonly occurs in deep leg veins or pelvic veins after immobilization following surgery. In fact, any sort of immobilization will predispose to this type of 'low-flow' thrombosis in deep veins. This gives rise to a high risk of thrombo-embolism to the lung. Venous thrombus tends to be soft, and resembles clot.

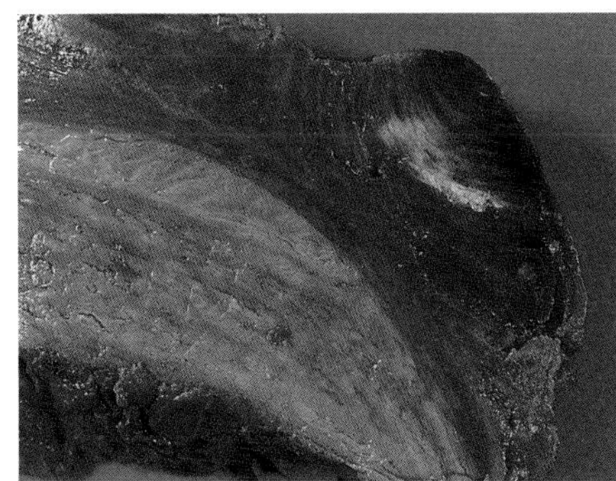

Fig. 1.18 Laminated thrombus.

Arterial thrombosis

This by its nature forms in regions of high blood flow, particularly over atherosclerotic intimal plaques. It is laminated in view of the alternating layers of white appearing platelets, and red blood cells mixed with fibrin. These stripes are sometimes referred to as *lines of Zahn* (Fig. 1.18). One of the most important dangers of arterial thrombosis, particularly in areas where only one artery supplies one area of tissue (an *end-artery*) is occlusion of the lumen with *infarction* of the tissue supplied by that artery. Organs that are particularly prone to infarction due to thrombus are the heart and brain. Myocardial and cerebral infarcts are very common in Western populations.

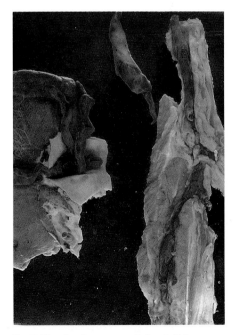

Fig. 1.19 A pulmonary embolus (left) has originated from a deep vein thrombosis (right).

Embolism

Emboli are solid, liquid, or gaseous collections which arise in one part of the circulation and travel to another part via the blood vessels. The majority of emboli are of thrombus (Fig. 1.19), but other less frequent types of emboli are listed below.

Gaseous

Air

- Entering through damaged vein or through intravenous line.
- Nitrogen bubbles in the 'bends' in divers ascending too rapidly.

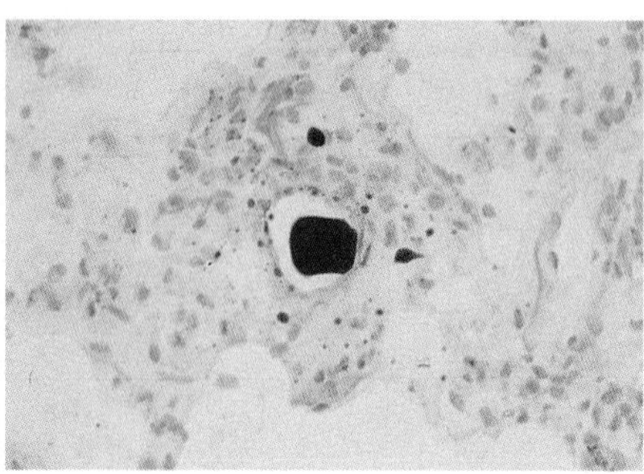

Fig. 1.20 Fat, stained red, in a pulmonary artery in the lung. The fat has come from a fractured femur.

Liquid

- Fat—this is liquid at body temperatures, and if a fracture of a long bone containing fat occurs, such as the femur, fat can escape into the venous circulation (Fig. 1.20).
- Amniotic fluid—this may escape into the uterine veins during delivery in view of the greatly increased intra-uterine pressure.

Solid

- Tumour—this is a mechanism of metastasis.
- Infective—vegetations containing organisms may break off and embolize in cases of infective endocarditis.

TISSUE DEPOSITIONS

Fat

All cells contain lipids, but in some cases, particularly in cell injury, there is a dramatic increase in lipids to give a clear or bubbly appearance to the cells on histology. Lipids are frequently seen in the liver and are described in the chapter on liver pathology.

Iron

There may be a local increase in tissue iron due to organization of blood clot with the release of iron from haemoglobin. An increase in iron in the whole body may be due to increased intake or absorption from the intestine. It may also be due to excessive release of iron in the circulation due to the breakdown of red cells in haemolytic anaemias, or multiple blood transfusions. Iron is very efficiently recycled in the body, very little being excreted. Iron is potentially a very toxic element in high concentrations. It can be seen in tissues as a brown pigment called *haemosiderin*. Iron is carried on a transport protein called transferrin. It is stored in cells as ferritin, which, when in large aggregates, is then visible on light microscopy as haemosiderin.

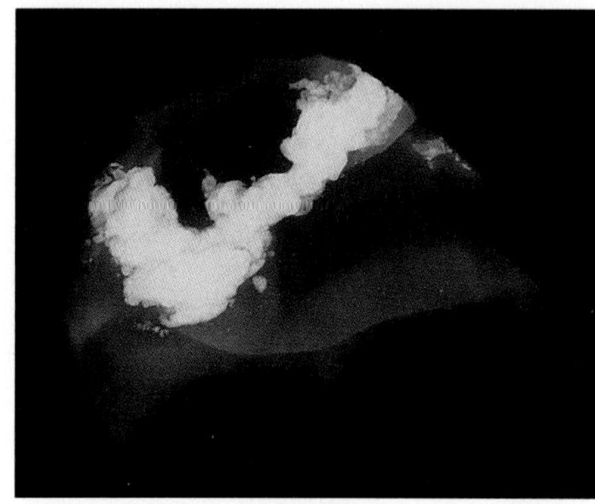

Fig. 1.21 Dystrophic calcification in a sclerotic aortic heart valve (radiograph).

Calcium

Calcium has a tendency to precipitate out of solution on damaged tissue, giving rise to abnormal or so-called *dystrophic* calcification. This occurs with normal blood levels of calcium and is seen, for example, in association with necrosis, atherosclerosis in blood vessels, damaged heart valves (Fig. 1.21), and in some tumours. Calcification of osteoid in the formation of bone, and dentine in the formation of teeth are, of course, normal processes.

Calcification of tissues, such as the kidney, lung, or blood vessels in the skin, may occur in the presence of raised blood calcium (hypercalcaemia). This is known as *metastatic* calcification.

Amyloid

This is an extracellular protein deposition which has a distinctive eosinophilic appearance on light microscopy (Fig. 1.22), a fibrillary structure on electron microscopy, and a 'beta-pleated' sheet molecular structure. It stains black with iodine (like starch), hence the name (Fig. 1.23). The beta-pleated sheet is a repetitive stacking of protein fibrils which gives amyloid its optical activity under polarized

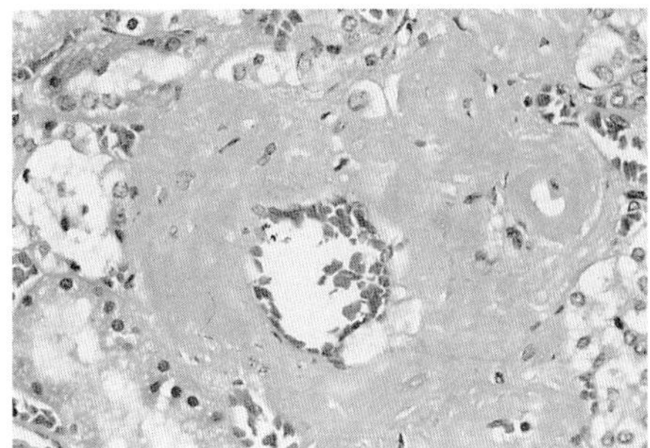

Fig. 1.22 Amyloid around a blood vessel is seen as pink amorphous material.

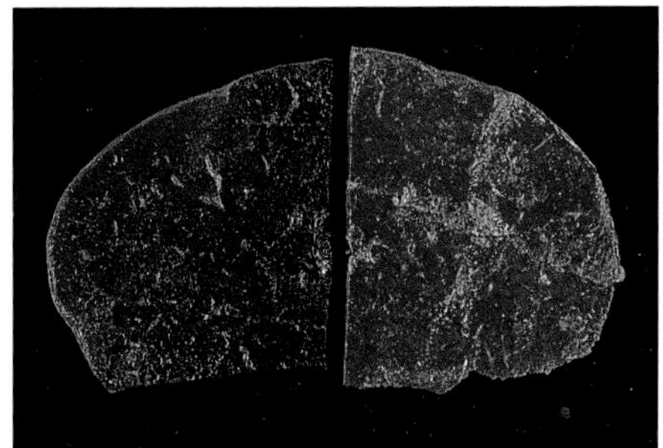

Fig. 1.23 How amyloid got its name; this amyloid spleen stains black with iodine, like starch (right, unstained).

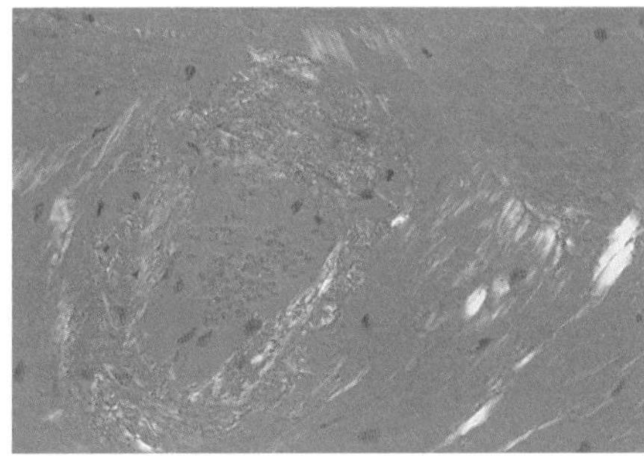

Fig. 1.24 Amyloid stained with Congo red and viewed with crossed polarizers showed green coloration.

light when stained with the dye Congo red (Fig. 1.24). About 10 per cent of amyloid is composed of a glycoprotein 'P' component. An important point to emphasize about amyloid is that it represents a variety of substances with similar morphological structure but a great variation in chemical structure.

Amyloid is formed from an aggregation or complex of a variety of precursor substances. Once formed, it is insoluble and difficult to degrade.

The deposition of amyloid gives affected organs a waxy appearance; the organs stain black with iodine in a similar way to starch (amyloid = starch-like). Affected organs are enlarged and cells become atrophic. Amyloid develops in a number of clinical situations, and its biochemical structure varies depending on the cause. These situations are summarized below.

Systemic amyloid

Immunoglobulin light chain-derived (primary amyloid) This is associated with an underlying abnormal proliferation of plasma cells, such as myeloma or B lymphocytes, which produce an excessive amount of immunoglobulin light chains. In view of the monoclonal proliferation involved, the immunoglobulin is of one specific type and forms a prominant monoclonal 'band' on a serum electrophoresis strip. The light chains are most commonly of lambda type. The amyloid is derived from deposits of this light chain material and is referred to as being of AL type. The term, primary amyloid, is applied when no plasma cell neoplasia can be found; it is possible that in these cases there is also a plasma cell disease, but it has not yet caused signs or symptoms.

Organs frequently involved with light chain-derived (primary amyloid) are the kidneys, spleen, heart, and liver. The tongue is a well-recognized site of primary amyloid; it presents as tongue enlargement.

Serum amyloid-associated (SAA) protein-derived (secondary amyloid) This occurs in association with chronic inflammatory and autoimmune diseases. Examples include chronic bacterial infection, and autoimmune disease such as rheumatoid arthritis.

Amyloid is also seen in patients with renal failure who are on long-term renal dialysis. This is due to an accumulation of beta-2-microglobulin in the circulation.

Finally, there are a number of rare hereditary types of amyloid which relate to an abnormal gene product called transthyretin (prealbumin).

In light chain- and SAA-derived amyloid, the deposits tend to occur in the kidney, spleen, liver, gastrointestinal tract, and the heart.

Localized amyloid

Amyloid can occur as local deposits in organs. Nodules of amyloid can occur in the lung, skin, mouth, and larynx, for example.

Amyloid occurs in association with some endocrine tumours such as medullary carcinoma of the thyroid (derived from calcitonin-producing 'C' cells, and beta cell islet tumours of the pancreas (producing insulin).

Amyloid is seen occasionally as an isolated phenomenon in the heart of very elderly people. Deposits of amyloid are found in the brain of patients with Alzheimer's disease.

Amalgam

Deposits of amalgam may be seen in the soft tissue of the gum if it becomes implanted, usually by trauma. It frequently causes a foreign body-type granulomatous reaction.

Tobacco

Heavy and long-standing tobacco smokers, particularly pipe smokers, may show impregnation of soft tissues by brown pigment. Microscopically, there is often discoloration of elastic tissue.

SUMMARY

Disease processes can be classified in the following way—*congenital* or *acquired*:

–infective
–nutritional
–environmental
–neoplastic
–inflammatory
–immunological
–vascular
–metabolic
–degenerative

Processes that occur at a cellular level manifest themselves at a clinical level. Cells are strongly influenced by the extracellular matrix. This consists of:

–collagen
–basement membrane
–elastic fibres
–proteoglycans

Differentiation: this occurs when a cell undergoes specialization in structure and function.

Cellular injury and death: this may occur with trauma, extremes of temperature, toxic agents and drugs, in association with severe immunological reactions, and accumulation of metabolic byproducts in some genetic disorders. Cellular injury may also occur with infection, reduced blood supply (ischaemia), hypoxia and radiation.

Necrosis: death of tissue.

Infarction: this is necrosis due to ischaemia.

Apoptosis: this is a process of active cell death, important in development and as a process of cellular growth control.

Atrophy: reduction in cell size.

Hypertrophy: increase in cell size, without increase in cell number.

Hypoplasia: abnormal development of an organ.

Hyperplasia: increase in cell number without increase in cell size.

Metaplasia: the change of one type of differentiated tissue into another.

Dysplasia: a cellular manifestation of abnormal growth with a high risk of malignant change. It is a process that is on the path to the development of cancer.

Thrombus: this is a solid mass formed from all blood constituents within a living blood vessel. It occurs with abnormalities of the:

–blood
–blood flow
–blood vessel

Embolism: a solid liquid or gaseous collection which arises in one part of the circulatory system and travels to another. Most are thrombi.

Tissue depositions: the most important tissue depositions are iron secondary to haemorrhage, calcium, and amyloid.

2 Inflammation and repair

2 Inflammation and repair

ACUTE INFLAMMATION

AN INFLAMMATORY response is an non-specific response to injury in vascularized tissue, in contrast to an immunological response which is characterized by specificity, memory, and diversity. Inflammation is classified into acute and chronic types. Acute inflammation is generally of short duration, lasting hours to days. The classical features of redness, swelling, warmth, and pain described by Celsus, a first-century Roman, reflect predominantly the vascular responses seen in acute inflammation. Loss of function is frequently added to this list. Blood vessels dilate and characteristically become leaky, allowing the exudation of fluid and plasma proteins. The cellular response is mainly of neutrophil polymorphonuclear leucocytes, resulting in the development of pus. The vascular and cellular responses are covered below.

An important point is that inflammatory reactions are stereotyped. The basic processes occurring in a periapical dental abscess are the same as those happening in acute appendicitis, for example. Another important point is that in most cases an inflammatory reaction is beneficial, but on occasions the reaction may have harmful effects. An example of this is in tuberculosis, where a lot of the tissue destruction is due to the inflammatory reaction rather than from toxic agents produced from the tubercle bacteria. Another point is that inflammatory reactions are extremely common in the mouth. Gingivitis has been said to be the most common inflammatory process, and perhaps even the most common infection in the world. A summary of the causes of inflammation is set out in Table 2.1.

Table 2.1 The causes of acute inflammation

Tissue necrosis
Trauma
Heat (burns)
Immunological reaction
Infection
Radiation
Ischaemia

Vascular response

Vascular changes are a typical feature of inflammation. The earliest change seen in blood vessels after injury is a short period of vasoconstriction of arterioles, which for mild injury may last a few seconds, whilst in more severe injury this may last several minutes. The next phase is that of dilatation involving initially the arterioles causing an increased blood flow through the capillary bed of the inflamed area. This is apparent clinically as the typical redness and heat of inflammation (Fig. 2.1). At this stage there may be a transudate of fluid which is *low* in protein due to the increased blood flow, blood vessels at this time retaining their barrier to large molecules. The next stage is a dramatic increase in the permeability of the blood vessels in the area of the inflammation, giving rise to a *high*-protein exudate. This results in *oedema*, the other classical feature of acute inflammation. Oedema is a term meaning increased fluid in the space between cells (the extracellular space). It is seen as a local effect in inflammation. There is reduction of the blood flow and stasis of blood cells. Neutrophils are then seen to adhere to the endothelial surface and emigrate between gaps in the endothelium (Fig. 2.2).

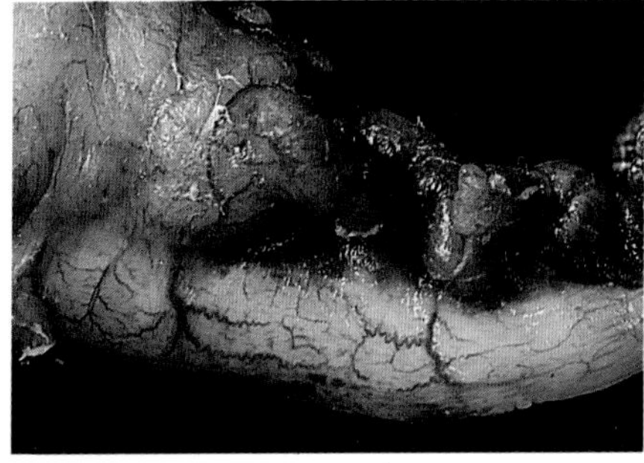

Fig. 2.1 Dilated blood vessels on the surface of an early acute appendicitis.

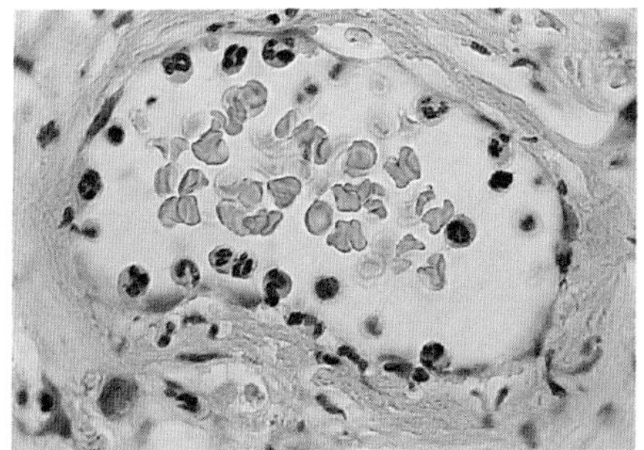

Fig. 2.2 Neutrophils adhering to the endothelium of a blood vessel.

There is normally a balance between the volume of fluid leaving the capillary bed at the arteriolar end and the volume absorbed at the venular end. There is a very small net loss which is drained by the lymphatic system. The hydrostatic pressure (the blood pressure in the capillaries) is balanced by the colloid osmotic pressure of the plasma proteins. In acute inflammation, because of the increased permeability of the endothelium with exudation of plasma proteins, there is an increased colloid osmotic pressure in the extracellular space. There is therefore a net outflow with retention of fluid in the space outside the vascular system (interstitium).

Patterns of vascular response

There are three main types of vascular response recognized in acute inflammatory reactions. The immediate-transient response is seen after mild injury due to, for example, heat. This response starts immediately after injury and lasts about 30 minutes. It has been shown that the response is due to a short-lived increase in permeability of post-capillary venules. The endothelial cells are seen to contract, creating gaps which allow the passage of large molecules.

The immediate-sustained vascular responses occur after severe injury. There is necrosis of endothelial cells and leakage continues until there has been endothelial repair. There is damage to all types of vessel in this type of injury.

The third type of vascular response is a delayed-but-sustained response in which there is a period of time after the injury before any vascular changes are seen. A typical example is radiation injury due to, for example, ultraviolet light, or other radiation. These changes are seen in both venules and capillaries.

Cellular response

The most striking histological feature of acute inflammation is the accumulation of large numbers of neutrophils, and to a lesser extent, macrophages. Both types of cell are derived from the blood, and therefore have to pass through the vessel walls to reach the interstitial areas of the inflamed tissue. The neutrophils go through a process of margination, adhesion, and migration before being available for phagocytosis.

Margination is a passive process in which cells are no longer kept in a central column in fast-flowing blood vessels separated from the endothelium by a layer of plasma. This central column breaks down at low-flow rates in dilated capillaries. Neutrophils and monocytes, in particular, cover the endothelial surface.

The next phase involves neutrophils sticking to the endothelial surface. This involves the physical interaction of adhesion molecules on the cell surfaces. When neutrophils are stimulated by certain inflammatory mediators, such as bacterial products, complement fragments, cytokines such as interleukin-1, leukotrienes, or tumour necrosis factor, there is increased surface expression of adhesion molecules. One group of adhesion molecules on leucocytes comprise three different types of glycoprotein termed LFA-1, MO-1, and P150. They are all composed of the same type of alpha-subunit but a variable beta-subunit. These molecules interact with endothelial adhesion molecules such as ELAM-1 (endothelial adhesion molecule-1) and ICAM-1 (intracellular adhesion molecule-1). Endothelium activated in an inflammatory response expresses platelet-activating factor which stimulates neutrophil function, and a group of adhesion molecules called selectins. Adhesion molecules and their actions are listed in Table 2.2.

The next phase is that of migration in which neutrophils and macrophages pass from the blood vessels into the tissues. The cells pass through gaps that develop between endothelial cells of mainly venules (Fig. 2.3). Endothelial cells are capable of contraction during acute inflammatory responses. The neutrophils and macrophages then pass through the basement membrane into the extravascular space. These cells follow a chemical gradient, a process termed chemotaxis. Chemotaxis factors include bacterial products, complement factors, such as C5a, and arachidonic acid metabolites, such as leukotriene B_4.

Table 2.2 Cell adhesion molecules

Family type	Function
Selectins	Neutrophil and lymphocyte adhesion to endothelial cells (leucocyte adhesion molecule, endothelial cell adhesion molecule-1)
Cadherins	Epithelial, neural, and placental cell adhesion. Component of desmosomes
Integrins	Adhesion between endothelial cells and neutrophils and lymphocytes. (Leucocyte function molecule LFA-1)
Immunoglobulin gene super-family	Neural cell adhesion molecule. Intercellular adhesion molecule (ICAM-1), vascular cell adhesion molecule-1 (VCAM-1)

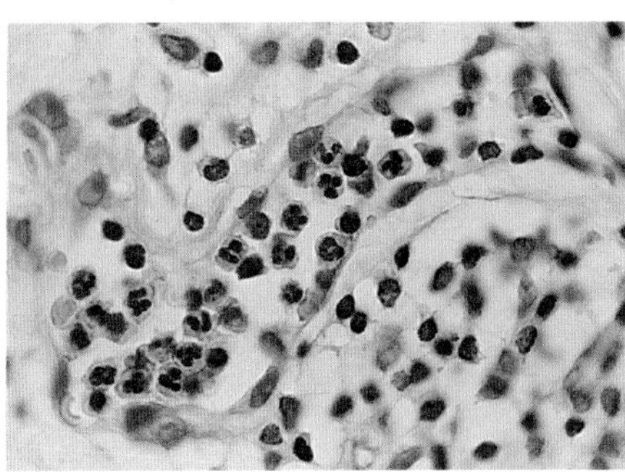

Fig. 2.3 Neutrophils migrating through the endothelium (bottom right).

When macrophages and neutrophils encounter a foreign particle, they go through a process of recognition, engulfment, and degradation of the material. Most bacteria are not recognized until they have been coated with immunoglobulin or complement, a process called opsonization. IgG and complement component C3b are very effective opsonins. The opsonized material then interacts with receptors on the surface of the neutrophils or macrophages, in particular IgG and C3b receptors. There is then engulfment of the foreign material and primary lysosomes in the cytoplasm fuse with the phagocytic vacuoles to form secondary lysosomes. The process of degradation then begins.

Engulfed bacteria are killed by either oxygen-dependent or oxygen-independent mechanisms—neutrophils being the most effective.

Oxygen-dependent mechanisms

These rely on the production of oxygen metabolites, mainly oxygen radicals and hydrogen peroxidase. The energy is obtained from the NADPH system (nicotinamide adenine dinucleotide phosphate) involving an oxidase enzyme. These bactericidal agents are produced in lysosomes. Although hydrogen peroxidase and oxygen radicals themselves can kill bacteria, the toxicity of these molecules is greatly increased by the enzyme myleoperoxidase. This is the substance that makes pus green. This enzyme functions in the presence of a halogen such as chloride.

Oxygen-independent mechanisms

These include the enzyme lysosyme, lactoferrin, bactericidal permeability-increasing protein, and major basic protein in eosinophils. The extracellular release of many of these products described above contributes to the tissue destruction seen particularly in an abscess, a common result of acute inflammation.

The importance of the function of neutrophils is demonstrated in a number of situations:

1. Neutropaenia—when the number of neutrophils in the circulation is low the person is at high risk of overwhelming infection, particularly from bacteria and fungi.
2. Congenital defects of leucocyte phagocytic function and killing ability occur in which affected individuals have a decreased defence against infection.

3. There is an inborn abnormality of the beta chain common to a number of leucocyte adhesion molecules in which affected people are prone to infection.

Chemical mediators

Many types of chemical messengers are involved in the acute inflammatory response.

Histamine and serotonin are the most important mediators contributing to the increased permeability of blood vessels seen in acute inflammation. Histamine is stored mainly in the granules of mast cells and serotonin is stored in platelets.

An important concept in acute inflammation relating to the plasma proteases is that interactions occur between the complement, clotting, and kinin systems. This explains, for example, the abundant fibrin seen in an abscess and the associated pain and vascular swelling. The cellular processes involved in acute inflammation are described in Fig. 2.4.

Complement

This is a group of plasma proteins that mediate reactions involved mainly in defence against microorganisms. They are activated by antibody–antigen complexes (the classical pathway) or bacterial products (the alternative pathway). The pathway is summarized in Fig. 2.5.

Complement is an integral part of the immune system and comprises about 30 proteins. They act in an amplification cascade to form active molecules. A proenzyme acts on an enzyme which then further produces another proenzyme. This goes on to act on another enzyme, and so on, hence having a marked amplification. Cleavage fragments are frequently produced.

Classical pathway

The classical pathway consists of C1–C9 which are all beta-globulins. C3 is the major component of the plasma. Circulating complement comes mainly from the liver, whilst local synthesis occurs in tissue macrophages. C1 may also be made by gastrointestinal and urogenital epithelium. The classical pathway is activated by immunoglobulin complexes. C1 can be activated by trypsin, plasmin, and lysosomal enzymes. A membrane attack complex is produced by the classical pathway which forms tubular structures which penetrate the cell membrane of the cell under attack. Activation of C3 is a very important step in the complement system.

Alternative pathway

This is activated by aggregates of IgG, IgA, bacterial endotoxin, viral infected cells, some tumour cells, and foreign particles. There is a continual generation of C3b in the circulation. C3b interacts with factors B and D to generate an enzyme called C3 convertase which produces more C3b creating an amplification cascade. C3b is constantly degenerated by enzymes in the circulation. The classical and alternative pathway then have a similar pathway involving activation of C3. There are genetic conditions that exist where there are deficiencies of complement components which predispose individuals to infection. Complement is involved in regulation of the immune system, and abnormalities of the complement system may predispose to autoimmune disease. Complement components are products of the class III major histocompatibility complex (MHC), together with tumour necrosis factor and the enzyme 21-hydroxylase.

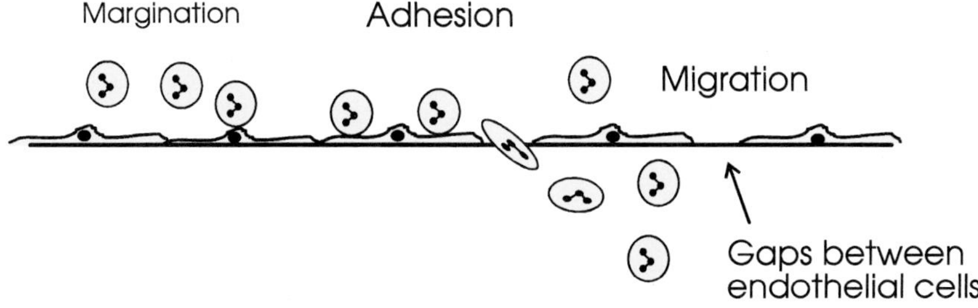

Fig. 2.4 A summary of processes involved in acute inflammation.

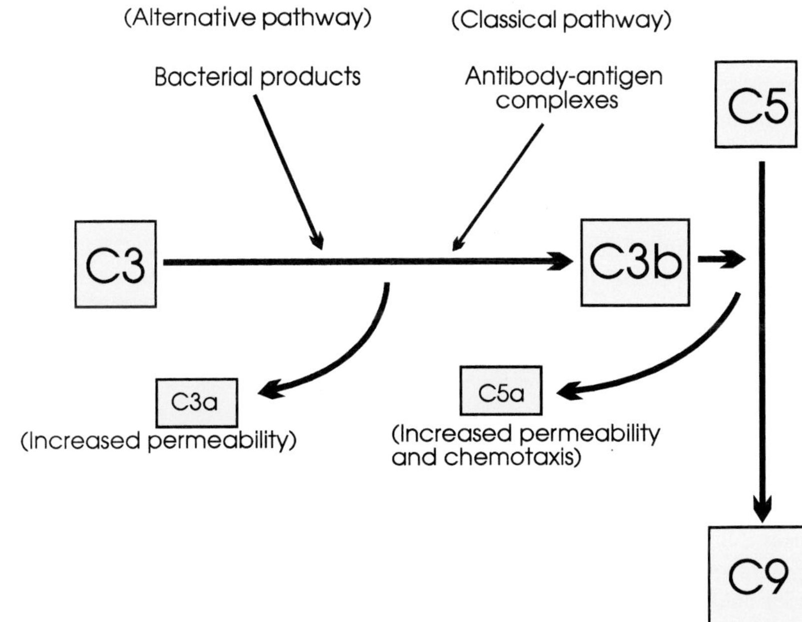

Fig. 2.5 The complement pathway.

The final result of the activation of both pathways is the production of C5b-9, the membrane attack complex, which can punch holes in cell membranes. Two complement components, C3a and C5a, have activity in inflammation. Both of these molecules increase vascular permeability; C5a also attracts neutrophils and macrophages.

Several of the complement proteins act as so-called acute phase proteins. These are a group of proteins that show an increased concentration in the circulation during acute inflammation, usually due to infection. They are important in innate, that is, non-specific, immunity. A well-known acute phase protein is C reactive protein. This, when bound to bacteria, increases the affinity of the organisms to macrophage phagocytosis.

The importance of complement proteins is emphasized by several congenital defects of complement components in which there is a marked susceptibility to bacterial infection.

Clotting cascade

The final part of this cascade is the production of fibrin (see p. 000), material prominent in acute inflammatory reactions. For example, inflammation in cavities, such as the pericardium or pleura, frequently is of fibrinous type. An enzyme called plasmin, which can break down fibrin, is produced from plasminogen (Fig. 2.6). Products derived from the breakdown of fibrin due to plasmin activation increase

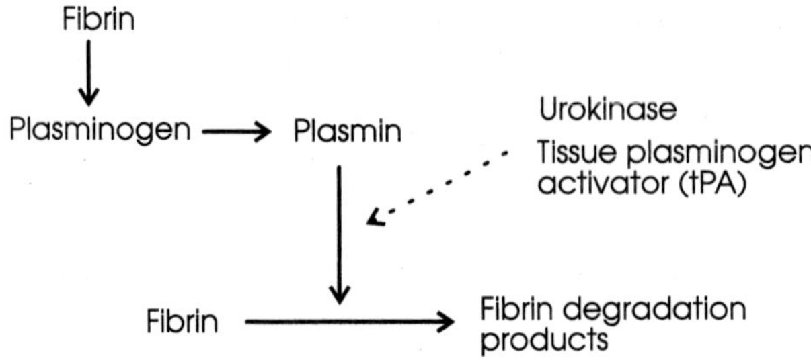

Fig. 2.6 Plasmin–fibrinogen pathway.

vascular permeability. Plasmin also induces the production of complement components and the production of bradykinin.

Kinins

These are produced by the activation of Hageman factor XII, the connection with the blood-clotting cascade being apparent. Bradykinin is the main product, and causes smooth muscle contraction, vascular dilatation, and pain. There is a group of short-acting local hormones involved in acute inflammation which are mainly products of arachidonic acid metabolism. The most important are the prostaglandins and leukotrienes. They have effects on vascular size and permeability, and on chemotaxis. Anti-inflammatory drugs act on this system. Finally, cytokines such as

Table 2.3 Inflammatory mediators

Mediator	Action
Vasoactive amines	
Histamine and serotonin	Vasodilatation and increased vessel permeability
Kinins	
Bradykinin	Pain, smooth muscle contraction, increased vessel permeability
Kallikrein	Chemotaxis; activates Hageman factor
Complement components	
C3a	Increased vessel permeability
C5a	Increased vessel permeability and chemotaxis
Fibrinolysis	
Fibrin degradation products (FDP)	Increased vessel permeability
Fibrin-related peptides (plasmin)	Activates Hageman factor, produces C3a and FDP
Arachidonic acid metabolism	
Prostaglandins (E_1, E_2)	Vasodilatation, fever, pain
Leukotrienes	Chemotaxis, increased permeability, smooth muscle contraction
Cytokines	
Tumour necrosis factor and interleukin-1	Adhesion molecule expression, fever, systemic effects
Platelet-activating factor	Smooth muscle contraction
Alpha-interferon	Fever

platelet-activating factor, interleukin-1, and tumour necrosis factor, are now known to be important inflammatory mediators. These also appear to be the cause of systemic features of inflammation, such as fever and leukocytosis and acute phase reactions including changes in plasma proteins. Cytokines and inflammatory mediators involved in acute inflammation and their actions are summarized in Table 2.3.

Some anti-inflammatory drugs act by inhibiting certain metabolic pathways or enzymes involved in the production of inflammatory mediators. For example, aspirin and non-steroidal anti-inflammatory drugs inhibit the production of prostaglandins (Fig. 2.7).

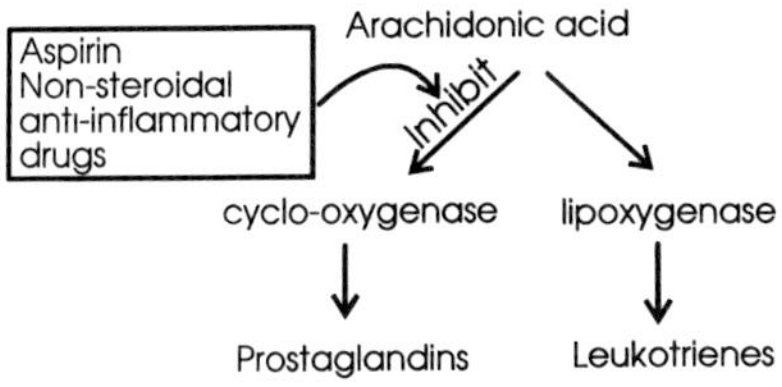

Aspirin
Non-steroidal
anti-inflammatory
drugs
Inhibit
Arachidonic acid
cyclo-oxygenase
lipoxygenase
Prostaglandins
Leukotrienes

Fig. 2.7 The action of anti-inflammatory drugs.

CHRONIC INFLAMMATION

Causes

Acute inflammatory reactions usually resolve, leaving little in the way of abnormality, particularly if the injury is mild. If, however, there has been a lot of destruction of tissue, there may be deposition of large amounts of collagen during the healing process resulting in fibrosis. Abscess development is another outcome of acute inflammation. This section will focus on another possible result, namely, chronic inflammation.

Chronic inflammation, in contrast to acute inflammation, is of long duration and associated with variable degrees of tissue destruction. It frequently occurs in conjunction with healing responses. It may follow some types of acute inflammation where there is persistence of the microorganism. It may also occur after repeated episodes of acute inflammation. In some cases, chronic inflammation appears to arise without any evidence of previous acute inflammation. These different situations are described below.

1. Persistence of the stimulus

This can be due to impaired healing due to poor blood supply or a foreign body such as insoluble stitch material, a metal prosthesis or necrotic tissue. There may be impaired drainage of pus. There may also be continuing infection resulting in increased tissue destruction and the development of a chronic abscess. In chronic osteomyelitis, the sequestrum of necrotic bone acts as a foreign body and a nidus for infection by pyogenic organisms.

2. Repeated acute inflammation

This is frequently due to multiple episodes of infection. An example of repeated acute inflammation resulting in chronic inflammation is chronic cholecystitis. Another example is chronic episodes of periodontal inflammation which leads to a chronic periapical granuloma relating to a tooth. A neutrophil-rich exudate may persist for a long time, for example, in a chronic abscess, empyema, or chronic osteomyelitis. This persistent protein loss via the exudate may result in hypoalbuminaemia. Pyogenic organisms, such as *Staphylococcus aureus* and *Escherichia coli*, are frequently involved.

3. Chronic inflammation *de novo*

This occurs without any evidence of previous acute inflammation. Some infections, typically tuberculosis, syphillis, or viral infections, are a cause of this. In general,

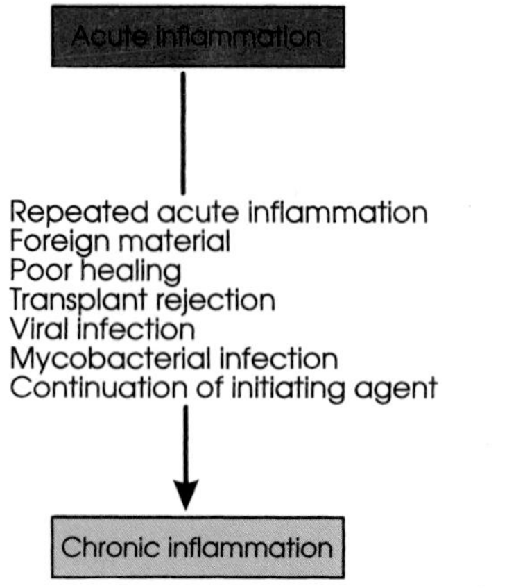

Fig. 2.8 The origins of chronic inflammation.

infections that are difficult to clear, in particular those caused by intracellular organisms, tend to generate chronic inflammatory responses. A frequent result of the response to a persistent antigen that is difficult to degrade is granulomatous inflammation. This is characterized by collections of cells of the monocyte–macrophage group. The granulomas are of foreign-body type; if the immune system is involved and lymphocytes are present the granulomas are of epithelioid cell type. For example, the histological hallmark of tuberculosis is the presence of necrotizing epithelioid cell granulomas.

Chronic inflammation is seen in association with autoimmune disease, such as rheumatoid arthritis, which is not organ-specific, or cryptogenic fibrosing alveolitis and Sjögren's disease of the salivary glands, which, in contrast, are organ-specific. In rheumatoid arthritis, for example, the synovium shows a heavy infiltrate of lymphocytes, lymphocytic aggregates, and plasma cells. There is synovial hyperplasia and fibrosis. In autoimmune disease there is a primary reaction of the immune system against the person's own tissues without an apparent cause. There is a loss of the mechanisms that keep the immune system tolerant of self-antigens. Other examples are Hashimoto's thyroiditis, with autoimmune destruction of the thyroid, or primary biliary cirrhosis where the immune attack is against the bile ducts.

Exposure to persistent non-degradable material is another cause of chronic inflammation, for example in silicosis, where fibrosis is the characteristic feature. Hypersensitivity-type immune reactions may result in chronic inflammation. This process is seen in, for instance, extrinsic allergic alveolitis due to exposure to organic dust resulting in lung fibrosis. The reaction seen in kidney or heart transplant rejection can be regarded as a chronic inflammatory response. Radiation is also a significant cause of chronic inflammation. Many of the changes seen in radiation injury are secondary to vascular damage. The causes of chronic inflammation are summarized in Fig. 2.8.

Cellular response

The cellular infiltrate in chronic inflammation consists primarily of mononuclear cells—macrophages, lymphocytes, and plasma cells. A proliferation of blood vessels also occurs. There is also associated collagen production by fibroblasts resulting in fibrosis. Tissue destruction with replacement by fibrous tissue is the usual result of chronic inflammation

1. The role of macrophages

Macrophages have primarily a phagocytic role in acute inflammation, acting as scavanger cells. They ingest and degrade foreign material and inflammatory debris. Macrophages are recruited from the circulation, the precursor cell being the monocyte derived from the bone marrow. Macrophages belong to the mononuclear–phagocyte system, and when present as fixed cells in tissues they are generally termed histiocytes. In chronic inflammation, macrophages also function as promoters of fibroblast and endothelial growth. They are capable of producing growth factors, resulting in fibrosis and vascular proliferation. The population of macrophages is maintained mainly by continued recruitment; local proliferation does not occur to a significant degree. Macrophages respond to macrophage imhibition factor (MIF) and macrophage activating factor (MAF), the latter increasing the phagocytic and killing ability of the macrophages.

Macrophages can be regarded as the prime movers in the immune response, in that they are involved in the presentation of foreign antigen to lymphocytes, particularly T helper (CD4-positive) lymphocytes. Macrophages express class II

HLA-DR antigens and are therefore important in the process of antigen recognition by lymphocytes.

Many factors are chemotactic for macrophages. These include complement fragment C5a, collagen and fibrin breakdown products, neutrophil-derived proteins, lymphokines, and platelet-derived growth factor (Table 2.4).

Macrophages produce enzymes responsible for much of the tissue destruction seen in inflammation, particularly elastase and proteases. Complement, coagulation factors, and other chemotactic molecules can be produced by these cells. They also produce growth factors for fibroblasts and blood vessels. Interleukin-1 and tumour necrosis factor are examples of cytokines produced by macrophages. Macrophages are therefore important in the development and modulation of chronic inflammatory processes.

Granulomatous inflammation is a form of chronic inflammation seen as a response to agents that are persistent and difficult to degrade. In this form of inflammation, macrophages are recruited into the site of inflammation and activated by cytokines produced by lymphocytes.

Table 2.4 Macrophage products

Inflammatory mediators
Complement components
Prostaglandins
Leukotrienes
Radicals
Cytokines
Interleukin-1
Interleukin-6
Tumour necrosis factor-alpha
Enzymes
Elastase
Lysozyme collagenase

2. Plasma cells and lymphocytes

Plasma cells are derived from B lymphocytes and produce immunoglobulin, representing the humoral arm of the immune system. T lymphocytes are involved in cell-mediated immunity. They are, however, considered as chronic inflammatory cells in the context of this discussion (Fig. 2.9). Activated lymphocytes, particularly T cells, produce lymphokines such as gamma-interferon that activate monocytes and macrophages. Macrophages produce cytokines, particularly interleukin-1, that have a stimulatory action on endothelial cells and fibroblasts. There is, therefore, a great deal of cellular interaction.

Eosinophils are frequently seen in chronic inflammatory reactions. They are involved in the inactivation of inflammatory mediators, using enzymes such as arylsulphatase. Eosinophils are also typically seen in type 1 allergic hypersensitivity reactions, together with mast cells. Eosinophils are also seen in association with parasites.

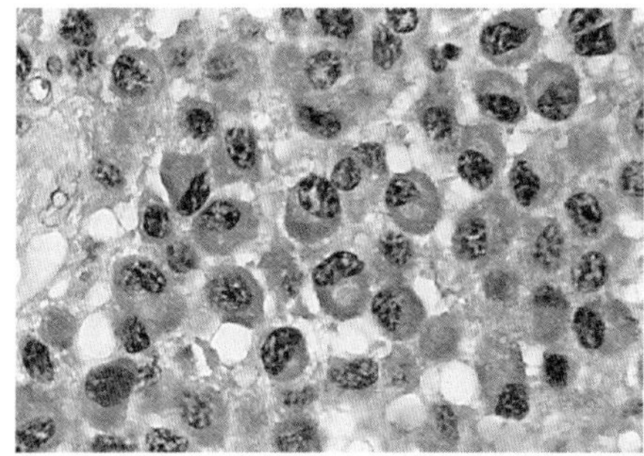

Fig. 2.9 Plasma cells and lymphocytes are seen in chronic inflammation.

3. Fibroblasts and blood vessels

Many cytokines produced in chronic inflammatory reactions, for example, growth-promoting factors from macrophages, stimulate fibroblasts to produce collagen, the hallmark of chronic inflammation. Vascular proliferation also occurs, and both this and fibroblast activity occur in tissue-healing. Granulation tissue develops as part of the healing response. This consists of groups of proliferating capillaries associated with inflammatory cells within a stroma containing myofibroblasts (Fig. 2.10). There may be marked distortion of tissue architecture in chronic inflammation (Fig. 2.11).

Systemic effects

The systemic effects depend on the nature of the cause of the inflammation. In some infections due to intracellular organisms there may be generalized macrophage activation resulting in splenomegaly, for example. Lymphadenopathy may occur in a chronic immune response together with a polyclonal increase in immunoglobulins. A frequent result of chronic infection as in chronic osteomyelitis or bronchiectasis is a sustained increased serum amyloid A protein (SAA) and as a consequence reactive systemic amyloidosis. Most of the other systemic effects of chronic inflammation are mediated by cytokines. Chronic pyrexia is associated with

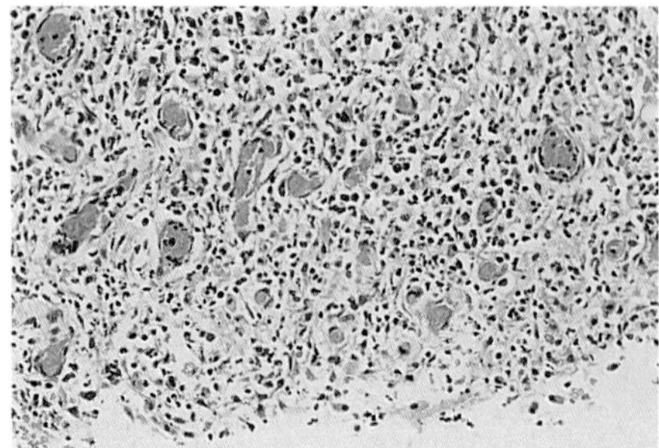

Fig. 2.10 Granulation tissue consists of abundant proliferating capillaries and inflammatory cells.

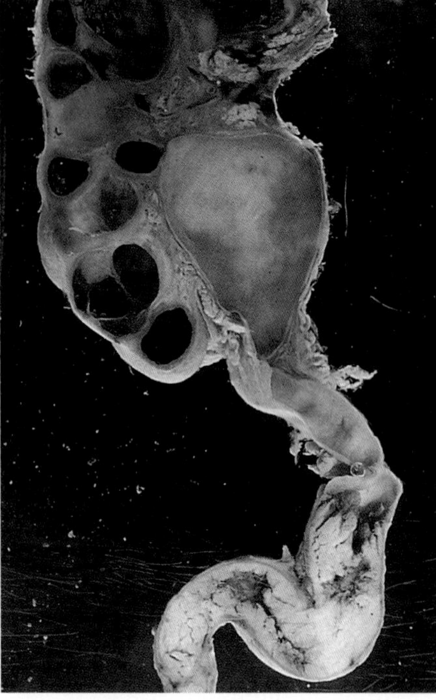

Fig. 2.11 A kidney shows marked chronic inflammation with distortion of architecture due to obstruction of the ureter by tumour (bottom).

increased levels of interleukin-1 and other pyrogens released from neutrophils and macrophages. Much of the wasting in tuberculosis is related to tumour necrosis factor-alpha. A normochromic normocytic anaemia is frequently seen as a result of chronic inflammation due to marrow suppression. As in acute inflammation, a persistent leucocytosis may occur with an increased erythrocyte sedimentation rate. The factors involved in a chronic inflammatory reaction are shown in Fig. 2.12.

INFLAMMATION RELEVANT TO THE MOUTH

Inflammatory conditions of the teeth, particularly gingivitis and periapical periodontitis, are common reasons for tooth loss apart from caries. The inflammatory reactions in the mouth and teeth are identical to inflammatory reactions anywhere else in the body. Another inflammatory condition of the teeth is pulpitis, which may be acute or chronic. In view of the high vascularity of the periapical and pulp tissue, there is also marked capability of healing if the underlying cause of the inflammation is treated. Chronic gingivitis associated with dental plaque can progress from the marginal gingiva, down the tissue surrounding the teeth and initiate periapical inflammation. Dental plaque appears to be the underlying initiating cause of periodontal inflammation. All the typical features of acute inflammation are seen in early gingivitis, including vasodilation, exudation of fluid, and acute inflammatory cell infiltrate, predominantly neutrophils. Repeated episodes of acute inflammation then progress to chronic inflammation, and there is infiltration by lymphocytes and fibrosis, with laying down of collagen from gingival fibroblasts. The adjacent squamous epithelium shows typically marked hyperplasia. Loss of epithelium, that is, ulceration of the gingival epithelium against the tooth, the so-called gingival pocket occurs. Lymphocytes and plasma cells increase in number and there is continued destruction of gingival tissue with fibrosis. In advanced gingivitis there will be healing responses, including development of

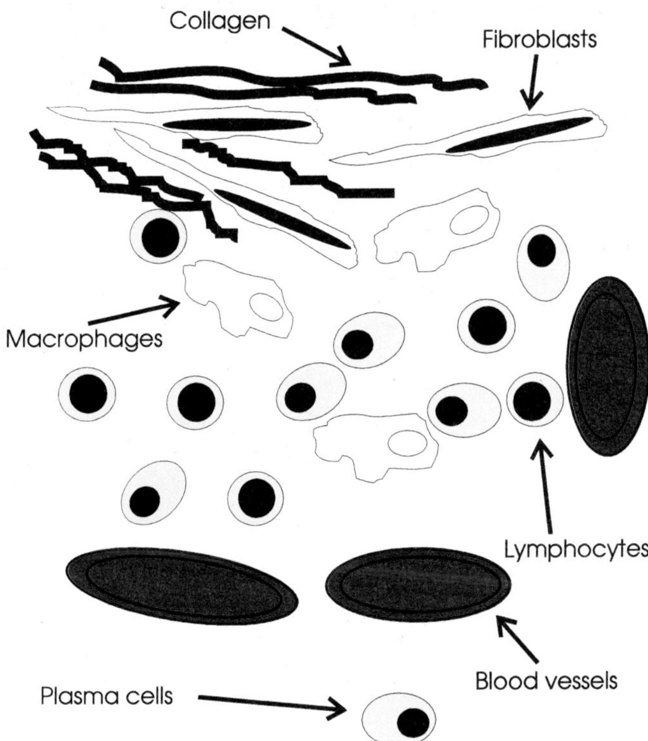

Fig. 2.12 The features of chronic inflammation.

granulation tissue and increased fibrous tissue. Immunological mechanisms then come into play, with evidence of cell-mediated immunological reactions. There is also evidence of humoral immune mechanisms in periodontal disease. With extension of periodontal inflammation down to the apex of the tooth, a frequent complication is the development of a periapical granuloma. The word granuloma in this sense is inappropriate in that epithelioid cell granulomas are not seen. It really describes the abundant granulation tissue and organizing blood clot that is seen in this condition. An abscess develops with organization. Abundant granulation tissue develops and there is also resorption of adjacent bone which is replaced by chronic inflammatory tissue. There is frequently a marked foreign-body giant cell reaction to cholesterol material derived from the chronic haemorrhage. There is also frequently hyperplasia of epithelial rests of Malassez. These epithelial cell rests are small inclusions of squamous epithelium commonly seen near the root of the tooth with tissue of embryonic origin. In effect, a periapical granuloma is an abscess with marked organization and attempts at repair. These squamous epithelial cells may eventually line the cyst and form a well-circumscribed radicular cyst. Periapical disease may progress to form a very large abscess with possible erosion into underlying bone and pointing of the abscess externally or into a nasal sinus. Also, inflammation may spread into the underlying and surrounding connective tissue forming a cellulitis. Rests of Malassez are formed by fragmentation of the epithelial root sheath during development of teeth.

Acute inflammation of the salivary glands (sialadenitis) due to bacterial infection is well-recognized. It is usually associated with duct obstruction, for example, due to a calculus. Chronic sialadentis may follow repeated acute inflammation, particularly in the submandibular gland. Sarcoidosis, a granulomatous disease of unknown origin, typically involves the salivary glands.

Viruses, such as mumps, affect the salivary glands, most frequently the parotid.

GRANULOMATOUS INFLAMMATION

Definition

A granuloma is a focal collection of activated macrophages forming a distinct microenvironment in the tissue. Granulomatous inflammation is usually seen as a response to an antigen that is persistent and irritant. This process is usually classified as a type of chronic inflammation. Granulomas vary in size from a collection of a small number of cells to many thousands of cells forming a nodule several millimetres or more in diameter. It can be regarded as a rather non-specific primitive response in the case of a foreign-body reaction. In the case of a hypersensitivity granuloma, however, the reaction is more sophisticated in that there is involvement of the cellular immune system. Lymphocytes are seen in association with the macrophages. This gives the granulomatous reaction specificity and memory for the antigen. This type of granuloma is usually called an epithelioid cell granuloma.

Causes

Foreign-body granuloma

Any insoluble particulate material is capable of inducing a foreign-body reaction. The pattern of response is generally very similar whatever the cause. The immune system does not show significant involvement, macrophages showing non-specific phagocytosis. In surgical pathology, common causes of a foreign-body granuloma are suture material, cotton fibres, mineral debris, hair fragments in a pilonidal sinus (Figs 2.13 and 2.14), dead bone in chronic osteomyelitis, and necrotic tissue in the tract of a fine-needle aspiration biopsy or site of previous surgery. Keratin, urate crystals in gout, and cholesterol frequently evoke this response, cholesterol clefts being seen in organizing blood clot. Foreign-body granulomas are also seen in the prostate following a trans-urethral resection. Granulomas can be seen as a reaction to ruptured thyroid follicles after palpation. In lymph nodes, granulomas can be seen as a reaction to lipid; the cystic lymph node in a cholecystectomy specimen frequently shows a foreign-body reaction to fat derived from bile. Even air can induce foreign-body granulomas, for example, in surgical emphysema or *Pneumatosis coli*.

Epithelioid cell (hypersensitivity) granuloma

The differential diagnosis of the underlying process when hypersensitivity granulomas are seen is very wide (Table 2.5). The common link is that cell-mediated immunity is required against the antigen for the development of epithelioid cell granulomas. In general, intracellular organisms incite this form of inflammation, a classic cause being tuberculosis and other mycobacteria. Substances causing this type of inflammation have some degree of solubility and are capable of

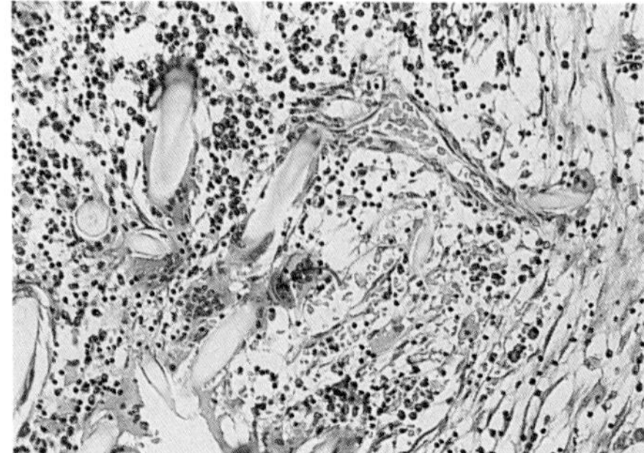

Fig. 2.13 Hair fragments causing a foreign-body giant cell reaction (left).

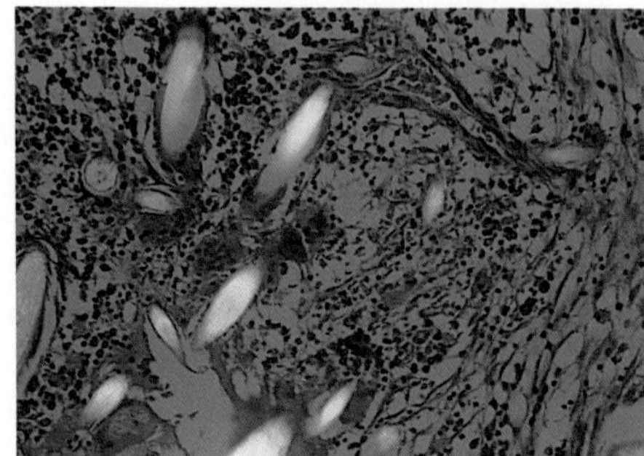

Fig. 2.14 Hair is more visible under crossed polarizers (left).

immunological recognition. Small molecules may induce such a reaction, but only when bound to a larger molecule termed a hapten. The involvement of the immune system explains why one person may develop granulomas to an antigen such as zirconium, and show the same reaction repeated over a long time period, whilst another will show no reaction. There are some diseases, however, where granulomas are seen, such as sarcoidosis and Crohn's disease, where the agent giving rise to this inflammation is not yet known.

Table 2.5 Causes of epithelioid cell granulomas

Intracellular infection
- Mycobacteria: tuberculosis, leprosy, atypical mycobacteria
- Histoplasmosis
- *Leishmania*
- *Toxoplasma gondii*

Other organisms
- *Listeria monocytogenes*
- Cat scratch fever
- Brucellosis
- Syphilis
- Pneumocystis

Fungi
- *Aspergillus*
- Cryptococcus

Hypersensitivity
- Allergy to foreign protein: extrinsic allergic alveolitis
- Aspergillosis
- Beryllium
- Silica
- Zirconium
- Drug reaction
- *Schistosoma* eggs

Response to tumours
- Hodgkin's disease
- T cell lymphomas
- Tumour antigens

Unknown
- Sarcoidosis
- Crohn's disease
- Primary biliary cirrhosis
- Wegener's granulomatosis

Pathology

Foreign-body granulomas

In a foreign-body reaction, macrophages are recruited from the circulation and the surrounding tissue and phagocytose the foreign material. Macrophages are a member of the mononuclear–phagocytic series of cells, along with, for example, Kupffer cells in the liver, Langerhans cells in the skin, and dendritic cells in lymph nodes. Lysosomal enzymes act to attempt to degrade the material. This process is usually associated with a degree of acute or chronic inflammation. In a histological section, the macrophages appear large, with abundant cytoplasm, and the foreign material can be often seen within the cells. Macrophages frequently fuse when attempting to ingest the same particle, and a foreign-body giant cell develops.

Epithelioid cell granulomas

At light microscopy, an epithelioid cell granuloma appears as a cohesive collection of large macrophages with abundant cytoplasm. These cells are frequently termed epithelioid cells because of their similarity to epithelial cells (Fig. 2.15). These cells show very close interaction on electron microscopy. They frequently show cytoplasmic interdigitations and intercellular junctions, explaining the cohesive nature of the epithelioid cells in granulomas. The cytoplasm of epithelioid cells is filled with secretory vacuoles instead of phagocytic vacuoles as are usually seen in macrophages. The macrophages in epithelioid cell granulomas therefore show a switch from a phagocytic role to a secretory role.

An important feature distinguishing a foreign-body granuloma from an epithelioid cell granuloma is the presence of lymphocytes. In an epithelioid cell granuloma, these lymphocytes can be seen closely interacting with the epithelioid cells. There are frequently surrounding fibroblasts, particularly if the granuloma has been present for any length of time.

Epithelioid cells frequently fuse to form multinucleated Langhan's giant cells. These may have 50 or more peripherally placed nuclei in each cell.

Central necrosis and cavitation of the granulomas, seen naked-eye as so-called caseation, may be present, particularly in mycobacterial infections. In surgical pathology, necrotizing granulomatous inflammation is tuberculosis until proved otherwise.

Immunology of epithelioid cell granulomas

The role of T lymphocytes

Epithelioid cell granulomas are initiated and driven by T lymphocytes which are mainly of helper (CD4-positive) subtype. This explains why patients with acquired immunodeficiency syndrome with a lack of CD4 lymphocytes are so prone to infections, such as tuberculosis, that are normally controlled by granulomatous inflammation. Granulomas are a manifestation of cell-mediated immunity. B lymphocytes are rarely found in granulomas, the humoral arm of the immune system showing little involvement. For example, in tuberculosis, serum antibodies

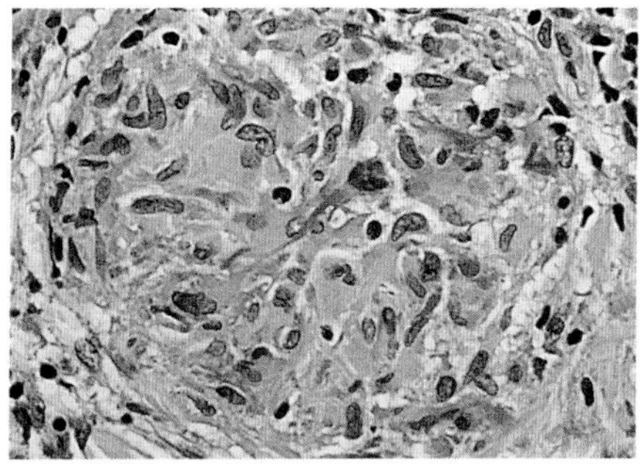

Fig. 2.15 An epithelioid cell granuloma.

to the myobacterium are not seen at significant levels. The indication of recent or previous infection with tuberculosis is a delayed hypersensitivity reaction to mycobacterial antigen in the skin in the form of a positive Mantoux test.

Macrophages present antigen to CD4-positive (CD4+) T cells. Activated T cells then produce cytokines, for instance, migration inhibition factor and gamma-interferon, which recruit and activate macrophages, transforming them into epithelioid cells which have increased ability to kill and degrade the causative organism or antigen. In an established granuloma, the CD4+ (helper) lymphocytes are found at the centre of the granulomas. CD8+ (suppressor) lymphocytes are found at the periphery and probably have an immunoregulatory role in granulomas.

The role of macrophages

Almost all the cells in epithelioid cell granulomas are derived from the circulation. Mononuclear cells derived from bone marrow stem cells are recruited from blood vessels and transform into activated macrophages and epithelioid cells under the influence of cytokines produced by lymphocytes. These macrophage-derived cells also act as antigen-presenting cells to sensitized T lymphocytes; epithelioid cells strongly express HLA class II. They also express cell adhesion molecules such as intercellular adhesion molecule-1 (ICAM-1).

Epithelioid cells, although derived from macrophages, show reduced phagocytic activity but increased secretory activity. The onset of hypersensitivity with macrophage activation dramatically alters the evolution of the immune response. For example, the onset of hypersensitivity indicates the change from primary to secondary tuberculosis with subsequent control of the infection. An idealized epithelioid cell granuloma is shown in Fig. 2.16.

The role of cytokines

Cytokines—hormone-like compounds produced by one cell to act on another or itself—are of primary importance in the development of a granuloma. This is why corticosteroids, which inhibit cytokine production by lymphocytes, supress granulomatous inflammation. Cytokines are usually small proteins. In some granulomatous inflammation, a side-effect of high cytokine concentration is cell necrosis. Caseation in tuberculosis is a cytokine 'burn' rather than being due to ischaemia. Release of toxic macrophage products, such as lysozyme, also contributes to this necrosis.

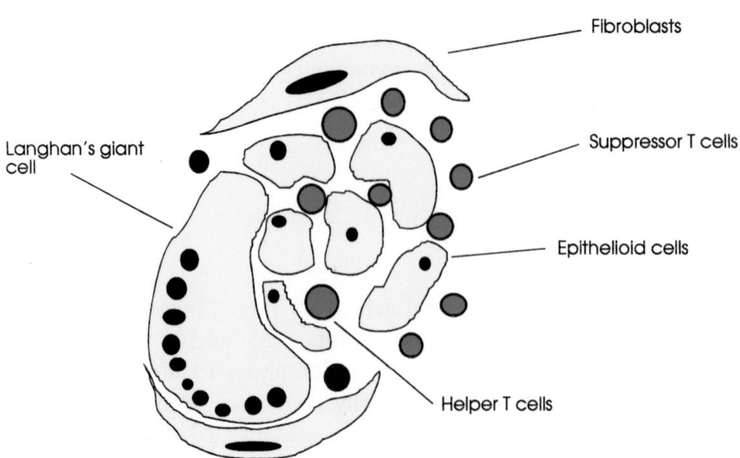

Fig. 2.16 An idealized epithelioid cell granuloma.

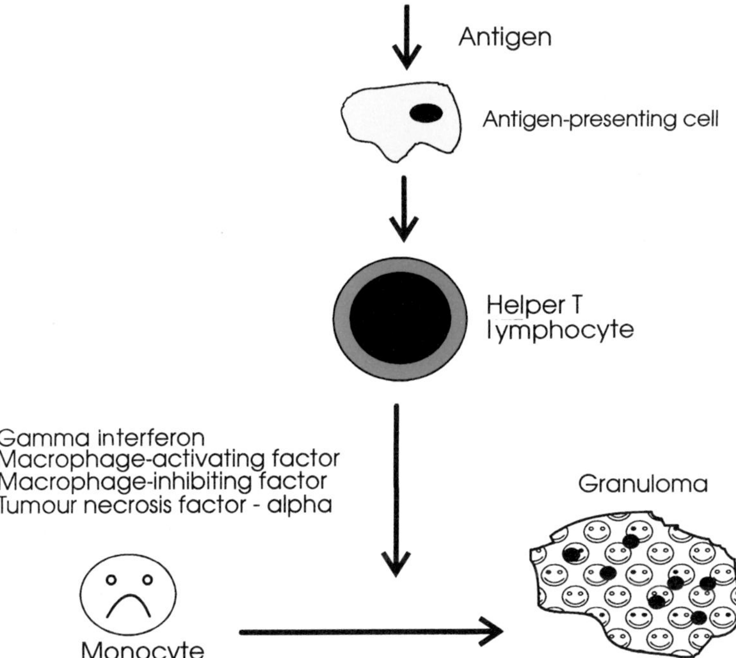

Fig. 2.17 Formation of an epithelioid cell granuloma.

As mentioned above, cytokines, such as gamma-interferon, are important in macrophage activation. Interleukin-2 stimulates the growth of activated T lymphocytes. It is now apparent that tumour necrosis factor, produced by macrophages, is an important mediator in granulomas, in synergism with interleukin-1. The severe wasting and fever in tuberculosis ('consumption') is due to tumour necrosis factor. The production of interleukin-1 and tumour necrosis factor is inhibited by interleukin-6 from many cells, including macrophages and lymphocytes. It can be seen, therefore, that many of these cytokines interact with each other. It has been recently shown that granulomas can be induced by some proteins alone, one of which is termed 'granuloma initiation factor'.

Increased fibroblast activity, which is cytokine-mediated, is a frequent response to epithelioid cell granulomas. The resulting fibrosis is manifested clinically, particularly in diseases such as Crohn's disease and sarcoidosis. The development of an epithelioid cell granuloma is shown in Fig. 2.17.

HEALING AND REPAIR

The main aim of all inflammatory responses is to return the tissues back to the state that they were before the onset of the injury, that is, resolution. If there is no destruction of tissue architecture, and in particular no necrosis, this may be possible. However, in many situations this does not occur and the hallmark of the reparative processes that result is the formation of granulation tissue and fibrous tissue, the latter manifesting as scarring.

The response seen is determined particularly by the nature of the tissue involved. *Regeneration* is a process which involves replacement of the damaged tissue by a proliferation of cells of the same type found in that tissue. In many cases, this returns the tissue to the state it was before the injury. If regeneration is not possible, then *replacement* of the tissue by collagenous scar tissue occurs.

Regeneration

Cells have different abilities to regenerate; generally the more specialized a cell is the less ability it has to proliferate. Cells fall into three main groups; labile, stable, and permanent.

Labile

These are cells which are continuously proliferating in a controlled way to replace cells which are being lost due to normal physiological activity. These cells do not leave the cell cycle between mitoses. Examples of tissues in which such cells are found include squamous epithelium, which is a 'wear and tear' epithelium, hair, the mucous columnar epithelium of the gastrointestinal tract, the bone marrow, and the lining of ducts of exocrine secretory glands. Tissue of labile type can undergo hyperplasia, and heal by regeneration.

Stable

These are cells which are normally in a very low or absent proliferative state, but can proliferate when called to do so. They can regenerate very rapidly. Examples include cells of most solid organs such as the liver, kidney, and connective tissue cells such as fibroblasts. They are held in the G_0 phase of the cell cycle (see p. 000) until called upon to enter the cycle again and divide. They re-enter the cell cycle in the G_1 phase of the cell cycle. As with labile tissue, stable tissue can become hyperplastic when called to do so, and it can heal by regeneration.

Permanent

Neurones, cardiac, and skeletal muscle cells are examples of very specialized cells which are incapable of division and cannot regenerate if lost. Muscle is capable of hypertrophy if increased demands are made on it. The cells are held in the G_0 phase of the cell cycle, and cannot re-enter the G_1 phase again. These types of tissue heal by repair only.

With tissues that have labile and stable cells, regeneration is generally possible if there is preservation of the architecture or connective tissue structure that underlies the tissue. This is usually provided by basement membranes, specialized protein gel-like sheets to which all epithelial cells are attached. This provides a framework or template on which the cells can regenerate. If, however, this framework is lost, the cells regenerate in a disordered fashion, and fibrosis is a frequent result with the development of a scar.

Repair

If regeneration is not possible, repair with eventual replacement by collagen is the result. Cells involved in the repair mechanism are macrophages, endothelial cells that form capillaries, and fibroblasts that synthesize collagen.

Macrophages are recruited early in the acute inflammatory response, and phagocytose cellular debris, fibrin, and degenerate material, contributing to organization and repair even at that early phase. The formation of granulation tissue, named because of its red granular appearance, is the next phase and it is characteristic of the onset of the healing process. It is formed by a proliferation of endothelial cells which develop from small blood vessels adjacent to the inflamed, damaged tissue. Chemical messengers or cytokines are involved that signal the blood vessels to form these buds, termed 'angiogenic' factors. Fibroblast growth factor is one such growth factor. Fibroblasts also begin to proliferate at this time. They are already present in connective tissue and are recruited by the action of cytokines. They can undergo a type of metaplasia into cells resembling smooth muscle which are capable of a degree of contractile activity, contributing to wound contraction. Fibroblasts lay down the extracellular matrix, including collagen, that is seen in repair following inflammation. The relationship of this process to wound healing is described below.

Collagen production

As collagen production, seen as scarring or 'sclerosis', is the hallmark of chronic inflammation and repair, it is of value to briefly cover collagen synthesis. Collagen is an abundant connective tissue substance, and is a polymer of high tensile strength. It is a group of related glycoproteins, different types being found in various tissues and sites in the body. It is produced by long, thin spindle-shaped fibroblasts. These cells also produce elastin and other matrix components. Fibroblasts have abundant rough endoplasmic reticulum and secrete collagen precursors into the extracellular environment. Procollagen, a spiral or helical molecule with three units, forms collagen in the extracellular space after secretion. Vitamin C is required for the synthesis of procollagen. Collagen molecules become cross-linked, contributing to its remarkable strength. There are different biochemical types of collagen. Type I is the most abundant collagen in the body, and type IV is only found in basement membranes. Type II is found in cartilage, and type III in blood vessels and skin (Table 2.6).

In healing wounds, a proportion of the fibroblasts acquire some features of smooth muscle cells in that they become contractile. The term *myofibroblast* is used for these cells and they contribute to the tissue contraction seen in healing wounds.

Other cytokines that are involved in wound healing include: (1) platelet-derived growth factor which causes the migration and growth of smooth muscle cells and fibroblasts; (2) epidermal growth factor (EGF) which causes proliferation of epithelium by binding to EGF receptors; (3) macrophage growth factor which stimulates fibroblast and endothelial growth; and (4) transforming growth factor-beta (TGF) which attracts inflammatory cells.

Wound healing

Two types of wound healing are generally recognized: 'first intention', otherwise known as primary union, and 'secondary intention', known as secondary union.

Table 2.6 Types of collagen and location

Type	Tissue
I	90% of collagen in interstitium, in particular, skin and musculoskeletal system
II	Cartilage, intervertebral disc
III	Skin, viscera
IV	Basement membrane
V	Interstitium
VI	Microfibrils
VII	Dermal–epidermal junction anchoring filaments

Primary union

This is best illustrated by a sutured surgical incision, in which there is no infection or other factors to delay healing. For example, in a clean sutured surgical incision of the oral mucosa, there is minimal damage to tissue. Fibrin fills the small space between the edges of the incision, which is eventually organized by macrophages. The adjacent squamous epithelium regenerates quickly by a proliferation of the basal cells and bridges the gap between the wound edges. In the underlying tissue there is growth of fibroblasts which produce collagen, and in 5 to 10 days the wound gains significant strength from this. Before this time, the sutures contribute most to the strength of the wound.

Secondary union

If there is reduced blood supply to a wound, poor nutrition, infection, extensive tissue loss, or other factors that may interfere with a healing wound, a large defect of tissue results. This heals with a much more striking inflammatory reaction in a process referred to as healing by secondary union. There is a marked proliferation of granulation tissue which grows into the fibrin filling the wound space. Epithelium bridges the gap in a similar way to that seen in primary union, growing over the surface of the granulation tissue. However, there is a more cellular inflammatory response and a larger amount of granulation tissue than that seen in a sutured wound. As mentioned above, cells are seen in granulation tissue that are a 'cross' between fibroblasts and smooth muscle, and are responsible for bringing the edges of a wound together by contraction. These healing processes are summarized in Fig. 2.18.

Bone heals in basically the same way; after the space between the bone ends fills with fibrin, there in reabsorption of clot by macrophages and bone by osteoclasts. New bone is laid down by osteoblasts from the periosteum and callus forms as the new osteoid calcifies. In about six weeks the major part of the healing process is complete.

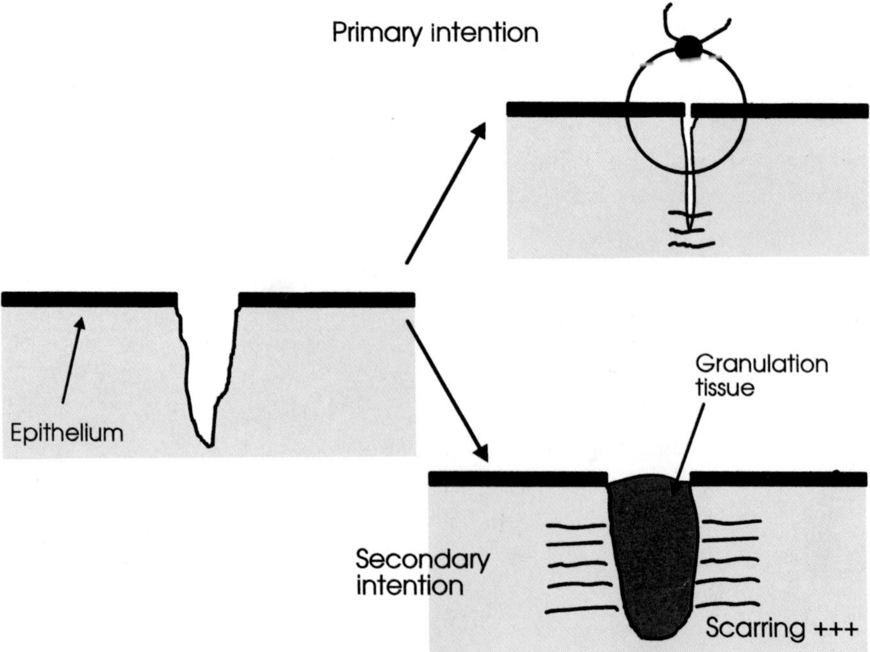

Fig. 2.18 Healing by primary and secondary intention.

Healing of a tooth socket

It is useful to consider the events occurring in a healing tooth socket. Many of the processes involved are very similar to those seen in other healing wounds. By the very nature of an extraction tooth socket, the wound heals by a process resembling secondary intention described above.

Initially, the socket fills with blood clot (fibrin) within a few minutes, forming a plug. Beneath this, after several days, there is a proliferation of granulation tissue, composed of endothelial cells, fibroblasts, and cells halfway between fibroblasts and smooth muscle cells (myofibroblasts). The bone of the socket is remodelled by osteoclasts (that remove bone) and osteoblasts (that lay down new bone). The surface squamous epithelium grows over the fibrin and granulation tissue plug, and completely covers the wound in about one to two weeks. After a few months the socket is eventually filled with connective tissue and bone.

Factors that influence wound healing

Local factors

Blood supply

A good blood supply is vital if adequate wound healing is to occur. Generally, this is not a problem in the oral cavity in view of the excellent blood supply and the extensive collateral circulation present in this area. A compromised blood supply leads to a reduced rate of healing. This may be seen in association with chronic inflammation, particularly if occlusion of small arteries is present (endarteritis obliterans). Poor healing in tissue that has been previously exposed to radiation for tumour treatment also occurs because of similar changes in such vessels.

Infection

This is a very important factor that delays wound healing. Wounds in areas exposed to the environment or in sites of the body which are colonized by bacteria are prone to such infection. If there are reduced numbers of circulating neutrophils and monocytes, the patient will be more vulnerable to infection. There may be inherited defects of neutrophil function or complement deficiency.

In an infected wound, there will be an increased acute inflammatory reaction with the production of pus and granulation tissue which may be seen by the naked eye. Infected wounds also tend to show increased scarring.

Foreign body

The presence of material that is insoluble and difficult to degrade will delay wound healing. Examples are fragments of suture material, mineral debris, such as glass, and bone fragments. The presence of foreign material greatly increases the risk of associated infection. In the presence of a foreign body, fewer organisms are required to initiate a wound infection compared to a wound that is free of such material. If epithelium becomes entrapped in the wound, it may continue to grow and form an epithelial cyst.

Instability

A wound in which there is excessive movement or separation of the wound margins shows delayed healing. This is one of the main reasons for wound suturing. Sutures also help a wound to heal by primary rather than secondary union.

Exposure

Wounds which are kept moist show improved regeneration of the covering epithelium compared to wounds that show surface drying, when a thick scab forms which may slow healing.

Systemic factors

Nutrition

This is one of the most important factors that influence wound healing. Protein deficiency, or a lack of certain trace elements or vitamins will slow wound healing. Examples include vitamin C deficiency, which results in scurvy due to production of abnormal collagen, and zinc deficiency, an element important for the function of some enzymes such as DNA and RNA polymerase.

Metabolic disorders

Diabetic patients in which the disease has been present for many years show poor wound healing. The pathology of diabetes is characterized by microvascular disease, with thickened but more permeable basement membranes. The delayed wound healing is primarily ischaemic in origin.

Drugs

Corticosteroids have a very marked affect on wound healing. They inhibit cytokine production, chemotaxis, bacterial killing by macrophages and neutrophils, and reduce collagen production. All these factors increase the incidence of wound infection and weaken the wound, particularly if it is not sutured. Steroids are frequently given to cause immunosuppression to treat autoimmune disease or as part of cancer treatment.

Abnormal wound healing

Over-production of granulation tissue

In some cases, there is abundant production of granulation tissue which delays healing. The cause for this phenomenon is not clear, but is usually treated by cautery of such lesions.

Over-production of collagen

This may cause contractures, particularly in burns, or obstruction in, for example, the gastrointestinal or urinary tract. Certain races of people, particularly negroes, young people, and wounds of the head and neck, are particularly prone to *keloids*, a form of inappropriate collagen production in a healing wound which persists.

Mechanisms involved in wound healing

The environment surrounding cells has an important influence in the healing of a wound. For example, extracellular substances, such as type IV collagen and laminin, which are present in basement membranes, influence the behaviour of epithelial and connective tissue cells. There is a specialized extracellular substance called fibronectin which is also important in this process. Cells have surface molecules which are involved in these interactions with the extracellular matrix called adhesion molecules. These were first mentioned in acute inflammation as being responsible for the adhesion of leucocytes to endothelium (p. 000), but they are important in all types of cell.

Epithelial cells, by producing growth factors, also influence the surrounding connective tissue. Epithelial and connective tissue cells produce extracellular

Table 2.7 Mediators involved in chronic inflammation

Mediator	Effect
Interleukin-1	Fibroblast recruitment and proliferation
Tumour necrosis factor	Fibroblast recruitment and proliferation; blood vessel proliferation (angiogenesis)
Gamma-interferon	Activates macrophages
Epidermal growth factor (EGF)	Epidermal, fibroblast proliferation
Platelet-derived growth factor	Fibroblast, smooth muscle growth
Transforming growth factor-alpha (similar to EGF)	Epidermal and fibroblast proliferation
Transforming growth factor-beta	Fibroblast recruitment and activation; inhibits collagen breakdown and macrophages
Fibroblast growth factor	Fibroblast, blood vessel growth
Prostaglandins	Growth inhibition

components that influence adjacent cells. Epithelium, in particular, produces basement membrane molecules. This process can be demonstrated in the skin, where the regenerating epidermal cells have a strong influence on the differentiation and development of the underlying connective tissue in the dermis. The epidermal cells themselves produce cytokines that influence the underlying connective tissue.

Locally acting chemical messengers are involved in the control of cell growth and function in chronic inflammation and healing. Cytokines and inflammatory mediators involved in these processes and their actions are summarized in Table 2.7.

An important concept is that inhibitory factors are produced in inflammatory and healing responses, including heparin, prostaglandin E_2, alpha-interferon, and transforming growth factor-beta. These are responsible for important growth control in wound healing.

Macrophages have an important role in wound healing in that they are capable of producing many of the growth factors mentioned above, particularly fibroblast growth factor, platelet-derived growth factor, interleukin-1, and tumour necrosis factor.

SUMMARY

Inflammation is a stereotyped, non-specific response to injury.

Acute inflammation: this is a short-lived phenomenon, often only days in duration.

Vascular response: blood vessels dilate and show increased permeability.

Cellular response: the hallmark of acute inflammation is the presence of neutrophils. Other cells seen include macrophages. Neutrophils are phagocytic, and break down bacteria, tissue debris, and foreign particles. They kill bacteria using either oxygen-dependent or oxygen-independent mechanisms.

Opsonization: this is a process by which bacteria are made more susceptible to phagocytosis. IgG, complement component C3b, and the glycoprotein fibronectin coat bacteria and bind to neutrophils via IgG and C3b receptors.

Complement: this is an amplification series of enzymes which are involved in defence against bacteria. Byproducts of complement have effects in acute inflammation.

Inflammatory mediators: chemical messengers are involved in acute inflammatory responses. They have an effect on:

–vascular dilatation
–increased vascular permeability
–recruitment of neutrophils
–production of pain associated with inflammation

Chemical mediators produced in acute inflammation have the following effects:

Vascular dilatation	–histamine –serotonin –prostaglandins –complement components –C3a, C5a
Increased vascular permeability	–complement components –C3a, C5a –kinins –prostaglandins
Neutrophil chemotaxis	–complement component –C5a –leukotrienes –fibrin degradation products

Chronic inflammation: this is a persistent inflammatory response. It may be a result of continued or repetitive acute inflammation, or it may begin as a chronic inflammation without acute phase. The response of chronic inflammation is mainly cellular and consists of lymphocytes, plasma cells, macrophages, and fibroblasts. The hallmark of chronic inflammation is fibrosis, the laying down of collagen by fibroblasts.

Granulomatous inflammation: this is a response to persistent material which is difficult to break down. A granulomatous response may either be non-specific (a foreign-body response) or specific (an epithelioid cell, hypersensitivity response). A granuloma is a rounded collection of cells derived from cells of the mononuclear–phagocytic system. A hypersensitivity granuloma is initiated by T helper cells.

Healing and repair: the ability to repair is dependent on the cell type injured. There are three types of cells:

–labile cells (can regenerate)
–stable cells (can regenerate when needed)
–permanent cells (incapable of regeneration)

If there is extensive tissue damage, granulation tissue (consisting of proliferating capillaries and fibroblasts) is formed.

3 Immunology

3 Immunology

INFECTION is the establishment and proliferation of a microorganism within a host which may lead to disease. A pathogen may either be virulent in that it has inherent ability to give disease or it may be opportunistic in that it only causes disease when the defence of the host is compromised. If the immune response is not effective there is disease and possible death of the host. The other outcome is elimination of the causative organism with protection from future infection. The organism may be eliminated but there may not be future immunity. Another possibility is that the organism remains viable but suppressed by the host immune system.

To cause infection an organism must enter the host through the skin, respiratory tract or gastrointestinal tract, for example, and then take up residence in a site in which there is access to nutrients to enable growth and reproduction. Microorganisms may be extracellular or intracellular in site. Organisms can release exotoxins which are heat labile proteins. Endotoxins are produced by Gram-negative bacteria and consist of heat stable lipopolysaccharides.

Immunological reactions differ from inflammatory reactions in that immunological reactions are specific to a particular inciting agent and have memory of previous exposure to the agent. We can acquire 'resistance' to specific infections. If you have had chickenpox, you will not get it again. However, unless you have not had it before if you have not been immunized, you can still get measles. The immune system gives protection against a great range of infective organisms, including viruses, bacteria, fungi, yeasts, and parasites. The basis of immunological reactions is the ability of recognizing molecules that do not belong to the person—the recognition of non-self. The immune system can also recognize unique molecules which are not naturally occurring.

The immune system can be divided into the pre-existing defence system which either involves cells or relies on non-cellular mechanisms, and the system which relies on mechanisms that can change, depending on the inciting stimulus, the so-called adaptive system. An important point is that the cells of the immune system are produced by the bone marrow.

An antigen is a substance which initiates an immune response. Most have a molecular weight of < 10 kDa. The best antigens are large proteins. A hapten is a small chemical group which, when chemically bound to a large molecule (carrier protein), will create a new antigen. A hapten on its own cannot initiate an immune response. However, it will combine with an antibody once this has been formed. Insoluble antigens are more immunogenic than soluble antigens. The three-dimensional structure in antigens is very important in the initiation of the immune response. Antigens can be proteins or carbohydrates.

Complement is an important part of the immune system and comprises about 30 proteins which make up about 15 per cent of plasma proteins.

INNATE IMMUNITY

The 'innate' system is an immunological defence system that we are born with. It is always functioning, but its effectiveness is not increased by a repeated infection some time in the future. This is in contrast to the 'adaptive' immunological system which has memory for previous invaders.

Non-cellular innate immunity

Chemical barriers to infection include acidity, secretions by sebaceous glands, serum beta-lysins which can disrupt bacterial membranes, and interferons which are a first line response to viral infection produced by infected cells leading to inhibition of viral application. Bacteria must be able to adhere to mucous membranes to cause an infection. Normal flora can also protect from invasion by pathogens. They may compete for available nutrients and produce inhibitory factors.

There is a first line of defence for the body to such organisms in the form of non-specific mechanisms. Examples include the skin, which forms an excellent barrier to infection, and ciliated respiratory epithelium which creates a 'mucociliary escalator' in the lung to clear foreign material. The cilia in the nasopharynx, trachea, and bronchi move rapidly (about 10 times a second) in a co-ordinated fashion to 'waft' foreign particles upward away from the lung. Many secretions of the body, including saliva, contain an enzyme called lysozyme which is capable of disrupting the cell wall of many types of bacteria. This enzyme therefore acts as a form of non-specific 'disinfectant'. Some sites of the body, such as the gastrointestinal tract and the vagina, are colonized by harmless bacteria called commensals. These organisms compete successfully against harmful bacteria and therefore have a protective effect. The stomach has high acidity to inhibit bacterial growth.

The complement system, when activated by bacterial products by the alternative pathway can be regarded as part of the innate system. This is an amplification cascade of enzymes which result in the production of proteins which disrupt the walls of bacteria. The complement system is also part of the adaptive immune system in that it is also activated by antibody–antigen complexes, by the 'classical' pathway. The complement system is described in the chapter on acute inflammation (p. 000). It can be seen in this example that the divisions between the innate and adaptive immunological system, inflammation and immunology can become blurred.

Cellular innate immunity

Members of this system are primarily phagocytic cells of the monocyte/macrophage series, termed macrophages when present in the tissues. In the liver they are called Kuppfer cells, in the skin Langerhans cells, and in lymph nodes dendritic cells. The main functions of these cells are phagocytosis with killing of bacteria and degradation of particles, and presentation of antigen to lymphocytes. Macrophages have receptors for the C3 component of complement, a series of proteins involved in defence against bacteria. C3 binds to bacteria, stimulating ingestion by macrophages.

Neutrophils, and a type of cytotoxic lymphocyte called a natural killer cell, can also be included in this immunological system. Neutrophils are phagocytic and capable of efficient bacterial killing; they are the predominant cell in an acute inflammatory response. Natural killer cells are able to detect some changes on the surface of virally infected cells and tumour cells and cause cell death of affected cells. This appears to be mediated by cytokines, including interferon, and toxic molecules such as nitric oxide.

ADAPTIVE IMMUNITY

This is a system which has memory and specificity for the inciting agent, and the response to the same agent at a future date is increased. This is the basis of vaccination or immunization. Adaptive immunological reactions generally only function after a foreign agent has entered the body. After a successful protective response against a potential pathogen, on further exposure, the immunological defence is so effective that usually the person has no symptoms.

This can also be divided into the non-cellular and cellular system, represented as the humoral antibody and the cellular arms of the immune system.

This system relies on a specialized group of molecules that are capable of recognizing antigen. An antigen is any molecule that can be recognized by and initiate an immune response. Antigens are generally large molecules, greater than a 1000 molecular weight, but the immune system usually only recognizes small regions of the large antigen molecule called 'epitopes' or antigenic determinant. There are two main types of these receptor molecules that recognize antigen molecules, immunoglobulins and the T cell receptor. There is tremendous diversity of these molecules, with an antibody or T cell receptor for any possible antigen. This vast diversity is generated by recombination of the genes that code for immunoglobulins or T cell receptors. This is covered in more detail below.

Non-cellular adaptive immunity

Antibodies

Antibodies are a group of specialized soluble proteins that are called immunoglobulins, which are found mainly in the gamma region of a serum electrophoresis strip, at the end towards the negative electrode, and are also known as gamma-globulins. They are produced by plasma cells, which are derived from B lymphocytes. As well as a soluble form, antibodies are also found on the surface of B cells. There is vast diversity in antibody molecules, each molecule showing a binding affinity at two sites at one end for only one specific type of substance, termed an antigen. Each type of antibody is produced by only one type of plasma cell. In other words, an antibody has specificity for only one particular type of antigen. These antigens are usually infectious organisms, such as viruses and bacteria, or toxins produced by bacteria. This diversity of antibodies is produced by genetic recombination of the immunoglobulin genes in B lymphocytes.

Antibodies can inactivate viruses and bacteria by binding them together as immune 'complexes'. Antibodies can also coat an infectious agent and make it much more amenable to phagocytosis by macrophages. This is because macrophages have receptors on their cell membranes to the 'Fc' (fragment crystallizable) portion of the antibody. In this way, antibodies can give macrophages a form of specificity in their action.

Antibodies are formed from two 'heavy' protein chains, which are bound together in a Y shape by disulphide bonds and two 'light' chains which are attached to the outer parts of the arms of the Y. The stem of the Y represents the Fc portion of the antibody, and the tips of the two arms the variable region that binds to the antigen sites or epitopes (Fig. 3.1). The part of the immunoglobulin molecule that includes the variable end is known as the 'Fab' portion (fragment antigen binding). Two types of light chain are produced, called kappa or lambda. In any one molecule there is only one type of light chain, kappa or lambda. The 'variable' end of the antibody molecule involves the N-terminal (amino) terminal region of both the heavy and light chains. Five different types of immunoglobulin heavy chain are produced, termed G, A, M, E, and D. These characterize the major classes of antibody. The

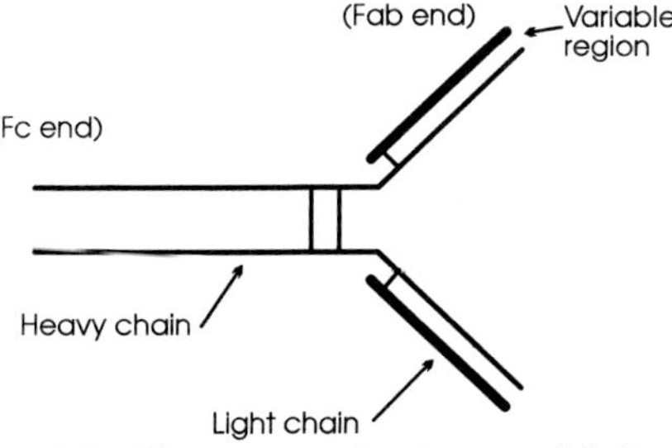

Fig. 3.1 The structure of an immunoglobulin molecule.

Table 3.1 Types of immunoglobulin

Class	MW	Binding sites	Features
IgG	150 000	2	75% of immunoglobulin in the blood. Four subtypes. Permeates tissues, crosses placenta, and gives passive immunity to the fetus. Neutralizes toxic agents. Seen in secondary response. Can be cytotoxic. Ig4 activates complement via alternative pathway. IgG 1–3 activate complement via the classical pathway. 1.5 g/100 ml blood
IgA	320 000	4	20% of immunoglobulin in the blood. Found in all secretions that have contact with antigens from the outside world, such as the gastrointestinal tract, saliva, and the respiratory tract. It is found predominantly as two molecules joined by a J chain forming a dimer. Secretory IgA is linked to a secretory fragment to resist breakdown by proteases
IgM	900 000	10	10% of immunoglobulin. Because of its large size this is normally only found in the circulation and does not escape into the surrounding interstitium. Five molecules are joined together by a peptide J chain. It is very good at complement activation. It is seen in a primary response to an antigen
IgE	200 000	2	This is almost entirely bound to mast cells and basophils, very little being found in the circulation. It is involved in allergy and parasite immunology. Eosinophils can bind IgE
IgD	180 000	2	About 1% of all immunoglobulin. Found on resting B cells. May have a role in lymphocyte maturation and activation. It does not activate complement

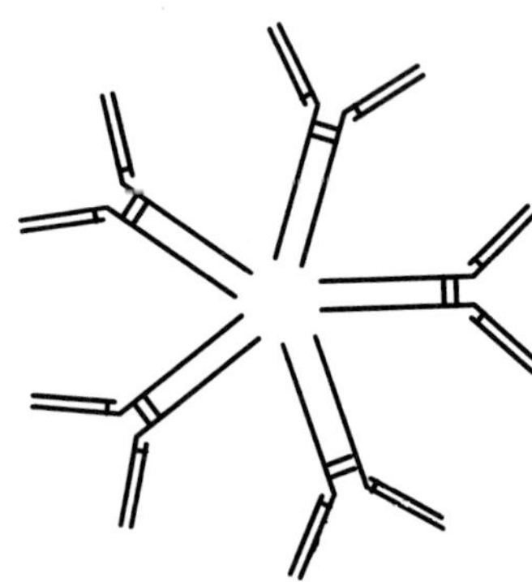

Fig. 3.2 IgM.

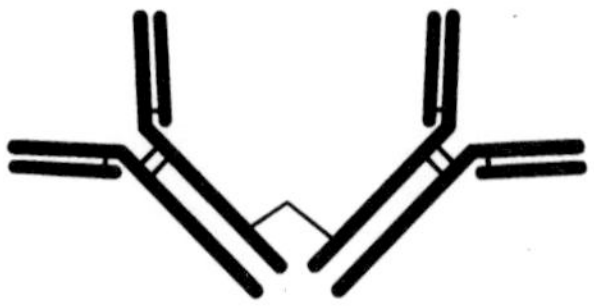

Fig. 3.3 IgA.

characteristics of these antibodies are summarized in Table 3.1. Immunoglobulins M and A are represented in Figs 3.2 and 3.3, respectively.

When the immune system is first challenged by an antigen, the first antibody to be produced is of IgM class. In view of its large number of binding sites in each pentamer, IgM is very good at activating complement by the classical pathway. IgG is produced later on repeated exposure to the antigen as a secondary response (Fig. 3.4). IgG is produced in much larger amounts and for a much longer time. The IgG produced has a much higher affinity for the antigen.

This memory for a previous antigen (which is the basis for immunization) is due to the increased number of circulating memory B cells produced after the primary exposure.

IgM can be synthesized more quickly than IgG because the IgM type B lymphocytes do not need T lymphocytes to stimulate them to mature into immunoglobulin-producing plasma cells. Also, IgM-producing cells do not go through a process of maturation in which high affinity antibodies are selected out by a process of further genetic rearrangement, as happens with IgG production. IgM therefore represents a rapid but less directed response to an antigen, and IgG follows up with a slower but much more specific action. Another reason for the higher affinity of the IgG response is that high-affinity B cells are selected out for proliferation, particularly at low concentrations of antigen. The switch from IgM to IgG production is under genetic and cytokine control.

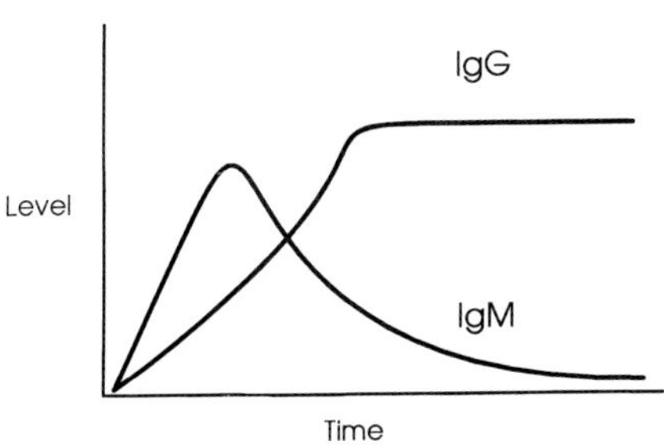

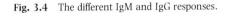

Fig. 3.4 The different IgM and IgG responses.

IgA receptors are found on polymorphs and macrophages. The gastrointestinal tract has the largest associated lymphoid tissue in the body. Membrane secretory component binds IgA which is then cleaved and then released as a complex along with free secretory component. IgA neutralizes antigens, particularly viruses, toxins and enzymes. It prevents antigen uptake from the gastrointestinal tract, it inhibits bacterial adherence, acts as an opsonin, and binds bacterial iron-binding molecules. There is homing of B cells to the gastrointestinal tract and mucosal immune system, probably involving homing receptors and vascular addressins. In the gastrointestinal tract there is, of course, discrimination between dangerous antigens and food antigens (there is oral tolerance). T helper-2 cells are predominantly found in the mucosa.

The specific binding of an antigen with an antibody relies on a combination of three-dimensional configuration, or 'fit'—like a key in a lock. Also, binding between the antigen is also dependent on appropriate binding by electrostatic, hydrogen, Van der Walls, and hydrophobic forces. The greater the forces holding the antigen and antibody together, the greater the *affinity* of the antibody for the antigen. This affinity has important implications; high-affinity antibody–antigen complexes are cleared quickly from the circulation, and are very good at stimulating complement, and at inactivating viruses and bacteria.

An important factor that plays a part in the strength of an antigen–antibody complex is the number of different binding sites involved. If there is the possibility of multiple antibody sites binding to a variety of different epitopes, as in the case of IgM, which has 10 antigen-binding sites, the resulting complex and strength of binding will be much higher.

A baby is susceptible to infection in the period from 10–14 weeks when maternal antibody has fallen but neonatal antibody has not yet risen.

Antibody responses

Primary response

Following exposure to a foreign antigen, there is an initial period of time when no antibody can be detected in the circulation. There is then a gradual increase in the level of immunoglobulin to reach a plateau. The level then gradually decreases as the antibody is cleared from the circulation. IgM is the antibody produced in the primary response.

Secondary response

This follows a repeated exposure to an antigen after an initial primary response. The secondary response shows a more rapid production of antibody compared to the primary response and the levels achieved are much higher; in some cases 10 times the initial concentration. The lag phase is shorter and the levels of antibody are more sustained. IgG is the antibody produced in the secondary response. In view of the selection of high-affinity clones of B cells that occur in the secondary response, the resulting antibodies have a higher affinity to the antigen compared to antibodies produced by a primary response.

The reason that the secondary response is so efficient is that there are already increased numbers of clones of B and T cells present after a primary response responsive to the activating antigen. These are available for activation following repeated exposure to the antigen.

Both T and B lymphocytes in co-operation are required for efficient antibody production.

B Cells

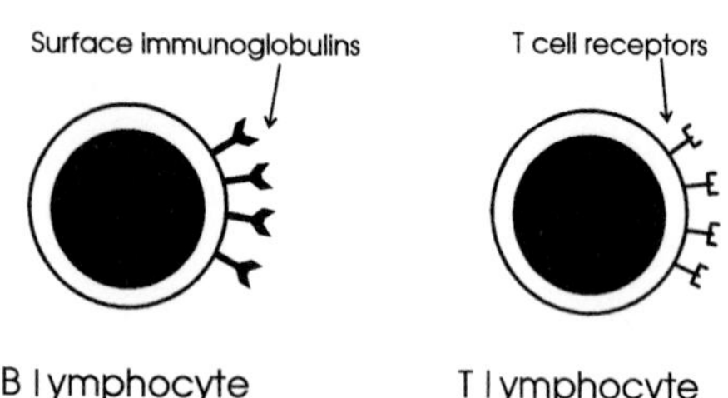

Fig. 3.5 Surface molecules on B and T cells.

These show surface immunoglobulin (Fig. 3.5) in contrast to T cells which have T cell receptors. The antibody molecules are embedded in the cell membrane and act as antigen receptors. The antibodies are made by the cells themselves. In a resting phase, most B cells in the circulation show surface IgD and IgM on the same cell. In other sites, different antibodies are expressed. For example, in epithelium which is in contact with antigens from the outside world, such as the gastrointestinal tract and the lung, B lymphocytes express IgA.

B lymphocytes also express receptors for the Fc portion of IgG immunoglobulin molecules (the non-variable end) and receptors for complement components C3b and C3d.

B cells recognize intact soluble antigens which, in contrast to the type of antigens that T cells recognize, are not processed. When a B cell encounters an antigen that is capable of binding to the immunoglobulin that it carries on its surface, it undergoes proliferation. Cross-linking of adjacent surface antibody molecules is required for B cell activation. Initially, the lymphocytes enlarge, become elongated, and show a large nucleus with a prominent nucleolus; they are then termed *immunoblasts*. The cells then undergo further maturation into immunoglobulin-secreting *plasma* cells (Fig. 3.6). Most plasma cells are found in lymph nodes and tissues, in particular the gastrointestinal tract.

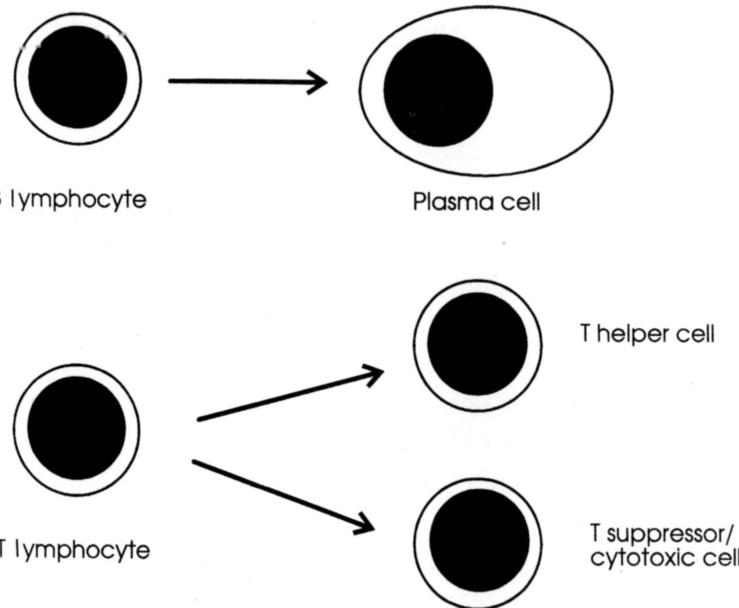

Fig. 3.6 B and T cell maturation.

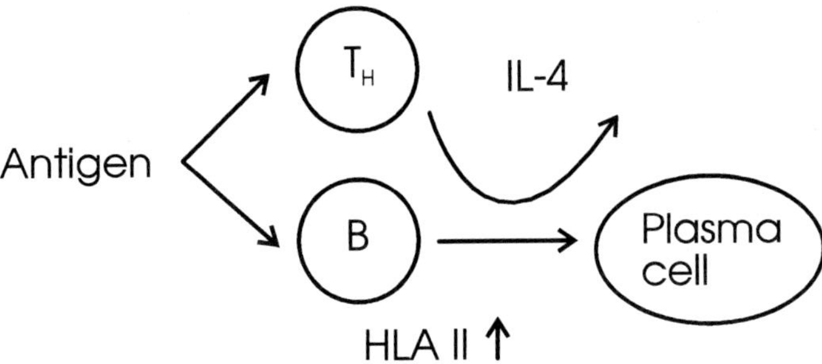

Fig. 3.7 T helper cell co-operation in B cell function.

B cells come into contact with trapped antigen in secondary lymphoid organs such as lymph nodes, the tonsils, the spleen, and Peyer's patches in the small intestine. They enter these organs from the blood through post-capillary venules, and specific B cells bind and process the antigen. The B cells also interact with specific helper T cells which have been activated by antigen, and migrate to lymphoid follicles. The B cells then interact with follicular dendritic cells (a form of macrophage), proliferate in germinal centres (see p. 000), and mature. Recombination of immunoglobulin genes occurs here, and clones of B cells producing high affinity antibodies are selected out; those clones with reduced affinity die by apoptosis (see p. 000).

There is rearrangement of germline genes in primary lymphoid organs. There is also derived somatic mutation in peripheral lymphoid organs. This is in contrast to T cells where this does not occur.

It is apparent that in order to produce an efficient immunoglobulin response, B cells need stimulation by helper T cells. The interaction of T cells with B cells is major histocompatibility complex (MHC) class II-restricted. In order for this cellular interaction to occur, the receptors of the T cells have to recognize the same antigen. Some large molecules, however, do not need to activate T cells to stimulate a B cells response; they are T cell-independent. These large antigens are usually presented by macrophages. T cells produce cytokines involved in B cell maturation; one is interleukin-4 (IL-4) which induces IgG and IgE production in B cells (Fig. 3.7). IL-5 is involved in the induction of IgA synthesis.

Cell-surface adhesion molecules, such as the integrins and selectins, are involved in cell-to-cell communication between B and T cells. Two other molecules that are not adhesion molecules, CD40 and CD80 are involved in communication of the activation state of lymphocytes.

B cells can function as antigen-presenting cells as they are capable of taking in antigens bound by immunoglobulin. They can present it with human leucocyte antigen (HLA) class II in a similar way to other antigen-presenting cells, although less antigen processing occurs. It has been suggested that B cells act as a mechanism of concentrating antigens.

As mentioned above, the change of antibody class during primary and secondary responses is dependent on the expression of specific genes. T cells appear to be important in determining which antibody type is produced, probably by cytokine production. For example, interleukin-4 is involved in the production of IgG and IgE. Interleukin-5 favours the production of antibodies of IgA type.

The production of diversity

Each B cell or plasma cell produces only one type of immunoglobulin, and each T cell has only one type of T cell receptor. When an antigen is encountered, only those cells specific for the antigen react. This is called *clonal selection*. This diversity is generated by having separate genes coding for the constant and variable parts of the molecules. There are, in particular, a large number of variable genes available for possible expression. The different variable genes show different recombinations during the development and maturation of lymphocytes. Only when a number of genes are brought together is a complete immunoglobulin molecule or T cell receptor produced. There are also mutations and errors in DNA copying occurring during lymphocyte maturation and in later life that add to the diversity of molecules produced. The basic mechanisms for the production of immunoglobulin diversity and T cell receptor diversity are basically the same.

Immunoglobulins

Some diversity is acquired by the ability of any light chain to bind to any heavy chain. This amplifies the variation possible from the different genes available. The kappa and lambda light chains and the heavy chains are all coded by genes on different chromosomes. In cells producing antibody, these genes are brought closely together; in cells not involved in immunoglobulin synthesis these genes are further apart. It is now known that there are different genes coding for the variable (V) and constant (C) parts of the immunoglobulin molecule. Between the two genes, and attached to the V gene is a joining 'J' gene. There is a further diversity (D) set of genes in the chromosome carrying the genes for the heavy chain. In the maturation of a B lymphocyte, there is recombination of these 'germline' genes, that is genes that all cells of the body carry. There are about 300 V genes, about 5 J genes, 12 D genes, and 5 C genes. The C genes of the heavy chain code for either IgG, M, A, E, or D. B cells 'switch' the class of antibody production by expressing different C genes. Diversity is first acquired by different combinations of germline genes (Fig. 3.8). There is also variation in the way in which C-D-J and V-J segments combine.

The recombination of these immunoglobulin genes occurs by unwanted sequences of DNA (introns) being 'cut-out', the genes to be expressed (exons) then moving closer together on the DNA molecule. The method of selection of any one of the available V, C, and J, genes (plus D genes in heavy chain production) allows the synthesis of many hundreds of thousands of different types of immunoglobulin. Therefore, after this process, occurring in developing B cells in the Bursa equivalent in humans (probably the liver), an immunoglobulin-sensitized lymphocyte is available for any possible antigen that the person may come across. Lymphocytes developing that are reactive against 'self antigens' are deleted, avoiding 'auto-immune' disease. This eradication of self-reactive B cells (so-called negative

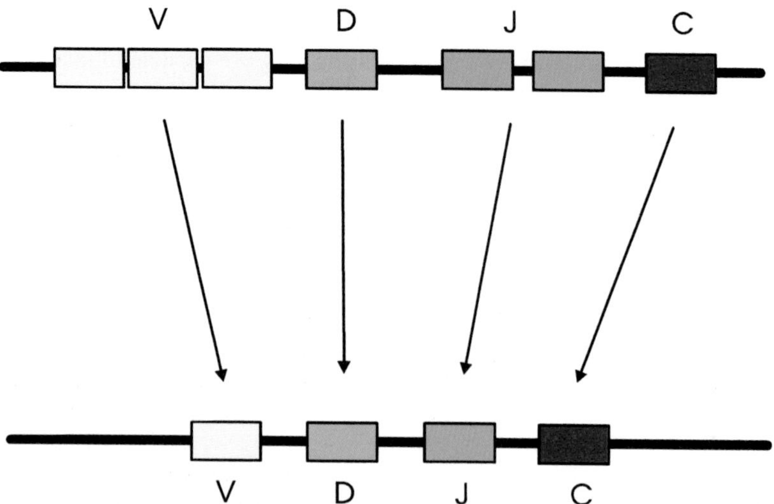

Fig. 3.8 Immunoglobulin gene rearrangement.

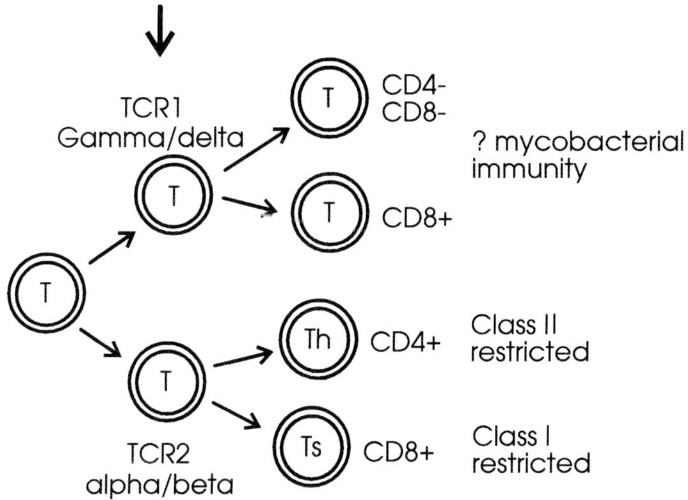

Fig. 3.9 T cell types.

selection) occurs if any of these immature cells react with self-antigens. When this occurs, the cell undergoes self-induced death by an active metabolic process under genetic control called *apoptosis*.

In the maturation of a B cell, further variation in immunoglobulin synthesis is acquired by mutations. There are areas of the V genes that have a tendency to have single base pair substitutions. This 'fine-tuning' of immunoglobulin production is responsible for the development of increasingly specific antibody production with time. This is known as 'affinity maturation'.

T cell receptors

Unlike immunoglobulin, the T cell receptor genes do not usually mutate somatically. T helper-1 cells make interleukin-2 and interferon gamma. T helper-2 cells make interleukin 4, 5, and 10. Gamma-delta T lymphocytes may be involved in defence against enterotoxins or mycobacteria (Fig. 3.9).

The mechanisms generating the diversity of T cell receptors are very similar to those involved in the generation of immunoglobulin diversity. As mentioned below, there are two types of T cell receptor, I, formed from gamma and delta chains, and II formed from alpha and beta chains (Fig. 3.10). Type II receptors are the most common type found. These receptors confer specificity on the T lymphocytes in the same way immunoglobulins do to B lymphocytes. There are D, J, and C loci in the genes coding for the different chains of the T cell receptor in a similar way to those coding for immunoglobulins. One difference is present, however, in that mutations do not occur after these genes have been selected in the way that occurs in the production of immunoglobulin diversity.

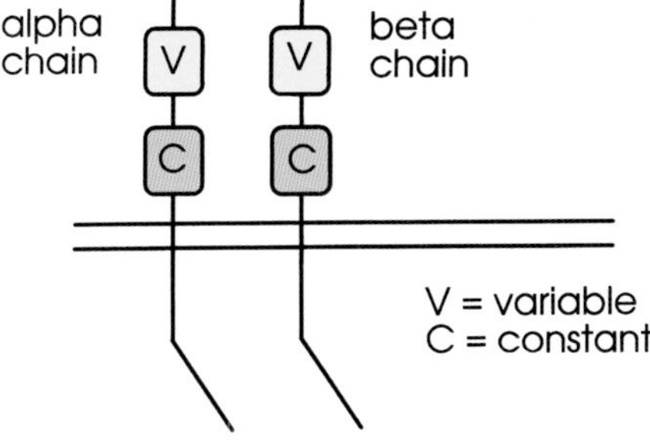

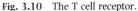

Fig. 3.10 The T cell receptor.

Cellular adaptive immunity

In summary, the cells involved in this aspect of the immune system are lymphocytes, plasma cells, cells of the macrophage–monocyte phagocytic system, and in some situations, eosinophils and mast cells. They are all derived from the bone marrow and are first seen at around the nine-week stage of fetal development. A relatively small number of precursor stem cells give rise to the vast number of cells that are involved in the immune system. At an early stage in development, lymphocytes become committed to only recognizing one particular antigen. One group of these lymphocytes are called T cells because they differentiate in the *T*hymus. They carry

T cell receptors on their surface. These represent about 80 per cent of lymphocytes. Another group are B lymphocytes which show surface immunoglobulin and probably differentiate in the fetal liver and bone marrow and can mature into plasma cells. B cells require interactions with specialized cells in the bone marrow called 'veiled' cells for normal development. B cells represent around 10–15 per cent of lymphocytes in the blood. They are called B cells in view of a unique organ called the *B*ursa of Fabricius found in birds where research into antigen sampling had originally been carried out. These lymphocytes, before they have been exposed to antigen, form a 'virgin' pool. The primary response is when the lymphocytes first detect an antigen. There is proliferation of the lymphocytes forming two main populations of cells; one group acts as the actual cells functioning in the immune response, the 'effector' cells. The other group remains as 'memory' cells that are long-lived and ready to mount an increased immune response on future exposure to the antigen. A similar expansion of effector and memory cells also occurs on subsequent exposure to the antigen. The memory cells continually circulate in the lymphatic and blood vessels, tissues and lymph nodes, acting as a monitor of antigen exposure.

There are also lymphocytes called 'null' cells which do not have characteristics of either T or B cells. These lymphocytes are identical in appearance at microscopy; special immunological methods are required to identify different types of lymphocytes. Lymphocytes express a large number of molecules on the cell surface. Immunohistochemical staining methods take advantage of the differences that various cells of the immune system show. Different moleculues are seen in various populations of cells involved in the immune system, and also at different stages of development. A system has now been developed to give a consistency to the classification of immune cells, termed the cluster designation (CD) system. This system has been derived from the study of the behaviour of different antibodies raised to lymphocytes and other leucocytes.

The cellular immune system has a main role in defence against viruses, intracellular organisms, such as tuberculosis, and is also involved in the process of transplanted graft rejection. The immune system is capable of identifying virally infected cells and killing them. Although this, of course, sacrifices cells, the production of further virus particles is stopped. The cellular immune system is also involved in the development of pathology, for example, in autoimmune diseases where there is inappropriate attack by the immune system on the host. The term *cell-mediated immunity* is usually applied to immune responses in which there is a minimal systemic antibody response. Antibodies may, however, be involved in the induction and regulation of cell immune responses. The differences between various types of immune cells are summarized below.

T cells

T lymphocytes of *helper* type (expressing CD4 molecules on the surface) are the predominant cells involved in cell-mediated immune reactions. They recognize antigens in association with HLA class II found on specialized immune cells such as macrophages and lymphocytes. T *cytotoxic* lymphocytes (expressing CD8 molecules) are mainly involved in defence against intracellular organisms and viruses; these lymphocytes recognize the foreign antigen in association with HLA class I found on all nucleated cells. The CD molecules mentioned above are important parts of the T cell receptor molecule.

There is another group of lymphocytes called natural killer (NK) cells which show a granular cytoplasm. Up to 5 per cent of circulating lymphocytes are of this type.

T helper cells (CD4-positive) can be divided into T helper-1 and T helper-2 subsets (Fig. 3.11). This split appears in the response to infection, vaccination, allergy,

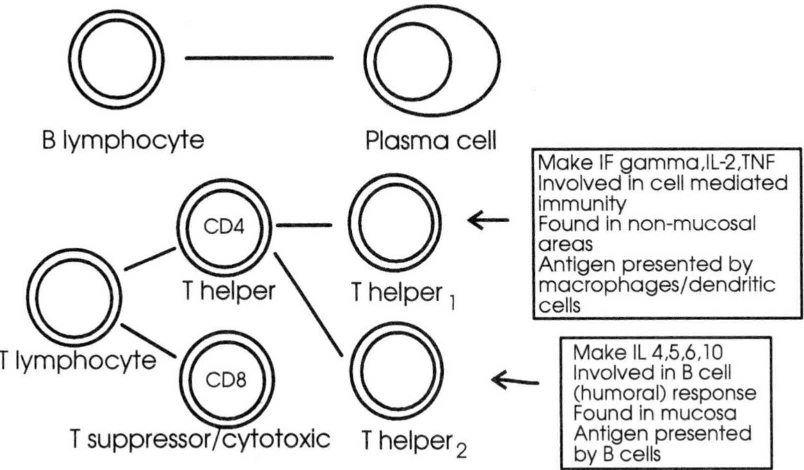

Fig. 3.11 T cell maturation.

response to tumours, and autoimmune disease. T helper-1 cells favour macrophages and dendritic cells as antigen-presenting cells. They produce interleukin-2, gamma-inteferon, and tumour necrosis factor. They affect cell-mediated immune responses and the B cells produce IgG2a, and Ig2B. They use interleukin-2 as an autocrine growth factor. They are preferentially found at non-mucosal sites, particularly lymph nodes and spleen. T helper-2 cells favour B cells as antigen-presenting cells and they produce interleukin-4, 5, 6, and 10. They effect humoral immune responses. They help B cells produce IgA, IgE, and IgG1. They use IL-4 and IL-2 as growth factors. They are preferentially found at mucosal sites (Peyer's patches). It appears that naïve T helper cells can mature either into T helper-1 or T helper-2 cells under the influence of cytokines. Both TH-1 and TH-2 cells produce IL-3 and TNF-alpha, which are cytokines. Interleukin-10 inhibits macrophage function and may involve nitric oxide. Interleukin-10 also decreases gamma-interferon production by T cells and natural killer cells.

As described previously T cells undergo development in the thymus, an organ situated in the anterior part of the mediastinum in the thorax. Severe immunodeficiency of the cell-mediated arm of the immune system develops if there is abnormality of thymic development.

T cells go through a number of stages before they are fully developed. At each stage there is selection of cells for further development. One of the first stages involves 'positive selection' when T cells that cannot recognize antigen in association with self-HLA are deleted; T cells that can recognize antigen are 'rescued' from programmed cell death. This is in contrast to the next stage of 'negative selection' or 'clonal deletion' at which T cells that are reactive to self-antigens in association with self-HLA are removed by induced self-destruction, so-called programmed cell death or *apoptosis*. There also appears to be suppression of autoreactive T cells in the periphery by other mechanisms. This is to prevent autoimmune reactions.

Another mechanism which acts as extra protection from attack by self-reacting T lymphocytes involves a molecule called CD28 present on the surface of T cells. A T cell has to interact with both a foreign antigen-HLA complex and involve the CD28 molecule before it can function. CD28 interacts with specialized proteins on the surface of macrophages, one being known as B7.

There are primarily three types of T lymphocytes, helper, suppressor, and cytotoxic cells. Helper cells derive from T cells that recognize class II HLA during early development. The helper lymphocytes, on stimulation with specific antigen for

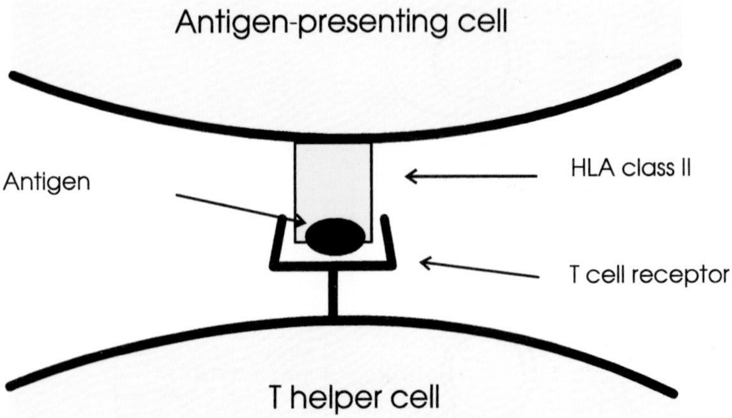

Fig. 3.12 The T cell receptor interacts with antigen on HLA.

a given cell, can produce cytokines which are involved in cellular communication and the activation and proliferation of cells of the immune system. Helper cells can induce B cells to produce immunoglobulin. Cytotoxic cells are involved in defence against viruses, and can kill cells with cytolysins, among other mechanisms.

Supressor cells are involved in the regulation of the immune response and develop from T cells that recognize HLA class I during early development. Generally, T cells are involved in the recognition of antigens on the surface of cells. The antigen undergoes processing before it is expressed on the cell surface.

The T cell antigen receptor (TCR) is similar to an antibody in that the molecule has a binding site which is specific for a given antigen. There are two types of TCR, TCR-1 and TCR-2. Both types of receptor are associated with the CD3 subunit, which is formed from three proteins, and are formed from a Y-shaped complex of two types of polypeptide linked together by disulphide bonds. The TCR-1 receptor is formed from gamma and delta chains, and the TCR-2 receptor is formed from alpha (the gene is on chromosome 14) and beta chains (the gene is on chromosome 7). Most (95 per cent) of T cells are of TCR type 2. In a similar way to immunoglobulins, the TCR has constant and variable regions. This group of T cells with type 2 receptors can be divided into T helper (CD4-positive) and T suppressor (CD8-positive) cells. There is subdivision even within the T helper cell population; some have the ability to increase suppressor activity in CD8-positive cells.

Lymphocytes with type 1 T cell receptors, so-called gamma-delta T cells, are of uncertain function. They are found in association with immune reactions to mycobacterial infections and a granulomatous disease called sarcoidosis.

The TCR has areas of reduced variability which interacts with the HLA proteins on antigen-presenting cells (complementarity determining regions, CDR-1 and -2). There is an area of higher variability (CDR-3) which interacts with the antigen.

T helper-inducer cells, which recognize antigen in association with class II HLA (Fig. 3.12), are able to induce B cell differentiation and increase the response of other T cells. T suppressor-cytotoxic cells, recognizing antigen in association with HLA class I, can modulate the immune response, and also cause cell killing. Cytotoxic T cells are able to bind to a target cell and release secretory products which result in cell death. This cell killing involves the induction of a form of programmed cell death called *apoptosis*.

There is as much diversity in the types of T cell receptor as there is in the diversity of antibody molecules; thc variety of T cell receptors is arrived at by a similar mechanism of genetic rearrangement. Each T cell has receptors for a specific antigen, in the same way that an antibody is specific for an antigen. There is

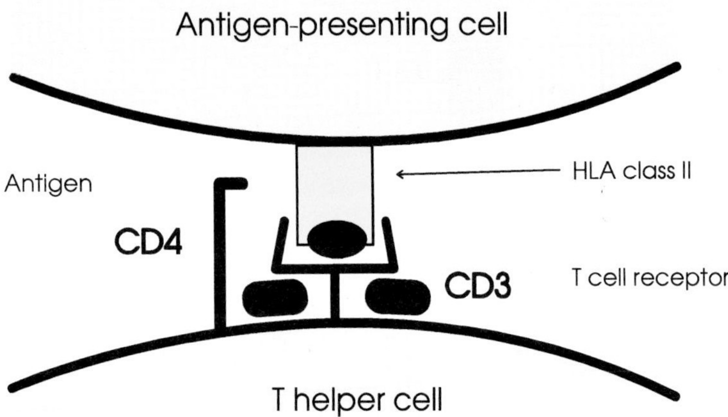

Fig. 3.13 The role of CD4 and CD3.

therefore a particular T cell primed and ready to detect any possible antigen in the environment.

Many of the surface molecules expressed on T cells have areas with similarities or 'homology' with those of the constant regions of immunoglobulin molecules and other molecules. This group of sequences has been termed the immunoglobulin gene 'superfamily'. They tend to be genes coding for cell-surface proteins. They include MHC proteins, T cell receptors, platelet-derived growth factor, intercellular adhesion molecules (ICAM, VCAM, N-CAM, and integrins), and the receptor for the Fc portion of immunoglobulin molecules.

The genes coding for the alpha chains of TCR-2 receptors on chromosome 14 are formed by variable (V) and constant (C) regions linked by a J region. Genes coding for the beta chains also comprise a V, C, and J region, but there is an additional 'D' region between the V and J region.

The vast diversity of T cell receptors is acquired by rearranging these genes. Selected genes are brought together, intervening DNA being spliced out. There are about 100 V and J alpha genes, 50–75 V, and 15 J beta genes, and 2 beta D genes. The selected genes combine with a C region. As can be seen, these mechanisms are very similar to those used in the generation of immunoglobulin diversity. However, further somatic mutation of the TCR genes does not occur, in contrast to the immunoglobulin genes.

In contrast to immunoglobulins, the T cell receptor does not recognize free whole antigen; it recognizes short peptides or *epitopes* that have been derived from the breakdown of larger protein antigen. This breakdown is performed by antigen-presenting cells such as macrophages. The other important difference between immunoglobulin and T cell receptor recognition is that T cell receptors only recognize antigen epitopes in association with HLA class II. The T cell will only respond if it sees a foreign antigen in association with its own HLA type.

The different types of lymphocytes have distinct functions. CD8-positive (mainly cytotoxic) suppressor lymphocytes recognize antigens in association with type I major histocompatibility antigens (HLA), for example, in viral infections. CD4-positive helper lymphocytes recognize antigens in association with HLA class II, and are important in the regulation of the immune reaction (Fig. 3.13). CD3 is expressed on all T cells.

The adhesion molecules mentioned in the chapter on inflammation are also involved in T cell antigen interactions (Fig. 3.14). These include the leucocyte function antigens (LFA), and molecules they bind to; for example, LFA-1 binds to intercellular adhesion molecule (ICAM-1 or ICAM-2).

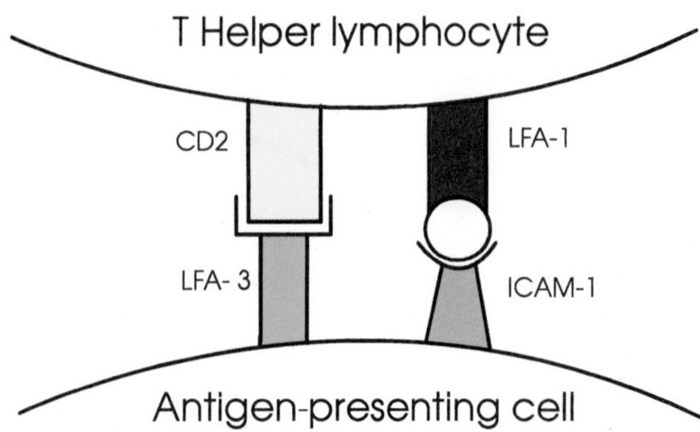

Fig. 3.14 Adhesion molecules.

T cells produce cytokines; an important one is gamma-interferon. This cytokine increases the function of antigen-presenting cells. It also activates macrophages to form granulomas in a similar way to interleukin-2. Gamma-interferon also induces B cell differentiation.

T lymphocytes acquire interleukin-2 receptors after activation, and also show increased numbers of interleukin-1 receptors and HLA class II molecules. Transferrin receptors also develop; these bind iron which is required for cell growth. T cells that react against self-antigens are deleted during development in the thymus.

Some antigens can activate a very high proportion of T lymphocytes, and bind to a specific site in the T cell receptor variable region, almost independently of the rest of the structure of the T cell receptor. These antigens are called 'superantigens'. Some bacterial exotoxins can act as such antigens. Superantigens also bind to class II molecules.

Macrophages

These cells belong to the monocyte–phagocytic group of cells. They include histiocytes in the tissues, Kupffer cells in the liver, microglial cells in the brain, and Langerhans cells in the skin. When activated by T cells they can form granulomas. They can function as non-specific scavangers or as processors and presenters of antigen to other cells of the immune system. This cell population is often referred to as the *reticuloendothelial* system. They are derived from the bone marrow and circulate initially as monocytes in the blood. The precursor cell in the marrow is the promonocyte; the stem cells involved are also involved in granulocyte production.

Macrophages contain membrane-limited packets of digestive enzymes called *lysosomes*. They contain enzymes that can break down proteins in an acid environment (acid hydrolases) and enzymes that are involved in the killing of ingested bacteria (peroxidases and lysozyme). There are oxygen-dependent mechanisms involved in the killing of microorganisms similar to those seen in neutrophils. Enzymes, such as elastases and other proteases, are present in macrophages which are involved in the ability of macrophages to move through and remodel tissue.

A prime role of the monocyte-phagocytic series of cells, as is suggested by the name, is *phagocytosis*. This function is encouraged if the antigen has been '*opsonized*' (the literal meaning: to make more palatable) by being coated by immunoglobulin or complement. Macrophages have receptors that bind to the Fc portion of the IgG immunoglobulin molecule and complement component C3b. Macrophages themselves produce complement proteins.

Macrophages can become *activated* under the infleunce of cytokines such as gamma-interferon, tumour necrosis factor, and macrophage-activating factor.

Cells of the monocyte–macrophage system which function as *antigen-presenting cells* express large amounts of HLA class II. These cells take up antigen, break it down into short peptides, and express it on the cell surface.

Exogenous antigens which enter the antigen-presenting cells by phagocytosis are processed within the acid environment of endosomes and react with class II molecules within this compartment. Selectivity may be provided by a specialized protein called the invariant chain which is associated with class II molecules inside the cell, which controls accessibility of the binding site. This invariant chain appears to keep the antigen class II complex inactivated. Class I antigens are primarily endogenous in that they are already located within the cell cytoplasm. Association of class I antigens occurs within the endoplasmic reticulum prior to transport to the Golgi. Transporter proteins TAP I and II are MHC-linked.

As well as processing antigen, macrophages and cells of the monocyte systems produce cytokines such as interleukin-1 (IL-1). IL-1 helps to induce B cell maturation, T cell proliferation, and the production of cytokines such as tumour necrosis factor from macrophages and cytokines involved in the production of neutrophils. IL-1 also induces the expression of IL-2 receptors on T cells. IL-1 and tumour necrosis factor are responsible for some of the systemic manifestations of macrophage activation such as fever and malaise.

Eosinophils

These cells can also be regarded as part of the immune system because they are associated in particular with allergic reactions (Fig. 3.15). They have low-affinity receptors to the Fc portion of IgE. They are phagocytic in a similar way to neutrophils. They are found as 2–5 per cent of the total of circulating white cells and show pink granules in a haematoxylin and eosin stain. The granules contain a toxic protein called major basic protein, which is important in killing parasites. Eosinophils can also be regarded as 'clearing-up' cells; they contain enzymes, such as aryl sulphatase and histaminase, which can inactivate inflammatory mediators.

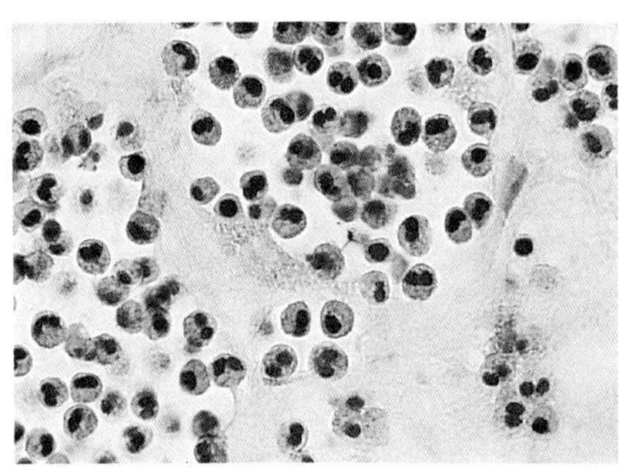

Fig. 3.15 Eosinophils in an allergic reaction.

Mast cells

There are two main groups of mast cells. They are either mucosal-associated or connective tissue-associated. They are particularly involved in immediate (type I) hypersensitivity reactions. Mucosal mast cells, which are very frequent in the lung and small intestine, appear to require interactions with T lymphocytes to proliferate, whilst connective tissue mast cells do not. Interleukin-3 (IL-3) causes mast cell proliferation. Mast cells are also involved in delayed hypersensitivity reactions. Mast cells are found particularly around blood vessels in the majority of tissues.

The cytoplasmic granules of mast cells contain very active inflammatory mediators such as histamine and heparin. Mast cells have high-affinity receptors to the Fc portion of IgE. This then acts as a receptor molecule for the mast cell. If an antigen cross-links two IgE molecules, the mast cell will degranulate, releasing inflammatory mediators into the surrounding tissue. Basophils, comprising of around 0.2 per cent of circulating white cells, are similar to mast cells in having high-affinity receptors to IgE.

Cytokines

Cytokines are chemical messengers that allow cells to communicate with each other. They are small proteins with a specific amino acid sequence and three-

Table 3.2 Cytokines

Tumour necrosis factor	Fever, cachexia, MHC I upregulated, tumour necrosis, inflammatory cells stimulated; induces ICAM
Alpha-interferon	Antiviral, NK cells stimulated
Gamma-interferon	Macrophage activation, MHC I and II, and ICAM expression increased
Interleukins	
IL-1	T cell activation, ICAM expression
IL-2	B, T, NK, cell, and macrophage stimulation
IL-3	Mast cells, haemopoetic cell proliferation
IL-4	B cell differentiation, MHC II on B cells IgE, IgG1 production
IL-5	B cell and eosinophil production, IgA, IgM production
IL-6	B, T cell production, production of bacterial-binding protein from liver
IL-7	B cell production
IL-8	Myeloid cell, chemotaxis
IL-9	Red cell and mast cell production
IL-10	Inhibits TH-1 cells
IL-11	Immunoglobulin synthesis
IL-12	T cell stimulation
IL-13	B and NK cell stimulation
Colony-stimulating factors	
G-CSF	Myeloid cell production
M-CSF	Macrophage activation
GM-CSF	Myeloid and macrophage stimulation
TGF-beta	Inhibitory to T, B, and NK cells

dimensional structure. Cells have a variable expression of specific receptors on their cytoplasmic surface to cytokines. The type and specificity of the receptors depends on the function of the cell. Cytokines involved in immunological reactions are listed in Table 3.2.

THE HLA SYSTEM

The *H*uman *L*eucocyte *A*ntigen system is primarily involved in the initiation and regulation of the immune system, by the recognition of self-antigens from non-self-antigens. The system has relevance in the development of autoimmune disease and in the relatively new field of organ transplantation. It is a large set of surface molecules coded by several hundred genes found on chromosome 6. This area is called the major histocompatibility complex (MHC). In view of the large number of genes and the vast number of possible combinations, there is a great variety of HLA in the population. Both alleles are expressed in a co-dominant fashion, that is, both maternal- and paternal-derived HLA is expressed. There may be recombination of HLA during development, which creates even more variety than would be expected from family studies.

As mentioned above, there are two types of human leucocyte antigens (HLA) involved in the immune response, class I (A, B, and C) and class II (DR, DP, and DQ). The molecules are embedded in the cell membrane and project from the cell surface.

They have a similar structure in that they are composed of two molecules joined together forming a pocket that binds the antigen. The class I molecule has a binding groove that is blocked at both ends; this limits the size of the antigen that can be bound, to about 8–9 amino acids length. HLA class I is associated with beta$_2$-microglobulin. Class II molecules have, in contrast, open ends to the binding site so that large antigenic peptides can be bound. Both types of molecule have a component that lies within the cell membrane (the 'transmembrane' portion) and a 'tail' that projects into the cell cytoplasm.

There is also a class III set of genes that are involved in the production of complement, tumour necrosis factor, and heat shock proteins. Beta$_2$-microglobulin is associated with the heavy alpha chain in the structure of HLA class I, coded by a gene on chromosome 15. It is a very important part of the class I molecule.

Heat shock proteins (HSP) are a family of proteins which function in stressed cells. They are protective. They are very highly conserved in nature and are coded by the MHC. In man, HSP70 is found in the class III region between complement and tumour necrosis factor (TNF). They frequently form the dominant antigens recognized in the immune response to a wide range of pathogens and in autoimmune disease. T cells expressing the gamma-delta T cell receptor which predominantly reside at peripheral/mucosal sites may be important in the recognition of HSP and may represent a primitive, non-specific form of initial defence against some organisms.

HLA molecules have areas that show increased variability associated with the antigen-binding sites.

The main types of HLA class I are A, B, and C. They are found on all nucleated cells and platelets and are mainly involved in protection against viral infection. HLA is expressed in particularly high concentration on lymphocytes. Cytotoxic T cells recognize foreign antigen in combination with HLA class I. The main types of class II antigens are DP, DQ, and DR. HLA class II are found on cells involved in immunoregulation, such as T and B lymphocytes, antigen-presenting cells including macrophages, and thymic epithelial cells. Helper T cells recognize foreign antigen in combination with HLA class II; interactions with B cells also occur to induce immunoglobulin production. Helper T cells are able to release cytokines which can activate macrophages to form granulomas.

In summary, class I antigens are presented along with antigen derived from products of the secretory mechanism of the cell—endogenous antigen. Class II antigens are presented along with antigen derived from material from outside the cell and processed before expression on the cell surface—exogenous antigens.

Class II human leucocyte antigens (HLA) are cell-surface molecules formed from two units called heterodimers, alpha and beta. These are synthesized independently and associate with another protein called the invariant chain, derived from a gene on chromosome 5. The invariant chain is probably important in the processes of antigen presentation in that it inhibits antigenic peptides from binding to class II antigens until required. It probably has a role in how a cell decides to express an antigen either in association with class I or class II antigens. They are found on the surface of cells that are involved in the presentation of antigens to helper T cells. Types of cells that are capable of antigen presentation include macrophages, dendritic cells, Langerhans cells, and B lymphocytes. The antigens are ingested by these cells, processed, broken down, and presented as peptides in association with the HLA antigens.

HLA class II antigens show variation from person to person, different antigens showing a different ability to bind to variable groups of peptides. This appears to be the reason why different individuals show a variable response to the same antigen. It also explains the observation that certain types of HLA are linked to certain autoimmune diseases and other disorders.

The class II molecule has a portion that projects from the cell surface and has a three-dimensional grooved structure that binds the peptide antigen as it is presented to other immune cells. It appears that the HLA class II molecule can cross-link two adjacent T cell receptor molecules. The CD4 molecule on the suface of helper T cells can bind to this structure; activation of the T cells results from cross-linking of the T cell receptor. The result of this activation is the production of cytokines and cell division.

HLA molecules are strongly expressed on cells that are involved in the initiation and regulation of the immune response. They are also expressed in cells that are involved in the process of T cell maturation and the deletion of T cells that have developed receptors to 'self-antigens'. This process occurs in the thymus; the epithelial cells in this organ strongly express HLA class II. The expression of HLA by cells can be regulated by cytokines, such as gamma-interferon and tumour necrosis factor.

THE STRUCTURE OF THE IMMUNE SYSTEM

Cells of the immune system can be found at any site in the body. However, they are organized in certain areas in order that they can function and, in particular, communicate and mature. These areas are referred to as the immune system. Lymphoid organs are either primary or secondary.

Primary lymphoid organs are regions where primary production of cells of the immune system are produced. These include the bone marrow and thymus. The liver also functions as a primary lymphoid organ in the fetus. The thymus is a bilobed structure in the anterior region of the chest which is particularly prominent in infants and children. It atophies during adult life. It is composed of large numbers of epithelial cells which occasionally form clusters, frequently with keratin in the centre (Hassal's corpuscles). These epithelial cells strongly express class II histocompatibility antigens (self-antigens). There are large numbers of T lymphocytes in the thymus, and it is the site where T cells 'learn' self-versus non-self-antigens. T cells that have developed receptors against self-antigens are destroyed, therefore preventing 'autoimmune' disease. During T cell maturation, the epithelial cells become intimately associated with the lymphocytes.

If the thymus is absent, for example in a congenital condition called di George's syndrome, there is a serious lack of T cells and therefore loss of cell-mediated immunity.

Secondary lymphoid organs are areas where immunological cells can interact, and include lymph nodes, the spleen, Waldeyer's ring in the pharynx (the tonsils, adenoids, and lymph nodes in this area), and the lymphoid cells of the gastrointestinal tract and lung.

The secondary lymphoid organ which has the most organized connective tissue structure is the *lymph node*.

Lymph node structure

Lymph nodes are firm oval or kidney-shaped nodules varying in size from a few millimetres to several centimetres in diameter. Their size often depends on how much activity is occurring within them. Inactive, quiescent lymph nodes may only be a few millimetres in diameter; active or hyperplastic lymph nodes may be several centimetres in diameter. Lymph nodes are situated at sites where lymphatics converge, and act as 'gatekeepers' or 'sentries', for lymph draining from tissues. Lymphatics are blind-ending channels that drain excess extracellular fluid from tissues. Lymph nodes are found particularly in the head and neck region, axilla,

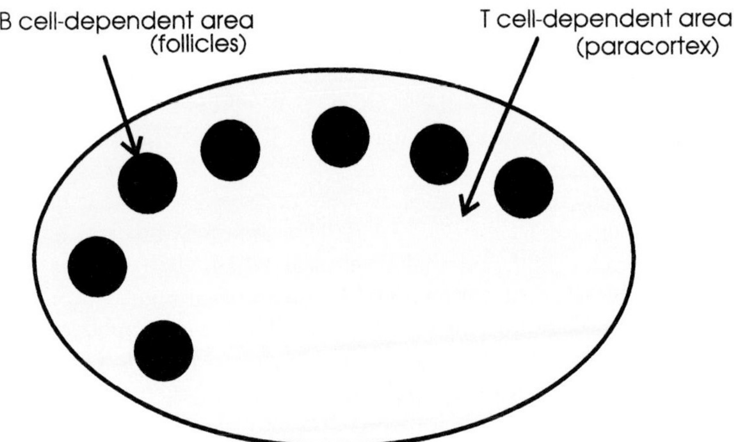

Fig. 3.16 Representation of lymph node architecture.

roots of the lungs, in the mesentery of the gastrointestinal tract, along the abdominal aorta, and the groins. They are 'in series' with the lymphatic flow, numerous lymphatics draining into the convex part of the node (afferent lymphatics), and a smaller number of lymphatics draining from the concave hilum of the node (efferent lymphatics, namely, effluent). Blood vessels also enter at the hilum. Lymph drains by progressively larger lymphatics into a large duct draining into the left subclavian vein called the thoracic duct.

Lymph nodes have a thin fibrous capsule, with connective tissue channels running towards the centre or medulla of the node. The outer part of the node is called the cortex. The channels are lined by macrophages in a similar way to those seen in the spleen.

In a section of a lymph node, two main areas are apparent (Fig. 3.16). Rounded 'follicles' are seen in the cortex, representing spherical collections of proliferating B cells responding to antigen stimulation (Figs 3.17 and 3.18). These have macrophages in the centre which phagocytose cell debris and are also involved in antigen presentation. These specialized macrophages are called follicular dendritic cells. The more antigen occurring in the lymph node the greater the size of the follicles. The centre of the follicles, known as the 'germinal centre', contains lymphocytes in varying degrees of maturation. Smaller folded cells, called centrocytes, and larger cells, called centroblasts, are seen in the germinal centres.

Recognition of a foreign antigen by immunoglobulin on the cell surface causes activation of B cells and maturation into immunoglobulin-producing plasma cells or memory B cells. This process also requires the assistance of T cells, with the action of interleukins 2, 4, and 5. There is also physical contact of B cells with macrophage-

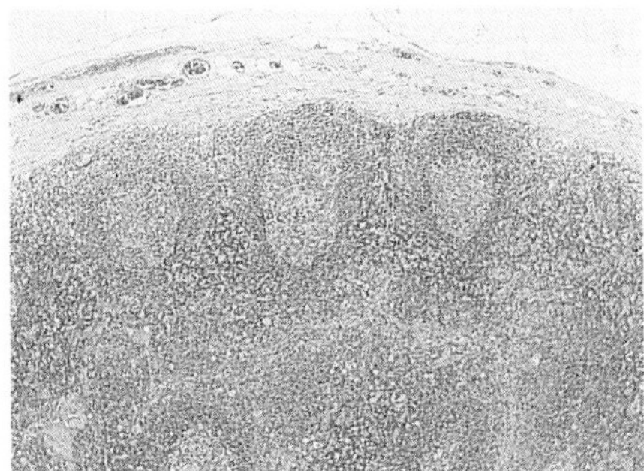

Fig. 3.17 Follicles in a lymph node.

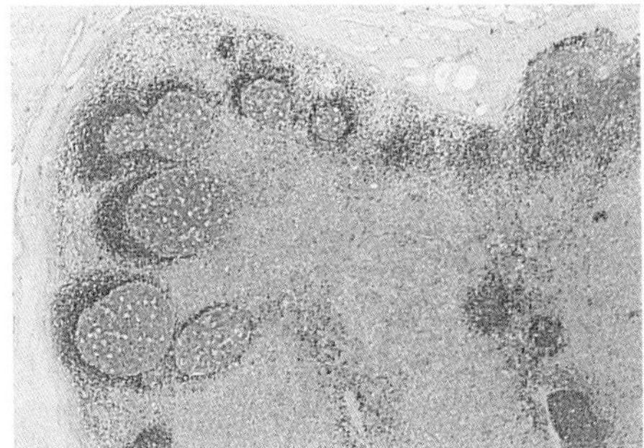

Fig. 3.18 The follicles stain brown for B cell markers in this immunoperoxidase stain.

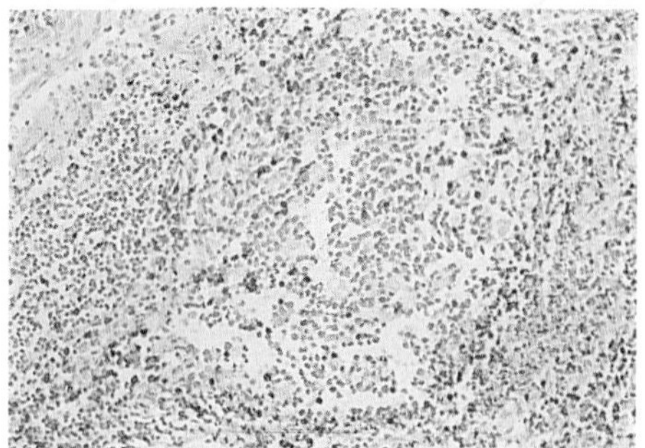

Fig. 3.19 T cells stained with an antibody are seen between follicles. The central follicle is negative for T cells.

like antigen-presenting cells and T cells in the lymph node. B cells interact with follicular dendritic cells and form recognizable germinal centres. It is during this time that they undergo somatic mutations of the variable (V) immunoglobulin genes to increase the specificity and affinity for the antigen. Cell adhesion molecules are involved in the movement of cells within lymph nodes. Two important molecules involved in T and B cell communication have been designated CD40 and CD80.

In between these B cell-derived follicles is the 'paracortex' which has a predominant cell population of T cells (Fig. 3.19). This area also has specialized types of post-capillary venules (high endothelial venules), which allow free passage of lymphocytes from the blood to the lymph node. Antigen-presenting cells are also present here, including interdigitating reticulum cells, a type of macrophage. The high endothelial venules are an important site of lymphocyte re-circulation from the blood into the lymphatic system. Although primarily found in lymph nodes, high endothelial venules can be induced in inflamed areas to allow the passage of lymphocytes.

At the interface between the follicles and the paracortex, called the mantle zone, there are a population of B cells which show surface IgD.

The spleen

The *spleen* acts as a 'filter' in the bloodstream, functioning as a protection against invading organisms that have managed to get past all the other innate and adaptive mechanisms that are present. It is composed of a large number of vascular spaces lined by macrophages, which phagocytose bacteria and break down degenerate red blood cells. An example of the importance of the spleen is that people who lose their spleen after splenectomy for traumatic injury are very susceptible to infection by, in particular, pneumococci. The spleen frequently becomes enlarged during systemic infection, for example in infective endocarditis. The spleen also contains frequent aggregates of lymphoid cells arranged around arterioles in the case of T cells, and budding off the lymphoid tissue surrounding blood vessels in the case of B cells.

Other lymphoid organs

Every organ at any one time has a resident immune cell population. In some organs, particularly those that are exposed to a lot of foreign antigens, there is a specialized permanent lymphoid presence. This is known as *mucosal-associated lymphoid tissue* (MALT). The gastrointestinal tract in particular has large amounts of this tissue. It appears that the lymphocytes that are present have surface receptor molecules that enable them to circulate out of the tissue and then find their way back. Adhesion molecules, such as *selectins* or *vascular addressins*, are involved in this traffic. The lymphocytes move in to the tissue through venules which are similar to those seen in lymph nodes. Lymphatics drain these organs, allowing continuous re-circulation of lymphocytes.

In mucosae, there is a high rate of IgA production by resident plasma cells.

AUTOIMMUNITY

Immunological processes involve the recognition of self- versus non-self-molecules. The cells of the immune system do not normally react against self-antigens; this phenomenon is known as *tolerance*. Several mechanisms appear to be involved in the development of tolerance:

1. Immature B cells are able to become tolerant to low concentrations of antigen, a process known as *clonal abortion*.

2. Repeated exposure of an antigen may cause all sensitive B cells to differentiate. There will therefore be reduced numbers of B cells available for further activation, a process of *clonal exhaustion*.
3. There may be removal of clones of helper T cells, which results in reduced B cell function. This process occurs in the thymus, where T cells that are reactive to self-antigens are deleted in the thymus.
4. There is no clonal deletion of auto-reactive B cells as seen with T cells in the thymus. Continued suppression of these potentially self-reactive B lymphocytes is provided by suppressor T lymphocytes.

The breakdown of this immunological tolerance is responsible for the development of autoimmune disease which is described below. In general, there is production of antibodies or T lymphocytes that react against host organs or tissues.

Autoimmune diseases fall into two main groups; they are either directed against a specific organ or they manifest as a systemic disease which is not specific for any organ. Examples are given below:

Organ-specific

Thyroid	–Graves' disease, Hashimoto's disease
Adrenal	–Addison's disease
Liver	–chronic active hepatitis; primary biliary cirrhosis
Stomach	–pernicious anaemia
Skin	–pemphigus; pemphigoid
Pancreatic islets	–diabetes mellitus

Non-organ-specific (often called connective tissue disease)

Rheumatoid arthritis
Systemic lupus erythematosus, discoid lupus erythematosus

Pathogenesis

Genetic factors

Autoimmune diseases that run in families are well described, particularly those diseases that affect individual organs, such as Hashimoto's disease. Genetic factors are implicated. For unknown reasons, autoimmune diseases tend to occur in females. There are also associations with autoimmune diseases and particular HLA types. Some examples are given below:

Addison's disease	DR3
Insulin-dependent diabetes	DR3/DR4
Rheumatoid arthritis	DR4, DRw
Graves' disease	DR3
Hashimoto's disease	DR5
Systemic lupus erythematosus	DR2 (weak association)
Coeliac disease	DR3
Sjögren's syndome	DR3, B8

Genes coding for HLA antigens may be linked to genes involved in the regulation of the immune response. This may explain the link between some HLA groups and autoimmune disease.

Some HLA antigens may initate antigens that the person is exposed to. If an immune reaction occurs to one of these antigens, there may then be an autoimmune response.

Autoantibody production

High concentrations of antibodies directed against self-antigens are associated with autoimmune disease. Examples are given below:

Organ	Tissue against which antibody is directed
Hashimoto's thyroiditis	Thyroid epithelium
Pernicious anaemia	Gastric parietal cell
Systemic lupus erythematosus	Nuclear proteins
Rheumatoid disease	IgG
Sjögren's syndrome	Nuclear proteins, IgG, salivary epithelium
Pemphigoid	Basement membrane
Pemphigus	Intercellular junctions

Antibody-dependent lymphocyte toxicity

Hashimoto's disease is a good example of this process. Antibodies bind to the thyroid epithelium, which then leads to cell-killing by cytotoxic T lymphocytes.

Auto-reactive T lymphocytes

In some stages of the development of insulin-dependent diabetes (type I diabetes) a lymphocytic infiltration of the islets of Langerhans occurs. This appears to be responsible for the destruction of the insulin-producing beta cells in the islets.

HYPERSENSITIVITY

In some immunological reactions, a side-effect of a successful immunological response is tissue damage. This phenomenon of apparent 'over-reactivity' is known as *hypersensitivity*. This occurs after initial sensitization by a specific antigen. Further exposure may induce the reaction in a particular individual. The result of a hypersensitivity reaction may be seen locally as severe inflammation or tissue destruction. Hypersensitivity may be life-threatening if circulatory shock develops or oedema obstructs the airway.

Hypersensitivity reactions fall into four main types (a classification system described by Gell and Coombs), shown in Table 3.3. These are covered in more detail below:

Type I hypersensitivity

This is relatively common and manifested clinically as *allergy*. The allergen is usually an antigen which in most people is harmless. Some conditions that are characterized by allergy are asthma, eczema, and hay fever. The term *atopy* is often applied to the features of allergy, particularly when it runs in a family.

Type I hypersensitivity reactions may be dangerous in some cases of insect bites or food allergy, and some drugs such as penicillin. These reactions are fortunately rare, and for a given individual, tend to be to a specific agent. The symptoms of such a reaction, called *anaphylaxis*, include a severe fall in blood pressure with disturbance

Table 3.3 Hypersensitivity

(i)	Type I	–Immediate hypersensitivity
(ii)	Type II	–Antibody-dependent cytotoxic hypersensitivity
(iii)	Type III	–Immune complex hypersensitivity
(iv)	Type IV	–Delayed hypersensitivity

of the circulation, respiratory obstruction, and collapse. Antihistamines and adrenaline are used to treat anaphylaxis, with other supportive treatments. The underlying mechanism involves:

1. IgE is produced by plasma cells following stimulation and maturation of B cells by an antigen.
2. This IgE binds to tissue mast cells via Fc receptors.
3. These sensitized mast cells then degranulate on exposure to the specific antigen, releasing inflammatory mediators such as histamine. There is also synthesis of inflammatory mediators from arachidonic acid with the production of prostaglandins and leukotrienes. Platelet-activating factor is also formed. These alter vascular permeability, smooth muscle tone, and glandular secretory activity. Agents that are chemotactic for eosinophils are also produced; eosinophils are seen in large numbers in allergic reactions.

The initial effect is local, the IgE and sensitization of mast cells occurring at the site of initial exposure. IgE released into the circulation then binds into circulating basophils and tissue mast cells. The hypersensitivity may then have a systemic effect.

IgE has a slightly larger molecular weight (188 000) than IgG (150 000), as it has a larger Fc portion. Almost all IgE is tissue-bound; very little is found in the circulation. The production of IgE is under T cell control. T helper cells with Fc receptors produce IgE binding factors in response to stimulation by T helper cells. These T helper cells respond to antigen presented by antigen-presenting cells such as macrophages. IgE binding factors either stimulate or suppress IgE synthesis.

Cytokines appear to be involved in the switch that B cells make in the production of antibody type to IgE. For example, interleukin-4 (IL-4) induces IgE production by B cells.

IgE is very important in defence against parasitic organisms. It may be that allergy is an unfortunate side-effect of having IgE in tissues and the circulation.

There are genetic factors involved in the development of immediate hypersensitivity. These effect, for example, total circulating IgE levels, the association of certain HLA types with allergy, and general 'responsiveness'.

The agent causing type I hypersensitivity in a person can be detected in many cases by skin testing in which an inflammatory reaction is induced by an antigen scratched into the skin. Circulating IgE to specific antigens may also be investigated.

Type II hypersensitivity

This involves an exaggerated or inappropriate response involving antibodies to antigens on the surface of cells in tissues of the body. The reactions are responsible for some 'autoimmune' reactions, but are also important in some forms of transplant rejection.

The term 'antibody-dependent cytotoxicity' is used because the binding of antibodies to surface tissue antigens is manifested by activation of complement components. This results in damage to cell membranes and cell lysis. The antibodies involved are IgG and IgM, classes of antibody that are good at causing complement activation. The activation of the classical complement pathway by antigen–antibody complexes is the formation of the membrane attack complex C5b–C9 (see p. 000). This causes pores to develop in the target cell membrane resulting in increased permeability and eventual cell lysis.

Another way in which binding of antibodies to the cell surface can result in cell damage is by activation of phagocytic cells. Cells such as macrophages, eosinophils, and neutrophils have receptors on the cell surface for the Fc component of immunoglobulin molecules. Phagocytic cells may also be attracted to the sites of antibody binding by the deposition of the C3b component of complement on the surface of target cells.

By mechanisms such as those described above, the binding of antibodies to tissues can result in inflammatory reactions. This induced inflammation can result in tissue damage. Examples of clinical conditions involving type II hypersensitivity are as follows.

Haematological

Incompatible blood transfusion reactions

These occur when a recipient has antibodies to transfused red cells. The ABO and rhesus blood group systems are the most important with regard to group matching of transfusions. If circulating antibody is present to the transfused red cells, it binds to the cell membrane, making the cells prone to lysis by complement or phagocytosis by macrophages in the spleen. Red cells may agglutinate, and the release of haemoglobin by the destruction of red cells in the circulation (haemolysis) may cause renal failure.

Autoimmune haemolytic anaemia

If antibodies are abnormally produced against an individual's own red cells, destruction of red cells occur in a similar way to that seen in a transfusion reaction. The cause of the production of these inappropriate antibodies is usually unknown, although they occur occasionally in association with other autoimmune disorders. Some drugs, such as penicillin or sulphonamides, may also induce autoimmune haemolytic anaemia. The circulating antibodies are detected by the *Coomb's test* in which rabbit antibodies against human immunoglobulin cross-link antibodies on the surface of the red cells. The cells then clump together forming large groups which can be seen with the naked eye as agglutination.

Autoimmune thrombocytopaenia

This occurs when circulating antibodies are present to an individual's platelets, inducing increased loss in the spleen due to phagocytosis. Removal of the spleen frequently reduces this platelet loss.

Haemolytic disease of the newborn

This develops when a rhesus (Rh) negative mother with anti-Rh IgG antibodies is pregnant with a Rh-positive baby. These monomeric IgG antibodies can cross the placenta to attach to the surface of the baby's red cells. This induces complement-mediated haemolysis in a similar way to autoimmune haemolyic anaemia described above. This causes chronic anaemia in the developing baby with a compensatory increase in red cell production in the bone marrow, liver, and spleen. Enlargement of the liver and spleen is therefore seen. There may be abnormalities of tooth development (enamel hypoplasia).

The mother develops these anti-Rh antibodies after exposure to fetal red cells at the birth of a previous Rh-positive baby. The first Rh-positive baby is not affected.

Anti-Rh antibodies can now be given to Rh-negative mothers at the time of delivery to clear the circulation of Rh-positive fetal red cells.

Specific tissue disorders

Systemic lupus erythematosus (SLE)

In this autoimmune disease, antibodies develop to a number of nuclear antigens in cells. The disease manifests itself in many tissues, including the skin, oral mucosa, and kidneys.

Goodpasture's syndrome

This is where antibodies are produced which react with basement membrane components, particularly in the kidney, but also in the lung. These antibodies are usually of IgG type, and when immune complexes develop in the kidney or lung, there is activation of complement and basement membrane damage.

Myasthenia gravis

These patients present with a progressive muscular weakness, made worse with exercise. This weakness is due to circulating antibodies which are directed against the acetylcholine receptor at the motor endplates in muscles. The antibodies bind to the acetylcholine receptors and compete with acetylcholine arising from the stimulated nerve. The function of the neuromuscular junction is impaired.

Transplant rejection

Hyperacute renal transplant rejection

This develops when there are antibodies circulating in the recipient to the donated organ. It is a very rapid reaction, with damage to the organ by a cellular reaction of neutrophils and platelets. This is an uncommon phenomenon, in view of the cross-matching performed before organ transplantation.

Type III hypersensitivity

This is characterized by persistent immune-complex formation, with deposition of these complexes in organs causing damage. Immune complexes can activate complement via the alternative pathway, and this is frequently the mechanism of tissue damage. In general, the underlying mechanism is the overload of systems that clear immune complexes from the circulation. Cells of the mononuclear–phagocyte system in the spleen, liver, and lungs play an important role in this clearance. Situations in which this overload by excess immune complexes occurs are:

Autoimmune disease—there is a continual formation of antibodies against host tissue with circulating immune complexes. Mechanisms involved in clearing the circulation of immune complexes, in particular the mononuclear–phagocyte system, are saturated, and complexes are deposited in tissues. The kidneys, arteries, and skin are sites frequently involved, and vasculitis may result.

Autoimmune diseases where immune complex deposition is a frequent problem are rheumatoid arthritis and sytemic lupus erythematosus.

Exposure to foreign antigen—injection of a protein from another species may result in immune complexes of induced antibody and the antigen being deposited in the kidney, resulting in glomerulonephritis. Arthritis may also occur. This phenomenon is called 'serum sickness'. Another example of immune complex-mediated hypersensitivity is extrinsic allergic alveolitis, where an antigen is inhaled by a previously sensitized host. For instance, a person may be sensitive to avian proteins and develop progressive lung fibrosis, called 'bird fancier's lung'.

Type IV hypersensitivity

This is characterized by a hypersensitivity reaction taking longer than 12 hours to develop, and is therefore also known as 'delayed hypersensitivity'. It involves the activation of previously sensitized T helper lymphocytes (CD4 cells). Histologically, the reaction is seen as a heavy lymphocytic infiltrate. In some types of hypersensitivity, epithelioid cell granulomas are seen. There is little or no involvement of the humoral immune system in the form of antibodies. Examples of delayed hypersensitivity reactions are given below.

Mantoux skin test (tuberculin test)—this develops about 48 hours after an intradermal injection of protein derived from killed *Mycobacterium tuberculosis* into a person with previous or active tuberculous infection. A red indurated papule develops at the site of injection, and if biopsied shows a heavy infiltrate of helper T lymphocytes.

Dermal macrophages present antigen to lymphocytes, and sensitized T lymphocytes exposed to this antigen proliferate.

Skin contact hypersensitivity—this is also known as contact eczema, and occurs 12–48 hours after exposure to a specific substance. It is seen clinically as a raised red skin rash at the site of contact with the antigen. People get sensitized to the antigen usually by repeated exposure. Examples of substances frequently implicated are certain plants, egg protein, certain chemicals such as epoxy resins, metals such as nickel, and rubber. Langerhans cells, the antigen-presenting cells in the epidermis of the skin, are particularly involved.

The antigens involved tend to be small molecules that by themselves are not capable of inducing an immune response. However, these small molecules, in this context termed 'haptens', bind to proteins in the skin to form a complex which then can initiate an immunological response.

Granulomatous reactions to intracellular infecting organisms—The most well known of these infections is tuberculosis. When hypersensitivity develops to the infective organism, the resistance of the host is increased and the infection can then be controlled.

TRANSPLANT IMMUNOLOGY

Mechanisms

As with all immunological reactions, transplant reactions in organ transplantation show specificity and memory. The transplant rejection reaction is specific for the organ transplanted, and in the experimental situation is accelerated in repeated grafts.

In human organ transplantation, the HLA system has the greatest influence over the type and degree of any rejection reaction. The survival of kidney grafts, for example, is the greatest with close matching of HLA types. Matching for ABO blood group types is also very important.

HLA molecules (major histocompatibility complex: MHC molecules) (see p. 000) are very effective at initiating an immunological response. It appears that HLA molecules can act as both antigen and as self-HLA, that is, the molecules do not have to be presented to T helper cells in association with self-HLA antigens. HLA types are inherited in a Mendelian fashion and are expressed in a co-dominant fashion, that is, genes on each chromosome are expressed together. Cells therefore have both expression of paternal and maternal gene products on the cell surface.

T cells are the predominant effector cell in transplant rejection reactions, and transplant rejection involves cell-mediated immunity. Although suppressor/cytotoxic lymphocytes are important in graft rejection, it appears that helper lymphocytes are primarily involved in the reaction. A large proportion of T cells in any person can respond to HLA molecules from any other individual who is genetically different. This is a so-called allograft reaction. The T cells either recognize determinants on the HLA molecules separate from any antigenic peptide that the HLA molecule may be carrying, or they also recognize some part of the antigen. There is evidence that macrophages recruited and activated by these lymphocytes are the cells that cause graft destruction. The mechanisms involved in transplant rejection are very similar to those involved in the elimination of cells infected by a virus.

Important cytokines involved in graft rejection are interleukin-2 (IL-2) and gamma-interferon. IL-2 causes activation of T cells, and gamma-interferon causes increased expression of HLA, increased function of antigen-presenting cells, and together with tumour necrosis factor-beta (TNF-beta) activation of macrophages. There is also increased production of antibodies to the graft by B cells.

Antibodies have less of a role in the mechanisms involved in graft rejection. Antibodies to graft antigens are certainly important in acute rejection, but are not so important in chronic rejection.

Different organs have varying abilities to initiate transplant rejection reactions. The bone marrow is the tissue most able to elicit a transplant rejection reaction, whilst the heart, liver, and kidney have less immunogenicity.

A tissue has to have a vascular supply, particularly lymphatic, to be rejected. For example, corneal grafts generally have a good survival after transplantation as the cornea is normally free of vessels. Only if the cornea develops blood vessels is rejection likely, if there is tissue mismatch.

Graft rejection may be very rapid (hyperacute) when there are antibodies already present to the graft which cause complement activation. Acute rejection takes weeks and is primarily caused by T cell activation. Chronic rejection takes months or years.

Complications of transplantation

Immunosuppression

Some degree of immunosuppressive therapy is required in all transplants, and therefore patients are made more susceptible to infection. If the immunosuppressive therapy is severe, microorganisms that are normally of low virulence and do not cause disease cause clinical infection. These are organisms that are usually in the environment or carried by the host, and are termed *opportunistic* pathogens in this context. Examples of microorganisms that cause opportunistic infections are some Gram-negative bacteria, fungi such as *Aspergillus* and *Nocardia*, *Candida*, atypical mycobacteria, toxoplasma, and pneumocystis. Viruses that are commonly seen in opportunistic infections, often representing a re-activation of a previously controlled infection, are cytomegalovirus and *Varicella*.

Graft-versus-host disease

This phenomenon happens when large numbers of cells of the immune system are transplanted along with a particular graft. A bone marrow transplant is a typical example. These immunological cells, in particular lymphocytes, when viable and functional (immunocompetent) attack tissue of the recipient. Organs which tend to be affected are the skin, gastrointestinal tract, the liver, and cells in the circulation. A lymphocytic attack on the epidermis, intestinal epithelium, bile ducts, and blood cells occurs.

IMMUNODEFICIENCY

This occurs when there is either a congenital or acquired abnormality of immunological function. Immunodeficiency may manifest itself in a person as a chronic infection with no other apparent cause for the persistence of the condition. It may also show itself as an *opportunistic infection*, as described above.

Congenital immunodeficiency (primary)

T and B lymphocyte deficiency (combined): severe combined immunodeficiency (SCID)

In this condition there is an abnormality in the development of the thymus and germinal centres in lymph nodes. There are therefore defects in T and B cell function, including reduced immunoglobulin levels.

T lymphocyte deficiency

In the most important example of this condition there is a severe abnormality of the development of the thymus, with a consequent severe reduction in T cell function. This is known as di George syndrome. Patients are prone to infections which are usually controlled by cell-mediated immunity, including viruses, fungi, yeasts, and intracellular organisms such as mycobacteria.

B lymphocyte deficiency

There is an X chromosome-linked abnormality of B cells called Bruton's agammaglobulinaemia in which there is a very low level of circulating immunoglobulin. Patients are particularly susceptible to bacterial infections.

IgA alone may be deficient in some cases, and presents as persistent respiratory or gastrointestinal infections.

Other conditions

There are also inborn abnormalities of neutrophils or complement components that may present as a general reduction in resistance to infection.

Acquired immunodeficiency (secondary)

General causes

Many chronic conditions induce some degree of associated mild immunodeficiency, such as diabetes mellitus, underlying malignancy, renal failure, splenectomy, renal failure, and nutritional deficiency. Some viral infections induce a temporary immunodeficiency. An example is influenza which is frequently followed by bacterial respiratory infection. Corticosteroid therapy induces general immunodeficiency as a side-effect. Cytotoxic chemotherapy or radiotherapy for malignant disease also commonly induces immunodeficiency.

Acquired immunodeficiency syndrome (AIDS)

This is a relatively recently described syndrome which is associated with the human immunodeficiency virus (HIV). The virus spreads by direct transmission of body fluids, particularly blood (so-called *horizontal* transmission, or from mother to baby (*vertical* transmission).

The HIV virus binds to the CD4 receptor on T lymphocytes and causes cell death. Patients show a severe reduction in circulation CD4 (helper-inducer) lymphocytes, and in established AIDS there is therefore reduced resistance to infections that are controlled by cell-mediated immunity. Examples of these infections include fungi such as *Aspergillus* and *Nocardia*, yeasts such as *Candida* and cryptococcus, and intracellular infections such as mycobacteria. Overwhelming virus infection, due to cytomegalovirus for example, may occcur. Malignant tumours such as lymphomas, squamous cell carcinomas, and Kaposi's sarcoma may develop. Some of these appear to be 'driven' by a virus. Epstein–Barr virus is associated with some lymphomas.

Acute HIV infection is sometimes manifested by an influenza-like 'sero-conversion' syndrome, when antibodies to the HIV virus develop. A persistent generalized lymphadenopathy can develop. AIDS-related complex develops before established disease and is defined by laboratory immunological testing and non-specific generalized symptoms. In the context of the dental surgery, control of possible transmission of infection is of paramount importance.

Finally, a summary of some immunological conditions relevant to dentists are listed in Table 3.4.

Table 3.4 Some immunological conditions of the mouth

Hypersensitivity
Lichen planus
Systemic lupus erythematosus
Pemphigus
Pemphigoid
Granulomatous disease (Crohn's, sarcoid, Wegener's)
Amyloid

SUMMARY

Immunological reactions, in contrast to inflammatory responses, are specific, have memory, and are capable of responding to wide and diverse factors.

Antigen: this is a substance which initiates an immune system.

Immune responses are either innate (inbuilt) or adaptive (can respond and change the response).

The immune response can be divided into the humoral system (immunoglobulins) and the cellular immune system (lymphocytes, plasma cells, and macrophages, including antigen-presenting cells).

Immunoglobulins:

–are produced from plasma cells derived from B cells
–they consist of heavy and light chains
–they are capable of opsonization in inflammatory responses
–they agglutinate and activate bacteria and viruses
–immunoglobulins activate the complement system to kill bacteria
–antibodies can initiate killing of cells by lymphocytes

There are five types of immunoglobulin:

IgG IgA IgM IgE IgD

Lymphocytes are derived from the bone marrow and either mature via the thymus (T lymphocytes) or a bursa equivalent (probably the bone marrow).

B lymphocytes:

–mature on stimulation to plasma cells which produce immunoglobulin
–share surface immunoglobulin
–have a major role in humoral immunity
–mature in the liver
–require T helper cells for normal function

T lymphocytes:

–are involved in cell-mediated immunity, particularly against virally infected cells
–mature in the thymus gland
–there are two types of lymphocytes, helper cells (CD4) and suppressor/cytotoxic cells (CD8)
–helper cells initiate the immune response and help the maturation of B cells
–suppressor/cytotoxic cells modulate the immune response and kill virally infected cells

Cells of the immune system communicate using cytokines.

The whole aim of the immune system is the recognition of self versus non-self. All antigens are presented to the immune system in association with self-antigens (HLA antigens). HLA antigens are coded by the MHC gene complex on chromosome 6.

Class I antigens: these are expressed on all nucleated cells. Class I antigens are linked to beta$_2$-microglobulin. Endogenous antigens are presented with HLA class I, that is, antigens that are produced by the cell itself. This is important in the detection of viral infection in cells. Suppressor/cytotoxic cells recognize antigen in association with HLA class I antigens.

Class II antigens: these are expressed on only specialized cells of the immune system, including T lymphocytes, B lymphocytes, and macrophages. Exogenous antigens are presented with class II antigens, that is, antigens derived from the outside of the cell. HLA class II is involved in the initiation and modulation of immune responses. T helper cells interact with class II antigens.

The macrophage and its derivatives, antigen-presenting cells including dendritic cells, are very important in the initiation of the immune response.

Diversity: the diversity of immunoglobulins and the T cell receptor is obtained by genetic re-arrangement of genes encoding these structures.

Hypersensitivity reaction: in some cases the immunological response is so severe that there are inappropriately excessive effects including tissue damage. Hypersensitivity reactions are classified as follows:

- Type I—immediate hypersensitivity. Examples include hay fever, eczema, and asthma. These involve IgE antibodies and mast cells.
- Type II hypersensitivity—cytotoxic. This involves damage to cells by the binding of specific antibodies to antigens on the cell surface. Examples include incompatible blood transfusion, autoimmune haemolytic anaemia, and rhesus disease of the fetus.
- Type III—immune complex hypersensitivity. This is when immune complexes form which produce tissue injury. Many autoimmune diseases manifest immune complex phenomena. Complement is frequently activated. Vasculitis may be induced.
- Type IV—delayed hypersensitivity. This response is mainly involved in intracellular infection, in particular viruses and mycobacteria. Contact dermatitis is an example of delayed hypersensitivity.

The immune system is also involved in autoimmune disease, graft-versus-host disease in bone marrow transplants, and organ transplant rejection.

Immunodeficiency may be primary (congenital) or secondary (for example, AIDS). Immunodeficiencies manifest as an abnormal sensitivity to infection and a susceptibility to organisms which normally are not pathogenic (opportunistic infection).

4 Neoplasia

4 Neoplasia

A TUMOUR is defined as a lesion arising from a proliferation of cells which is *autonomous* and *persists* after the initiating stimulus has been removed. It is a manifestation of an abnormality of the processes involved in the control of cell growth. The word *neoplasm*, meaning a new growth of cells, is sometimes used instead of the word *tumour*; tumour means a lump or swelling. A few basic concepts are summarized below:

- The underlying basis for cancer is cellular; if one cell in the body decides to stop growing, the effect is *negligible*. However, if one cell in the body decides to continue growing in an uncontrolled fashion, then the effect is serious and may be *fatal*.
- Following the above, tumours are generally considered to originate from one cell and are therefore *monoclonal* in character. Cells in a tumour have very similar genetic and biochemical features. Tumours have been shown to demonstrate the same chromosomal abnormality in all the cells, or the same particular enzyme type.
- A tumour is due to an imbalance between cell production and cell loss. A tumour does not necessarily have a proliferative rate that is faster than the surrounding normal tissue.
- The ultimate definition of malignancy is the ability to *metastasize*.
- Benign tumours *never* metastasize.
- There is a range of neoplastic change, with benign at one end and malignant at the other. There is generally a stepwise progression from one end of the spectrum to the other.
- As a cell *differentiates*, it tends to lose its ability to *proliferate* and vice versa.
- Cancer is primarily a *genetic* problem.
- The development of cancer is a *multistage* process.
- In general, cancers present clinically with symptoms very late in their biological history or life. There is a long period of time during which a cancer is growing and capable of metastasis, but in which the tumour is not large enough to produce symptoms. In comparison, there may be only a relatively short time before the tumour is fatal. One positive feature of oral tumours is that they are frequently visible at an early stage, and can therefore be diagnosed when effective treatment is still possible.

THE CELL CYCLE

The different stages that a cell goes through when it divides are grouped together and referred as the 'cell cycle'. Cells that are not within the cell cycle and 'resting' are described as being in the G_0 phase. Cells that are fully differentiated and incapable of further division, such as neurones, are in this state permanently. Most cells only spend a limited time in G_0 phase. Cells enter the cell cycle at a stage termed G_1 (gap 1). It is this stage that varies with slowly or rapidly dividing cells. After the G_1

phase, the cell then starts synthesizing DNA (the S phase). At the end of this phase the cell has twice the amount of DNA it had before the S phase. The cell then enters a G_2 phase, and then undergoes mitosis (M phase), the phase of nuclear division. Cytoplasmic division then occurs, and the resultant cells then enter G_1 again (see p. 000).

CONTROL OF CELL PROLIFERATION

There are specific genes that are responsible for controlling the processes involved in the different parts of the cell cycle. There are also genes that act as regulators of cell proliferation, particularly if abnormalities occur. Cell proliferation can be stopped until the correct processes have occurred. Proteins, such as cyclins, and factors influencing protein kinases and growth factor receptors are involved in this regulation (p. 000). Cyclins in particular bind to and influence protein kinases that regulate the phosphorylation of molecules involved in cell cycle control.

External influences are particularly important in the initiation of cell proliferation. Chemical messengers known as cytokines are involved in cell-to-cell communication. There are an increasing number of *growth factors* that have been discovered. Examples are included in Table 4.1.

Table 4.1 Growth factors

Growth factors
Platelet-derived growth factor
Epidermal growth factor
Fibroblast growth factor
Transforming growth factor-alpha
Interleukin-1

Hormones, such as thyroxine and corticosteroids, can also act as stimulators of cell proliferation.

Factors that inhibit cell proliferation are also described. Examples are shown in Table 4.2.

Table 4.2 Growth inhibitors

Growth inhibitors
Tumour necrosis factor
Interferon
Transforming growth factor-beta

Cells have *receptors* which are specific for particular hormones or growth factors. These have been covered in the cell pathology chapter (p. 000), but are summarized below.

These receptors are proteins that are inserted into the cell membrane and they have binding sites that are specific for a given growth factor or hormone. The receptors have a part that projects outside the cell, the *extracellular domain*. There is part of the receptor that is within the cell membrane, and part that projects into the cell, the *intracellular domain*. In general, once the receptor has bound to its respective factor or hormone, termed a *ligand*, this sets a train of events into action which is similar irrespective of the ligand. This involves specific enzymes, such as kinases and phosphorylases, which alter cell biochemistry, sending signals to genes involved in cell proliferation. When a receptor binds with its respective ligand, the tyrosine kinase activity of that receptor is increased. Proteins called G- and N-proteins are involved in intermediate stages and they control adenylate cyclase activity, altering intracellular cAMP (cyclic adenosine monophosphate) concentrations. The intracellular calcium levels change and the phosphorylation of metabolites occurs altering, for instance, the ADP:ATP ratio and the concentration of GTP (guanosine 5′-triphosphate).

Steroid receptors are different in that the receptors are free within the cytoplasm, and when bound to the respective ligand the receptor–ligand complex then migrates to the nucleus.

Similar mechanisms to those described above are involved in other receptor-mediated cell processes such as activation of a lymphocyte after binding of surface receptors, or hormone secretion by an endocrine cell.

CELLULAR DIFFERENTIATION

The process of cellular specialization is called differentiation. It is primarily under genetic control, although the local environment of a cell can cause a change in differentiation. For example, basement membrane components and the extracellular matrix have an influence on cell differentiation. Cytokines and hormones also influence cell growth and differentiation. All cells have a complete complement of genetic information and the process of differentiation involves the selective expression of certain genes, with suppression of others. There is generally an inverse relationship between cell differentiation and cell proliferation. If a cell becomes differentiated, it generally loses the ability to divide.

In a tissue that is undergoing a continual and controlled proliferation and differentiation, such as the bone marrow or skin, cells pass through different developmental stages. There is a *stem cell* population in which a small proportion of cells are proliferating at any one time. Most of the proliferation needed to produce the large numbers of cells required occurs within the next stage where cells are also beginning to specialize. There is a later stage where cells are fully specialized and stop dividing. An important point is that there is a careful balance in normal tissues between the numbers of cells being produced by a particular tissue and the numbers of cells being lost. Cells are lost by death (for example, neutrophils in acute inflammation), by desquamation (in the case of the skin), or by apoptosis (programmed cell death).

ABNORMAL CELL PROLIFERATION

Cellular responses which involve a stimulation of cell growth such as *hyperplasia* or a change in cell type as in *metaplasia* do not in themselves predispose to malignancy. Abnormal cell proliferation which has a high probability of malignant change shows itself as visible changes down the microscope in the forms of *dysplasia*, literally meaning 'disordered growth'. This is a recognizable manifestation of an underlying genetic problem which has resulted in an increased risk of malignant change. Dysplastic cells are some way along the pathway to malignant change. It can be shown that the presence of abnormal growth factors and other proteins can result in disturbances to the cytoskeleton of cells, resulting in abnormal shape. This sort of correlation goes some way towards explaining the underlying reason for the appearances of neoplastic cells. Dysplastic cells show the following features:

- Enlargement.
- A nucleus which is abnormally large for the given size of cell.
- The nuclei vary in size and shape and are darkly staining
- Frequent and abnormal mitoses.
- Loss of normal maturation and differentiation.
- Loss of normal orientation to other cells.
- Increased numbers of cells in the tissue and loss of the normal tissue architecture.

Dysplastic cells are part of the way along the multistep pathway to overt malignancy. Until these cells have developed the ability to invade through connective tissue, in particular the basement membrane of epithelium, and metastasize, they are not defined as 'malignant'. If, however, these dysplastic cells are studied in isolation, for example in tissue culture, they will show some of the features of 'transformed' cells.

The progressive changes of mild to severe dysplasia, and then the development of invasive activity are best seen in epithelial tissue. The dysplastic cells involve the lower, middle, and then the full thickness of the epithelium (Fig. 4.1), and eventually invade through the basement membrane. The term 'severe dysplasia' is usually synonymous with carcinoma *in situ*. The changes are not as well categorized

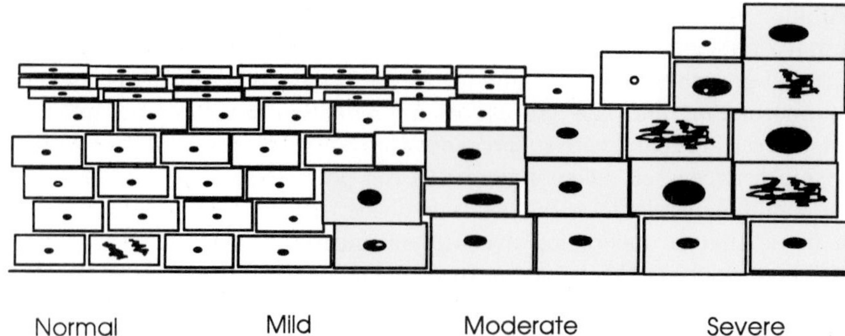

Fig. 4.1 The progression of dysplasia in the epithelium.

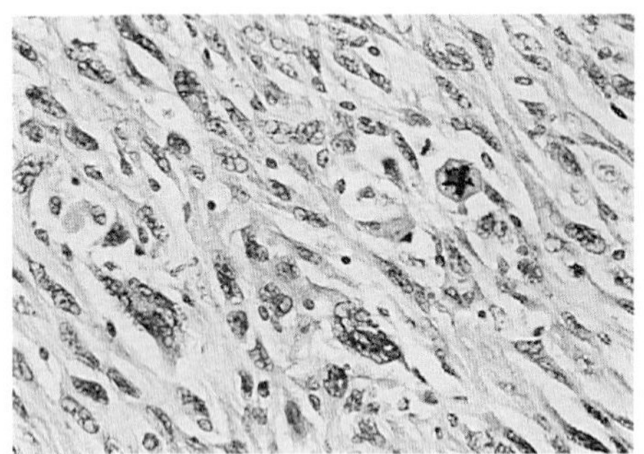

Fig. 4.2 A malignant tumour showing marked nuclear variability (pleomorphism) and abnormal mitoses.

in connective tissue, where there is no basement membrane to define an '*in situ*' phase of the disease. Other criteria, such as invasion of adjacent tissues, mitotic rate, and the presence of necrosis are used (Fig. 4.2).

THE MULTISTAGE DEVELOPMENT OF CANCER

The development of cancer is a *multistage* process, involving a number of steps. A number of changes accumulate in a cell before it becomes malignant. The development of a tumour is therefore a multistage process. This is consistent with the observation that there is usually a long 'latent' period between the exposure to a substance well recognized as a cause of cancer, that is, a carcinogen, and the development of a tumour.

The concept of 'initiation' and 'promotion' was developed some years ago. This idea involves a model in which a stimulus initially causes a change which by itself does not induce neoplastic change, but requires a further stimulus to be manifested. Initiating agents induce genetic mutations in the cell. This concept can be applied to the current idea that cancer initiation is a *genetic* event. Promotion can be either an accumulation of genetic errors, a stimulus to proliferation, or an alteration to the cell which eventually results in overt malignant change.

GENETIC CHANGES IN CANCER

The underlying change in cancer cells occurs at a molecular level, and involves an alteration or mutation in the genes themselves or in the expression of single or multiple genes. It is apparent that there are many genes that are involved in cell proliferation and changes in these are particularly relevant in the development of neoplasia, in particular *oncogenes*. There are also genes which produce factors that appear to supress the development of a tumour. These are known as *tumour suppressor genes*, and mutations in these genes are also relevant in the initiation of cancer. These alterations are dealt with in more detail below.

Chromosomal (karyotypic) abnormalities

These may be *congenital* or *acquired*.

Congenital abnormalities are usually discovered as part of the investigation of families with a high risk of a particular tumour. Examples are:

1. *Retinoblastoma*, a malignant tumour of the retina occurring in children. In individuals carrying the abnormality, there is a family history and the tumour develops at a very young age. The tumour tends to involve both eyes. It has been

shown that in the tumours there is deletion or mutation of both suppressor genes Rb1 in chromosome pair 13. All other cells in the patient (the 'germline' genetic make-up) show a pre-existing abnormality of one of the Rb1 genes. The concept is that it only takes one 'hit' of genetic damage to the remaining normal Rb1 gene to cause tumour development. Up to 40 per cent of retinoblastomas occur with a family history of the disease. In patients with retinoblastoma with no family history and no inborn genetic abnormality, the tumours occur at an older age and are unilateral. Two genetic 'hits' are required on both *Rb*1 genes (alleles) to cause development of retinoblastoma, and this takes more time to occur. It has been shown that the product of the retinoblastoma gene can be inactivated by certain small proteins.

2. *Familial polyposis coli*, a condition in which numerous polps occur in the colon, with the development of malignancy at a young age. There is loss of a tumour suppressor gene in chromosome 5 (the *APC* gene).

3. *Wilm's tumour* (nephroblastoma), a malignant tumour of the kidney in childhood. This is associated with loss of a gene in chromosome 11. This gene is called *WT*-1.

These deletions are either visible in stained chromosome spreads down the microscope, or detected by molecular biological techniques. Individuals with inborn genetic abnormalities associated with tumours develop these neoplasms at a younger age than individuals without these abnormalities. This supports the hypothesis that sequential mutations are required in the development of cancer; if you are born with a mutation, it takes less time to accumulate the other abnormalities required to develop the tumour associated with this mutation.

Acquired chromosomal abnormalities are very common in a very wide range of tumours, and are not always of a specific type. However, there are some abnormalities that appear more frequently than would be expected by chance and some common ones are described below.

- Chronic myeloid leukaemia: a *translocation* or 'exchange' between part of chromosome 9 and part of chromosome 22, t(9;22). The Philadelphia chromosome is a short chromosome 22, and the translocation is equal or 'balanced'.
- Burkitt's lymphoma: a *translocation* between parts of chromosomes 8 and 14, t(8;14).
- Mixed parotid tumour: a *translocation* between parts of chromosomes 3 and 8, t(3;8).
- Colonic carcinoma: a *deletion* of part of chromosome 17 (del 17p).

Gene mutation

There is evidence that genetic alterations are relevant in neoplastic change.

- The majority of carcinogens are capable of causing genetic mutations.
- There is a higher incidence of skin cancer in patients with the condition xeroderma pigmentosum, a congenital defect in the repair mechanism involved after DNA damage due to ultraviolet light.
- Cells with mutations in their 'oncogenes' show malignant behaviour. Oncogenes are genes found in normal cells which code for growth factors and other important products involved in cellular function. When mutations occur, the abnormal gene product is associated with malignant change. There may be an increased expression of the gene product due to an increased number of copies of the gene.
- Malignant cells frequently produce abnormal proteins not normally seen by that particular cell type, for example carcino-embryonic antigen in colonic carcinoma or alphafetoprotein in liver carcinoma.

CARCINOGENESIS

Chemical carcinogenesis

A large proportion of cancer is related to some form of environmental exposure. In man, environmental factors, such as chemical carcinogens and radiation, are associated with the development of cancer. The feature common to these carcinogenic agents is the ability to alter cells at a genetic level by inducing abnormalities in DNA. An important concept, as mentioned above, is the 'multi-hit' hypothesis of carcinogenesis. Chemical carcinogens either act directly or require metabolism before becoming biochemically active (known as procarcinogens). In general, they are highly reactive molecules which react with electron-rich areas of proteins and DNA in the cell. Mutations inducing inappropriate activation of proto-oncogenes with oncogene expression are relevant in carcinogenesis. Examples of carcinogens and situations where exposure occurs are listed in Table 4.3.

Viruses associated with cancer—the discovery of oncogenes

Although many viruses are associated with malignancy in animals, few have been shown to be related to cancer in man. The most well-known viruses associated with human cancer are the Epstein–Barr virus (EBV), the hepatitis B virus, and the human papilloma virus (HPV).

Viruses exert their carcinogenic effect by a number of mechanisms. In DNA viruses, the virus genome becomes incorporated into the cell's DNA. Some viruses, for example the human papilloma virus, contain genes that have product that can cause transformation of a cell, in a similar way to activation of a proto-oncogene. Viral genes which are expressed early in the infection appear particularly important in the transformation of an infected cell.

RNA viruses differ from DNA viruses in that they convert their RNA into DNA using a viral enzyme called reverse transcriptase. Many of these viruses can cause cancer in animals. The human T cell leukaemia virus is the only RNA virus closely associated with cancer in man.

It has been found that in these cancer-producing viruses are abnormal genes that have replaced genes normally involved in virus production. These abnormal genes code for transforming factors and have become known as *oncogenes* (viral-oncogenes: v-*onc*). It is of interest that identical and well-conserved genes are found in normal cells in many species, including man. These normal genes are known as proto-oncogenes, but when they are abnormal, as in some tumours, they are also known as oncogenes (cellular-oncogenes: c-*onc*). It is an important point that the term 'oncogene' has been applied for historical reasons and that, in fact, normal cells have proto-oncogenes which code for normal physiological factors such as growth receptors or enzymes involved in cell proliferation.

Many of these cellular oncogenes are expressed in normal cells, particularly during cell proliferation. However, in many cancers there are abnormalities of these oncogenes. There may be mutations of these genes, caused by carcinogens. Over-expression of oncogenes may be seen, caused either by active virus promoter sequences that stimulate cellular-concogene expression, or by translocations to an area close to other active cell genes. There may be multiple copies of the gene which also leads to over-expression of the gene product.

Oncogenes of either ceullar or viral type have been given three-letter names, often after the species or type of tumour they were found in. Some well-known oncogenes are summarized in Table 4.4.

As mentioned in Table 4.4, some specific products coded for by proto-oncogenes are growth factors such as epidermal growth factor, platelet-derived growth factor,

Table 4.3 Chemical carcinogens

Anti-cancer cytotoxic drugs—cyclophosphamide, chlorambucil, busulphan

Organic chemicals—benzene, benzopyrene

Polychlorinated biphenyls—previously used in electrical industry

Chemicals used in dye, rubber, and plastic industry—naphthylamines, biphenyls, vinyl chloride monomer

Dietary exposure—nitrosamines, amides, aflatoxins from fungi, Betel nut chewing

Metals—chromium salts, nickel

Table 4.4 Oncogenes

Oncogene	Tumour	Function
bcl-2	Follicular lymphoma	Inhibits apoptosis
erb-B	Squamous cell carcinoma	Epidermal growth factor
erb-B2	Breast carcinoma	Tyrosine kinase
myc	Burkitt's lymphoma	Nuclear protein
L-*myc*	Lung carcinoma	–
N-*myc*	Neuroblastoma	–
ras	Colon, lung, bladder cancer	GTP-related proteins (H, K, N)

and transforming growth factors. Also, protein kinases involved in the regulation of cell proliferation, and receptors for growth factors are also under proto-oncogene control.

Three important DNA viruses that are associated with human cancer are described below.

Epstein–Barr virus (EBV)

This is a DNA virus in the herpes virus family which is implicated in the development of nasopharyngeal carcinoma, a type of rapidly growing (high-grade) B cell lymphoma called Burkitt's lymphoma, and possibly other lymphomas such as Hodgkin's disease.

The EBV virus is the cause of infectious mononucleosis (glandular fever) in which B cells are infected and proliferate, but do not produce a lymphoma. Environmental factors are therefore also relevant in the development of these tumours, but as, for example, all nasopharyngeal carcinomas can be shown to contain EBV DNA, the virus has a very important role in the genesis of these tumours.

Hepatitis B virus (HBV)

There is a strong association between hepatitis B virus (HBV), which is a DNA hepadenovirus, and hepatocellular carcinoma (also known as hepatoma). Hepatitis B virus induces a chronic hepatitis which can go on to produce a cirrhosis, predisposing to the development of carcinoma. The HBV becomes incorporated into the infected cell's DNA and then exerts a transforming effect. As with the other viruses described here, there are additional factors such as the increased proliferative activity of the liver in chronic liver disease and cirrhosis. Environmental factors appear important, such as exposure to carcinogens such as aflatoxin B_1 produced by *Aspergillus flavus*, a fungus growing on grain.

Human papilloma virus (HPV)

This is a papovavirus and is responsible for the common skin wart, but is also associated with other neoplastic lesions, particularly laryngeal and genital warts, cervical intra-epithelial neoplasia, (CIN), and cervical carcinoma. There are at least 50 different types of HPV, but some types are strongly associated with specific lesions, as listed in Table 4.5.

In the case of cervical carcinoma, HPV is found in association with CIN. However, as with EBV, the virus is not the whole story as HPV DNA is found in up to 70 per cent, or more, of normal women. Other environmental factors, such as smoking, are associated with cervical carcinoma.

Table 4.5 Types of human papilloma virus (HPV)

Type	Lesion
1	Benign plantar warts
2, 4, 7	Benign skin warts
6, 11	Genital and perineal warts (condyloma acuminata)
16, 18, 30, 31, 33	Cervical carcinoma, oral carcinoma

Tumour suppressor genes—p53

Tumour suppressor genes are genes that, if absent, are associated with an increased risk of developing cancer. Examples are the retinoblastoma and familial polyposis genes. An important tumour suppressor gene that has relatively recently been characterized is the so-called p53 gene. The name of the protein gene product relates to its molecular weight, and the gene is located on chromosome 17. There are mutations in the p53 gene in up to 60 per cent of cancers. The p53 protein normally functions as an inhibitor of cell division in the G_1 phase, and it can induce apoptosis (active cell death). It is called into function if there has been genetic damage which requires repair or genetic changes putting the cell at risk of neoplastic change. Two genes called GADD-45 and *mdm*-2 relate to the function of the p53 gene. GADD-45 expression is increased in DNA damage, and the p53 gene may 'monitor' the levels of this gene. The gene *mdm*-2 may be used to allow cells to re-enter the cell cycle in the S phase.

If there are abnormalities in the p53 gene or reduced levels of the p53 protein due to complexing with an abnormal product, mutations or amplifications of genes, particularly those involved in the control of the cell cycle, are allowed to accumulate.

Other genes

Genes are also involved in the control of apoptosis, a process that can be regarded as an 'antidote' to mitoses (see p. 000).

It is now also apparent that genes are involved in the process of metastasis. One such gene is called nm23.

FEATURES OF BENIGN AND MALIGNANT NEOPLASMS

Benign tumours

Macroscopic appearances

Benign tumours are localized and well circumscribed with a smooth boundary. They do not show any invasive activity at the periphery and frequently have a well-formed capsule. They usually have an even cut surface with no areas of softening due to necrosis; benign tumours do not generally outgrow their blood supply. The are slow growing and, by definition, there will be no clinical evidence of metastases. For instance, local lymph nodes will be normal. Although benign tumours do not cause harm in most cases, if the tumour is in an enclosed space, such as in the brain, or if the tumour is secreting a large amount of hormone such as insulin, there may be serious consequences.

A special case where the cells have malignant characteristics but will not metastasize is in the condition of *carcinoma-in situ*. In this lesion of epithelium the cells show disordered growth with *severely dysplastic* features, but no invasion through the basement membrane (Figs 4.3 and 4.4). If neglected, however, this condition has a high incidence of transformation into *invasive* carcinoma.

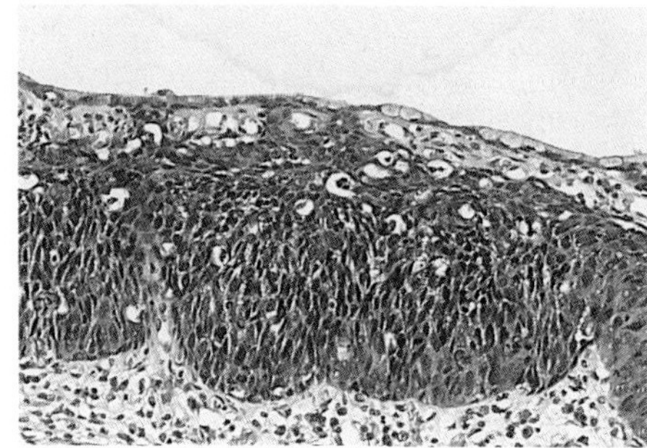

Fig. 4.3 Severely dysplastic epithelium compared to normal in Fig. 4.4.

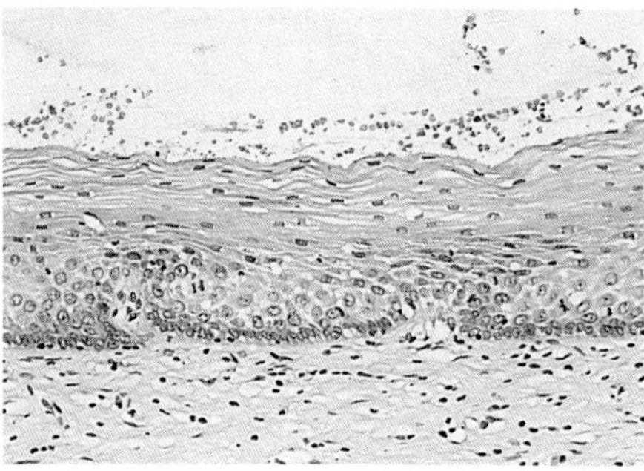

Fig. 4.4 Normal squamous epithelium for comparison with Fig. 4.3.

Microscopic appearances

Benign tumours show no evidence of capsular or vascular invasion (Fig. 4.5). The tissue is well differentiated, a term meaning that the tumour quite closely resembles the tissue that it has originated in. The cells in a benign tumour are regular, and show equally sized and evenly staining nuclei, indicative of their normal chromosomal and genetic structure. The mitotic rate, a guide to proliferation rate, will be low.

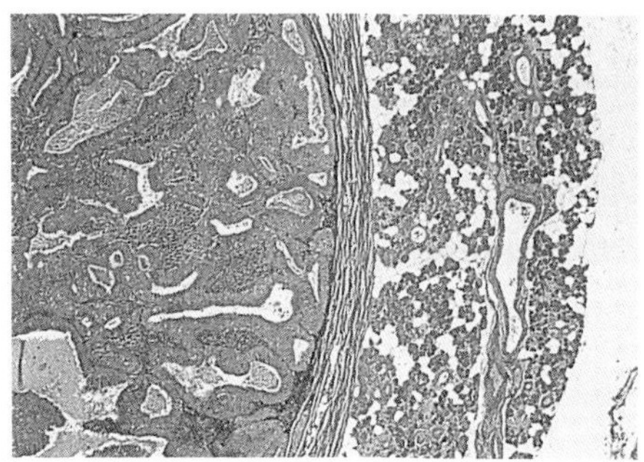

Fig. 4.5 A benign adenolymphoma (Warthin's tumour) of the parotid with a well-formed capsule and no invasive activity.

Malignant tumours

Macroscopic features

Malignant tumours, in contrast to benign tumours, show invasive activity at the margin (Figs 4.6 and 4.7), and infiltrate through basement membranes and any surrounding tissue. Malignant tumours are generally faster growing than benign tumours, although this is not always the case. There are influences, such as blood supply, nutrition, and hormonal factors, that affect cell proliferation. They have the capability to invade lymphatics or blood vessels, the main method of distant metastasis. The cut surface is often irregular because of different growth patterns, and necrosis is frequent due to the tumour out-growing its blood supply. This is despite the vascular proliferation that tumours induce by the production of *angiogenesis factors*.

Microscopic features

Through the microscope, the cells in a malignant tumour show less differentiation in that they only resemble the tissue of origin to a limited extent. If it is difficult to determine what sort of tumour is present the term *poorly differentiated* is used. In some cases, the tumour is so poorly differentiated that it is impossible to be precise about the type of tumour and the term *anaplastic* is used. If the tumour shows more of a resemblence to recognized tissue the term *well-differentiated* is applied.

The tissue is generally microscopically disordered, and shows invasive activity (Fig. 4.8). Blood and/or lymphatic invasion may be present (Fig. 4.9). The nuclei of

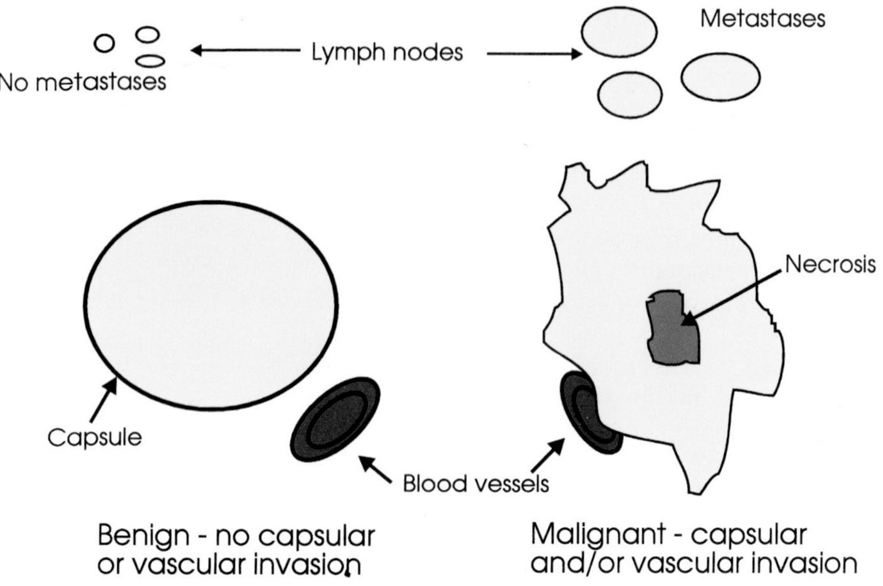

Fig. 4.6 A summary of features of benign versus malignant tumours.

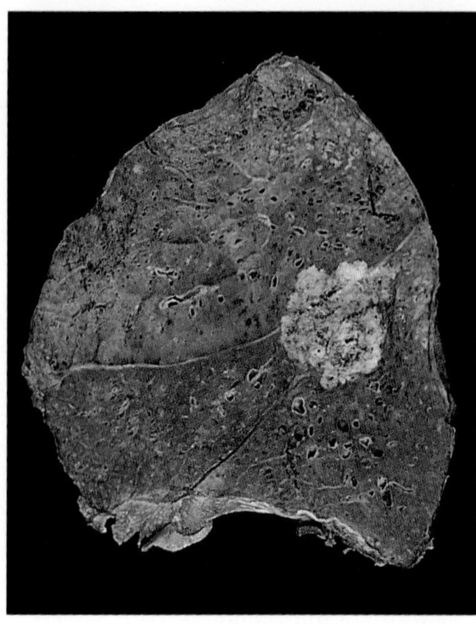

Fig. 4.7 A lung carcinoma invades across lobar fissures.

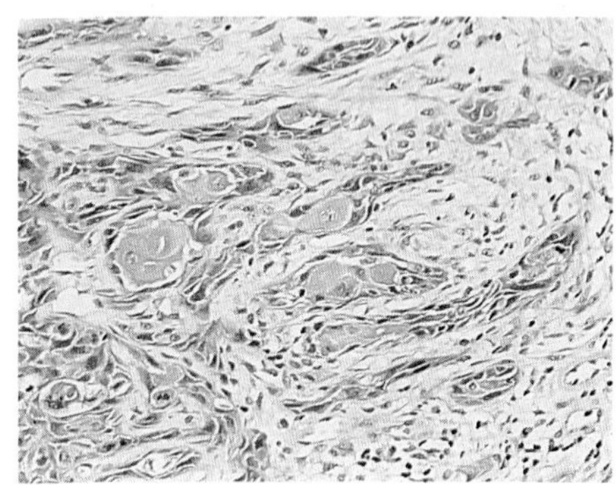

Fig. 4.8 Invasive squamous cell carcinoma. No basement membrane is seen.

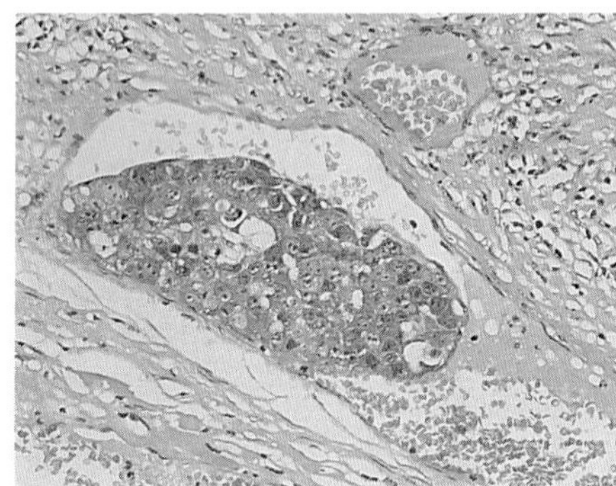

Fig. 4.9 Vascular invasion by tumour.

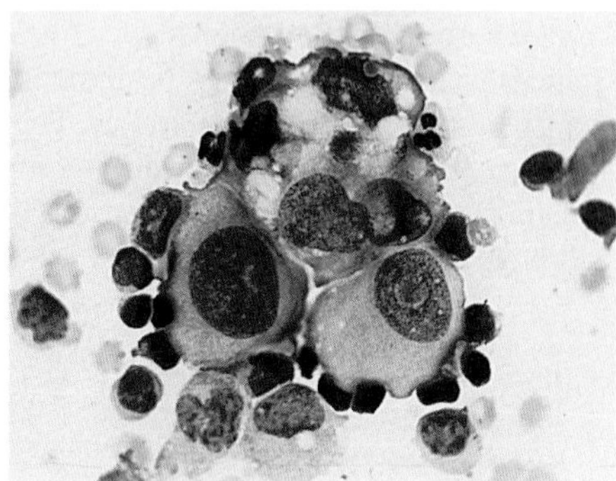

Fig. 4.10 A cytological preparation showing nuclear variation.

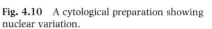

the cells in a malignant tumour are *pleomorphic*, a term meaning variation in size and shape (Fig. 4.10). The nuclei may also vary in staining intensity, and appear too large for a given size of cell (the nuclear-to-cytoplasmic ratio is increased). These nuclear features reflect the chromosomal and genetic abnormalities present in malignant cells. The term applied to these features of abnormal growth is *dysplasia*. The mitotic rate may be high, indicating a high rate of cell division. Also, the mitotic figures may be abnormal. The nucleoli, structures in nuclei involved in RNA production, are prominent, indicating a high rate of nuclear activity. It must be pointed out, however, that the problem with cancer is an imbalance between cell production and cell loss; cancers do not always have a higher proliferation rate than normal tissue.

TUMOUR BIOLOGY

In experimental conditions, malignancy is defined in a different way to that described above. Malignant cells are capable of continued growth in an animal which is either immunosuppressed or of the same species and histocompatibility (tissue type) as the host developing the tumour.

The term *transformation* is applied to cells that have developed these characteristics of malignancy. These cells show several characteristics:

1. Tumourigenicity. This is the ability to form tumours described above.
2. Enlargement of the nucleus.
3. They pile up on each other in culture instead of forming a single cell layer as is seen with normal cells. This represents a loss of *contact inhibition*, and represents a reduced response to factors that regulate cell proliferation.
4. Changes of surface molecules. There may be expression of new antigens on the surface of the cells.
5. The malignant cells show abnormal chromosomes.
6. Transformed cells show an extended life in culture, and sometimes show 'immortal' growth. They lose any tendency to differentiate.

Within a tumour there are generally two types of cells; cells that are undifferentiated and proliferating, forming a *stem cell* population, and cells which are *differentiating*. Cells which are differentiating lose the ability to divide.

An important point about the biology of tumours in the clinical situation is that by the time a tumour is evident, biologically it is at a very late stage. Assuming a tumour comes from one cell, to be detectable there has to have been about 25 to 30 cell doublings (about 2^{25} to 2^{30} cells). The tumour in some cases may have been present for several years before clinical presentation, possibly with a potential for metastasis during that time. There is usually only another 10 doublings before the result is fatal. This, of course, is a very rough approximation, and does not take into account factors that limit the growth of a tumour such as vascularization and nutrition.

Another feature of a tumour is that at any given time only a small proportion of the tumour cells are in the cell cycle and dividing. This dividing population is called the growth fraction. Generally, the faster a tumour is growing, the higher the proportion of the tumour cells found to be dividing.

MECHANISMS OF INVASION AND METASTASIS

Metastasis is the spread of tumour cells from the primary site in the body to one or more separate distant secondary sites.

Tumour spread

There are several methods of tumour spread which are summarized below:

1. *Direct local spread*: this involves direct invasion of surrounding structures.
2. *Lymphatic spread*: tumour may invade lymphatics and metastasize to local and distant lymph nodes.
3. *Blood spread*: tumour may invade veins and spread to distant sites. If tumour invades systemic veins, tumour may metastasize widely, in particular to the lungs or bones.
4. *Transcoelomic spread*: tumour may invade across the surface of cavities, such as the pleura or peritoneum, to cause fluid accumulation or involvement of other organs.

Sites of metastasis

The sites that a tumour spreads to depends not only on the vascular supply of that tissue or organ, but also on local microenvironmental factors. This is illustrated by the fact that although the spleen has a very large relative blood supply, metastases are rare. The liver, in contrast, also has a high blood supply and metastases are common.

In many cases the anatomy of the lymphatic or vascular supply is an important factor:

- Carcinomas have a high incidence of metastasis to local lymph nodes.
- Sarcomas tend to spread via veins and therefore frequently metastasize to the lungs, the next capillary network in the circulation.
- Cancer of the gastrointestinal tract frequently metastasizes to the liver via the portal vein.

However, some tumours show unusual behaviour, suggesting that there are local factors needed to sustain metastatic growth, possibly cytokines:

- Gastric cancer may show solitary metastases in the ovaries.
- Lung carcinoma has an unusually high frequency of adrenal metastasis.
- Renal carcinoma may show isolated metastasis to the thyroid.
- When a blood vessel is invaded by tumour, malignant cells are distributed in all sites of the body, but only a few of these will develop metastatic tumour.

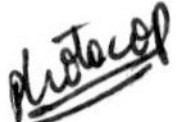

The process of metastasis

The development of a tumour metastasis can be considered as a multistep process, in a similar way to that of the development of cancer. It is a process is which a large number of criteria must be satisfied before metastasis can occur.

1. In a given tumour, only a small proportion of the tumour cells will have developed the potential ability to metastasize.

2. As a tumour develops and grows, genetic mutations occur which in some cases will give cells a growth advantage. For instance, a cell may have a greater ability to induce the development of blood vessels by expressing a gene for a blood vessel growth factor. In another case cells may develop that have an increased ability to invade into lymphatics. A form of 'evolution' appears to occur in a tumour, with selection of advantageous clones.

3. The tumour cells have to first develop the ability to invade through the adjacent tissues to penetrate a blood or lymphatic vessel. In the case of an epithelium, the cells have to be capable of invading through a basement membrane to make the transition from carcinoma-*in situ* to invasive carcinoma. Therefore, the cells have to have the ability to synthesize the relevant proteases and elastases to break down basement membrane and interstitial substances such as collagen and elastin. Interactions with extracellular matrix are very important in the progression to invasion and metastasis. Tumour cells have to interact with type IV collagen and laminin in basement membranes and extracellular components such as types I and III collagen, fibronectin and other proteoglycans. Adhesion molecules also play an important role in the behaviour of tumour cells. Two types of adhesion molecules are involved; one set is involved in cell-to-cell interactions and the other is involved in cell and extracellular matrix interactions (see p. 000). The main adhesion molecules involved are the integrins, cadherins, selectins, and molecules belonging to the immunoglobulin superfamily. Integrins are involved in cell-to-cell contact, and cadherins are involved in cell to extracellular matrix contact. In malignant change,

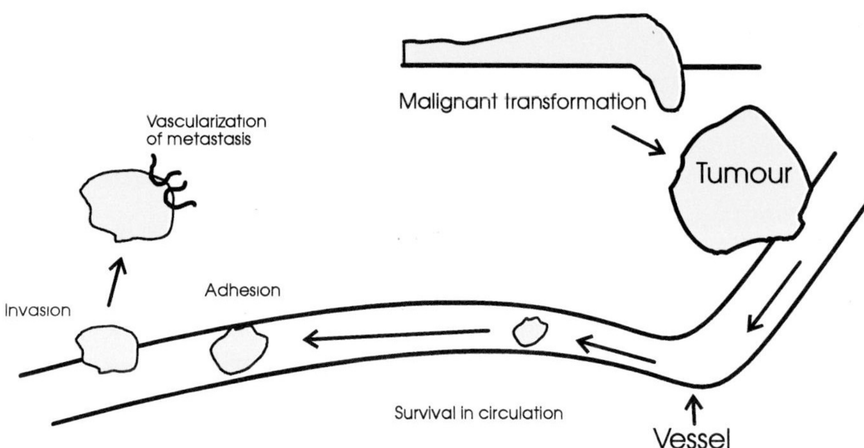

Fig. 4.11 The process of metastasis.

there are changes in the expression of these adhesion molecules to allow detachment and movement of tumour cells through tissues. Adhesion molecules are also important in interactions between tumour cells and endothelium in the case of vascular invasion.

A group of zinc-binding, calcium-dependent enzymes called metalloproteinases are relevant in the breakdown of connective tissue to allow tumour invasion. Metalloproteinases have a role in the development of tissues and organs in embryogenesis, and their function is disturbed in tumours. For example, increased activity of these enzymes is detected in invasive tumours. Other enzymes, such as plasmin, cathepsins, and elastase, are also involved in tumour invasion.

A recently discovered molecule that is also involved in tumour cell and lymphocyte adhesion and migration has been given the name CD44. This has the structure of a growth factor receptor, having a portion that interacts with the outside of the cell, and a portion that communicates with the cell cytoskeleton. The molecule binds to extracellular matrix components such as hyaluran, chondroitin sulphate, fibronectin, and collagen. The activity of the CD44 gene has been discovered to be abnormal in invasive tumours.

A very important point is that by the time a cancer has presented clinically with symptoms, the disease is already very late in its biological history. There is potential for metastasis at a very early stage, long before the tumour has been detected. The process of metastasis is summarized in Fig. 4.11.

CLASSIFICATION OF TUMOURS

Benign and malignant tumours are classified, usually by the histological appearance, because various types of tumours behave in different ways. The most important distinction to be made in any tumour is whether or not it is benign or malignant, because this will have a great affect on the treatment, and ultimately, the prognosis of the disease.

The term 'cancer' is a general term which applies to a *malignant* tumour of any type. The world derives from the crab-like extensions that many malignant tumours show at the edge. Tumours show differentiation either towards some type of epithelium when the term *carcinoma* is applied, or towards some type of connective tissue when the term *sarcoma* is applied. Tumours are classified with the concept that it is more important to look at what the cells are *doing* rather than to look at the type of tissue the tumour arose from.

Table 4.6 Tumour classification

Site	Benign	Malignant
Epithelium		
Squamous	Papilloma	Squamous cell carcinoma
Glandular	Adenoma	Adenocarcinoma
Transitional	Papilloma	Transitional cell carcinoma
Connective tissue		
Fat	Lipoma	Liposarcoma
Smooth muscle	Leiomyoma	Leiomyosarcoma
Skeletal muscle	Rhabdomyoma	Rhabdomyosarcoma
Collagenous tissue	Fibroma	Fibrosarcoma
Blood vessels	Angioma	Angiosarcoma
Lymphatics	Lymphangioma	Lymphangiosarcoma
Bone	Osteoma	Osteosarcoma
Cartilage	Chondroma	Chondrosarcoma
Melanocytes	Naevus (mole)	Melanoma
Lymphocytes	–	Lymphoma
Bone marrow	–	Leukaemia

Features that suggest epithelial differentiation in a tumour include cohesion of cells in groups, the formation of sheets or 'packets' of tumour cells, and the presence of junctions between the cells seen as fine lines or 'prickles' between the cells. These represent the 'rivet-like' desmosomes holding epithelial cells together and are particularly prominent in squamous epithelium, which by definition makes keratin. Another characteristic feature of epithelium is the development of basement membrane in association with the cells.

Features that suggest connective tissue differentiation are cells lying separated by a loose stroma.

The suffix '-oma' is applied to the word classifying the origin of a benign tumour, for example, a benign glandular tumour is termed an aden*oma*, or a benign bone tumour is called an oste*oma*.

Tumours that resemble tissue found in the fetus have the term blastoma applied to them. For instance, a tumour of the kidney in children that imitates fetal kidney is called a nephro*blastoma*. The classification of tumours is summarized in Table 4.6.

Although tumours are usually classified by light microscopic features alone, the development of techniques, such as electron microscopy and immunocytochemistry, have allowed more objective identification of tumours. This is of importance in tumours which appear undifferentiated at light microscopy.

COMMON TUMOURS

Benign

Common benign tumours are listed below:

–melanocytic naevi in the skin
–colonic adenomas
–uterine leiomyomas (fibroids)
–fibroadenomas of the breast
–lipomas
–haemangiomas (pyogenic granulomas)
–squamous papillomas of the mouth

–oral fibromas
–dermatofibromas of the skin

Malignant

These are in the order of frequency:

Males		Females	
Mortality	*Incidence*	*Mortality*	*Incidence*
Lung	Prostate	Breast	Breast
Colon and rectum	Lung	Lung	Colon and rectum
Prostate	Colon and rectum	Colon and rectum	Lung
Stomach	Bladder	Stomach	Endometrium
Lymphoma/leukaemia	Lymphoma/leukaemia	Ovary	Lymphoma/leukaemia
Stomach	Stomach	Pancreas	Pancreas
		Leukaemia/lymphoma	Cervix

CLINICAL EFFECTS OF CANCER

Local effects

Both benign and malignant tumours can cause clinical problems by the fact that they are space-occupying lesions. Even a benign tumour can be dangerous if it occurs in a confined space, such as the skull, as in the case of a meningioma. Both benign and malignant tumours can cause obstruction of a lumen, for example in the urinary tract or the gastrointestinal tract (Fig. 4.12). Malignant tumours are, however, locally destructive and invasive.

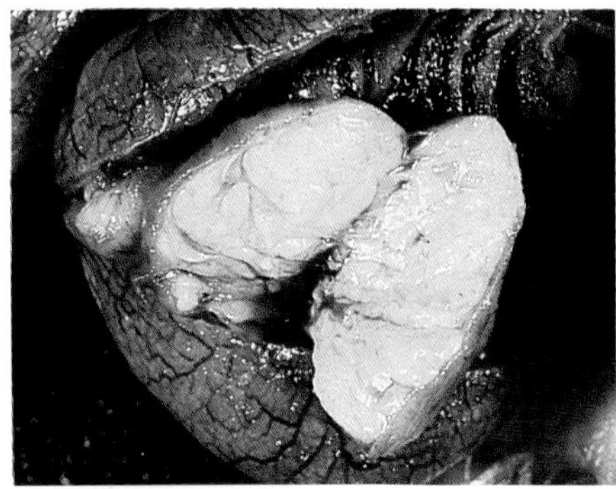

Fig. 4.12 This benign lipoma caused life-threatening obstruction of the colon.

Distant (systemic) effects

Non-metastatic

Both benign and malignant tumours of the endocrine system, and some other types of tumour can produce hormones which can have serious effects. Some examples are given in Table 4.7.

Some of these hormones can be used as tumour 'markers', to assess the effect of therapy or the presence of recurrence. Some tumours produce a specific protein which may not have any clinical effect, but may also be used as a tumour marker. Some common ones are listed in Table 4.8.

Table 4.7 Hormonal effects of tumours

Tumour	Hormone
Benign	
Thyroid adenoma	Thyroxine
Pituitary adenoma	Adrenocorticotrophic hormone
Parathyroid adenoma	Parathyroid hormone
Pancreatic islet adenoma	Insulin
Malignant	
Squamous cell carcinoma	Parathyroid hormone-like action
Small cell lung carcinoma	Adrenocorticotrophic hormone
Renal cell carcinoma	Erythropoetin

Table 4.8 Tumour markers

Tumour	Product used as marker
Prostate carcinoma	Prostate acid phosphatase Prostate-specific antigen
Choriocarcinoma Hydatidiform mole Testicular teratoma	Human chorionic gonadotrophin
Thyroid medullary carcinoma	Calcitonin
Alphafetoprotein	Hepatocellular carcinoma
Myeloma/plasmacytoma	Monoclonal immunoglobulin

Table 4.9 Intermediate filament proteins

Cytokeratins	All epithelium
Vimentin	Mainly connective tissue
Desmin	Muscle
Glial fibrillary acidic protein	Glial cells in brain, astrocytes
Neurofilament	Neurones
Nuclear lamins	All nucleated cells

Frequently, wasting (cachexia) is associated with cancer which is probably due to a cytokine or other metabolite produced by the tumour. There are also a number of clinical syndromes associated with some types of cancer, probably also due to the production of some factor by the tumour. A neuropathy, myositis, or periosteal proliferation of the fingers (hypertrophic osteoarthropathy) may develop in association with lung cancer.

There are different types of cytoskeletal filaments that are found in different cells which are of use in diagnostic pathology. Antibodies can be used to identify them. They are summarized in Table 4.9.

Metastatic

Complications frequently relate to local effects of metastases. The lung and liver are frequent sites of metastatic deposits. Carcinomas tend to spread via lymphatics to local lymph nodes, whilst sarcomas tend to spread by blood vessels, particularly to the lung.

ORAL TUMOURS

Connective tissue neoplasms

Common neoplasms of the connective tissue of the mouth include fibromas (fibrous epulides), fibroepithelial polyp, histiocytomas, malignant fibrous histiocytoma and fibrosarcoma. Connective tissue tumours of fat also occur in the mouth, the most common being a benign lipoma. Tumours of vascular tissue are also very common, in particular haemangiomas and lymphangiomas. The so-called pyogenic granuloma is a capillary haemangioma. Tumours of peripheral nerves also occur in the mouth, in particular neurofibromas. It is important to remember that malignant lymphomas of the lymphoid tissue around the back of the mouth and pharynx, so-called Waldeyer's ring are the most common site of extranodal lymphomas after the gastrointestinal tract. Burkitt's lymphoma, a high-grade lymphoma endemic to Africa and associated with the Epstein–Barr virus, presents as a jaw or maxillary tumour.

Epithelial neoplasms

Squamous cell papilloma

This common benign tumour of the oral mucosa frequently presents as a solitary raised polypoid lesion with a papillary or finger-like growth pattern. Histologically, there is marked over-growth of squamous epithelium, but with no dysplastic changes. Squamous cell papillomas are closely associated with the human papilloma virus.

Squamous cell carcinoma

Squamous cell carcinoma is the most common type of oral epithelial malignancy, and is seen in 90 per cent of all oral cancer (see p. 000). It is particularly associated with environmental exposure to carcinogens, particularly tobacco and Betel nut chewing. There is also association with alcohol, dietary factors, and possibly viral infections, in particular human papilloma virus. As with any squamous cell carcinoma at any site of the body, the tumour is defined histologically as an epithelial malignancy showing keratinization and evidence of intracellular junctions seen as 'prickles'. As with any malignant tumour, there is frequently local invasion and destruction of adjacent structures, and metastasis via lymphatics to local lymph nodes.

Basal cell carcinoma

This is mentioned because of its high frequency on the skin of the face and head, particularly in occupations with a long history of sun exposure. It is primarily a tumour of the skin and although it is termed a carcinoma it very rarely metastasizes unless it is very large.

Melanoma

It is important to remember that melanocytes are seen in the normal mucosa of the mouth. Melanocytic naevi frequently occur on the skin of the head and neck and are also occasionally seen in the oral mucosa. Malignant melanoma can also occur in the mouth.

Epithelial dysplasia

The term leukoplakia, which refers to a white patch on the oral mucosa, encompasses a large number of underlying causes. These include abnormal epithelial development, hyperplasia of the epithelium due to chronic trauma, infective lesions such as candida, skin conditions involving the mouth including lichen planus and lupus erythematosus. It also includes neoplastic lesions, including dysplasia, which may be severe and amounting to carcinoma-*in situ*, and overt squamous cell carcinoma. Frequently, leukoplakia is biopsied, not only to diagnose the underlying cause, but also to exclude the possibility of neoplasia. Epithelial dysplasia, as with any other dysplasia of epithelium anywhere on the body, is characterized by abnormal epithelial maturation and keratinization. The epithelium is frequently hyperplastic, but also shows nuclear and cellular pleomorphism. Nuclei are of abnormal size and shape and of abnormal staining pattern. Nuclei are also too large for a given size of cell. There may also be abnormal mitotic figures, with abnormal forms. Mitoses should only normally be found in the basal layer of the oral mucosa, and in the case of dysplasia these mitoses are found higher in the epithelium. Cells also show loss of polarity in that they show an abnormal orientation with regard to the epithelial surface. The degree of dysplasia is often classified by the proportion of the epithelium that is involved with the dysplastic change. It may be mild, moderate, or severe. The term severe dysplasia is synonymous with carcinoma-*in situ*. It is only when there is penetration of the basement membrane that the term invasive carcinoma is used. Carcinoma-*in situ* does not have metastatic potential because cells do not have access to blood or lymphatic vessels. In many ways the progression of dysplasia through carcinoma-*in situ* to invasive carcinoma reflects the multistep progression that appears to occur in the development of carcinoma.

SUMMARY

The fundamental problem of cancer is an imbalance between cell production and cell loss. Cancer is a group of conditions. A cancer involves cells showing loss of normal growth control which show invasive and metastatic potential.

Benign tumours: typically slow growing, encapsulated, resemble the parent tissue (are well differentiated), and show little cellular atypia and few mitoses. There is no necrosis, vascular or lymphatic invasion.

Malignant tumours: typically show rapid growth, invasive activity at the margin, poor resemblance to the parent tissue (poor differentiation), and frequently show central necrosis. There is frequently striking pathological atypia with frequent mitoses.

The word cancer is a generic term for all malignancy.

A *carcinoma* is a tumour which is differentiating towards epithelial structures. Common carcinomas are squamous cell and adenocarcinomas.

A *sarcoma* is a tumour which differentiates towards connective tissue such as bone.

Normal tissue: as normal tissue differentiates, the proliferative ability of the specializing cells is reduced. There is a balance between the cells proliferating in the tissue forming the functional cells and the cells being lost or dying.

Neoplastic tissue: in tumours, cells do not differentiate properly and maintain proliferative ability with faiure to fully differentiate. There is therefore an imbalance between the constant proliferation of the cells and lack of loss of cells through differentiation and death.

The underlying problem of carcinogenesis is *genetic*.

Carcinogenesis: an important concept is that the development of cancer is a process that involves multiple steps. Cancer is inherently a molecular or genetic problem and multiple abnormalities accumulate within a cell before it becomes overtly malignant. These changes are frequently manifested through the microscope as *dysplasia*. In epithelium, for example, carcinogenesis goes through a multiple process of dysplasia of increasing severity, with the development of pre-invasive carcinoma (carcinoma-*in situ*) before overt invasive carcinoma occurs. It is only when it is invasive that it has metastatic potential.

A cancer is derived from a *single* cell. Cancers are therefore *monoclonal*.

Many of the genes involved in the development of cancer are involved in the production of growth factors or growth factor receptors. The genes that code for growth factors and similar molecules involved in the control of growth and proliferation of cells are the *oncogenes*. These genes are found in normal cells which are not malignant. However, in many tumours there are abnormalities with oncogenes. It appears that inappropriate activation of the genes and mutations of oncogenes are involved in the development of cancer. It is important to emphasize that the products of normal oncogenes are involved in normal cell proliferation and regulation.

There are series of genes which are involved in the suppression of malignant growth and in the control of proliferation called *tumour suppressor genes*. In many ways, these genes oppose the action of oncogenes. Abnormalities of tumour suppressor genes or the absence of a tumour suppressor gene are strongly associated with the development of cancer. An important tumour suppressor gene is p53.

5 The cardiovascular system

5 The cardiovascular system

DISEASES of the cardiovascular system are responsible for almost one half of all deaths; a third of all deaths are caused by heart disease alone. A glossary of terms used in describing cardiovascular pathology is given in Table 5.1.

Table 5.1 Terms used for abnormalities of the circulatory system

Hypoxia	Reduced oxygen supply to tissue. Usually caused by ischaemia. May also originate from respiratory disease with reduced gas exchange, from anaemia, or metabolic abnormalities and toxic effects
Ischaemia	Inappropriate reduction in blood supply to an organ or tissues. Most frequently caused by atherosclerosis involving arteries
Thrombus	A solid mass composed of all blood constituents (platelets, fibrin, red cells) within a living blood vessel
Embolus	A solid, liquid, or gaseous mass or collection which originates from one site in the circulatory system and is carried to another site
Infarct	Necrosis due to ischaemia. Common sites include the heart, brain, spleen, kidney, and distal leg
Oedema	Abnormal collection of fluid within the interstitial space in tissues
Shock	Reduced perfusion of tissues. May be due to reduced blood volume (hypovolaemia), reduced peripheral resistance with venous pooling (endotoxic shock), or heart failure (cardiogenic shock)

SHOCK

This is a commonly used term, and in the context of clinical medicine it means a reduced perfusion of cells by the circulatory system. In view of this, the topic is included in this section. The consequences of shock are reduced metabolic and gas exchange. The mechanisms that cause and are involved in shock are summarized below.

Hypovolaemic shock

This occurs when there is a reduced volume of blood or plasma in the circulation. About 3.5 to 4 litres of blood is in the circulation, and the body has mechanisms to maintain blood pressure when there is loss of blood or fluid. However, there comes a point when blood pressure cannot be maintained after loss of 15–20 per cent of the blood volume, and the blood pressure falls. Organs such as the kidney and brain are particularly sensitive to reduced perfusion.

Causes of hypovolaemic shock include severe haemorrhage either internally or externally, and loss of plasma volume due to fluid loss from burns and the gastrointestinal tract.

Cardiogenic shock

Reduced cardiac output occurs when there is heart failure due to, for example, myocardial infarction or ischaemic heart disease. This occurs in the presence of a normal blood volume.

Bacteraemic (septic) shock

Metabolic products from bacteria, particularly so-called *endotoxins* from Gram-negative bacteria, and toxins from some streptococci are capable of inducing shock. In septic shock there is a marked pooling of blood in the veins which has an effect similar to blood loss. (This phenomenon also occurs in another form of shock associated with spinal cord or neurological injury, called *neurogenic* shock.) There is also a reduced resistance to blood flow through arterioles and capillaries, which causes a fall in blood pressure.

There is widespread activation of inflammatory mediators and cytokines which are associated with cellular injury, particularly to endothelial cells. Mediators involved in acute inflammation and cytokines such as tumour necrosis factor and platelet-activating factor are involved. Radicals and nitric oxide also appear to be relevant in the pathogenesis of some types of shock. Activation of complement and blood-clotting factors occurs, and extensive fibrin deposition may occur in small blood vessels, so-called disseminated intravascular coagulation (DIC).

Organs prone to damage in septic shock include the kidneys, brain, heart, and lungs. The diffuse microvascular damage in the lung may become the dominant clinical feature, and this condition is known as 'shock lung'.

ARTERIOSCLEROSIS

The term arteriosclerosis encompasses three basic conditions that affect arteries: (a) atherosclerosis; (b) arteriolosclerosis; and (c) medial sclerosis.

Atherosclerosis

This is primarily a proliferative condition that affects arteries, particularly the intimal layer. The underlying cause appears to be endothelial damage with an end result of intimal hyperplasia. It generally involves medium- and large-sized muscular and elastic arteries. It is a process which is seen mainly in the Western world, and the most important factors are a strong family history, often associated with hypercholesterolaemia. Hypertension, diabetes, smoking, and being male are also strong risk factors. Weaker risk factors include a high cholesterol and fat diet, obesity, and lack of exercise (Table 5.2).

Table 5.2 Risk factors for atherosclerosis

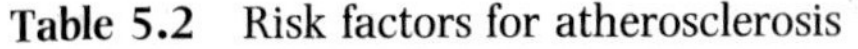

Risk factors
Raised lipoprotein (LDL) and cholesterol levels in the blood; relates to family history
Hypertension
Smoking
Diabetes mellitus
Being male
Age
High cholesterol diet
Obesity
Lack of exercise

The major complications of atherosclerosis are occlusion of the affected artery or associated thrombosis with embolism. The most clinically important arteries involved are the coronary arteries, the cerebral arteries, and vessels supplying the limbs, particularly the lower leg.

There are several complications of atherosclerosis (Fig. 5.1 and Table 5.3).

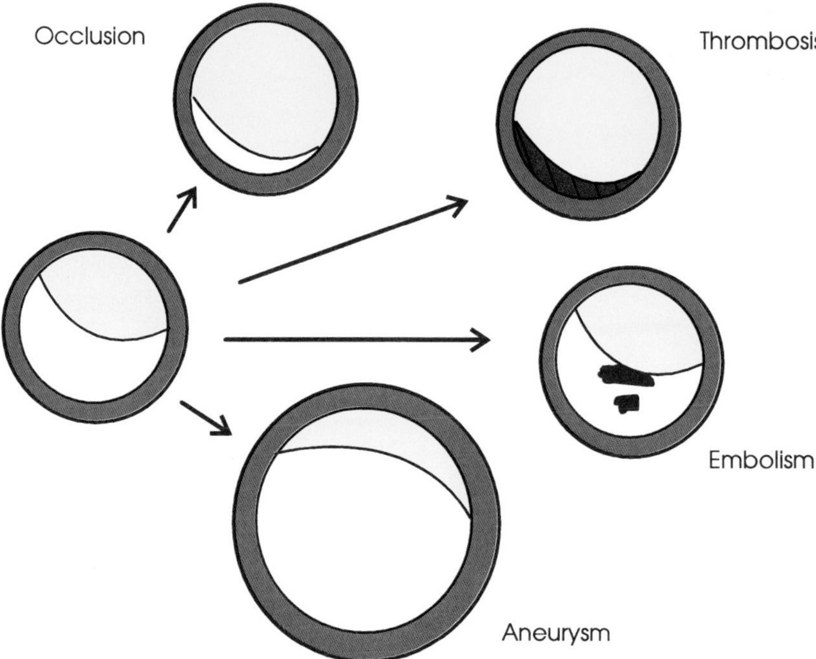

Fig. 5.1 A summary of the complications of atherosclerosis.

Table 5.3 Complications of atherosclerosis

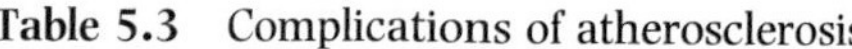

Complications of atherosclerosis
Ischaemic heart disease
Cerebral ischaemia and infarction
Peripheral vascular disease
Aneurysm
Embolus
Calcification
Small bowel ischaemia and infarction

Occlusion

Occlusive disease of the coronary arteries results in reduced perfusion of the myocardium with features of ischaemic heart disease (Fig 5.2). There may be sudden occlusion by thrombus with myocardial infarction (Fig. 5.3). Occlusion of leg vessels may result in reduced blood supply to the peripheral limbs with a development of muscle dysfunction and gangrene. Occlusion of cerebral arteries may result in cerebral dysfunction or infarction with the development of a stroke.

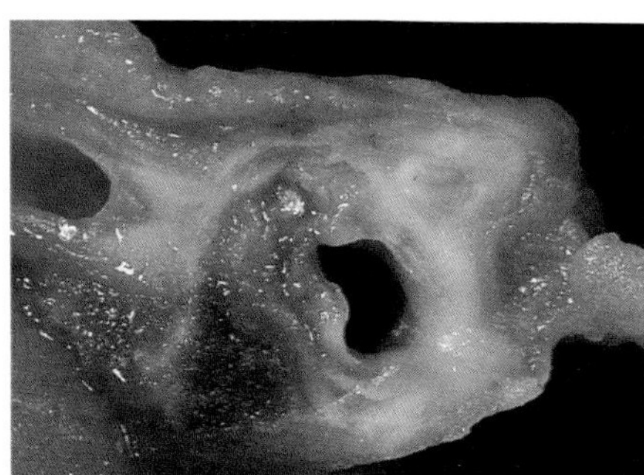

Fig. 5.2 Severe coronary artery atheroma near a branch.

Aneurysm

The development of severe intimal atherosclerosis may result in a weakening of the underlying media with subsequent dilatation of the vessel with a development of a sac-like aneurysm. There is frequently associated calcification with atherosclerosis. Large aneurysms have a high risk of sudden rupture with extensive arterial haemorrhage.

Thrombosis

Atherosclerotic plaques, particularly when well developed may show endothelial loss with ulceration and exposure of subendothelial connective tissue. This predisposes to thrombosis. Subsequent thrombi may break off from atherosclerotic plaques and embolize to distant sites in the arterial circulation.

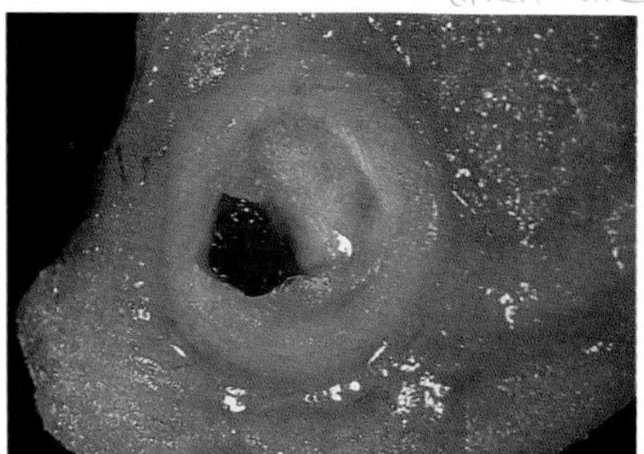

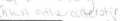

Fig. 5.3 Occlusion of a coronary artery by recent thrombus.

The morphology of atherosclerosis

The most apparent lesion of atherosclerosis that can be seen with the naked eye is the so-called fatty streak, which is seen as a slightly raised white streak on the intimal surface of arteries. Established atherosclerosis consists of marked fibrous or soft plaques of intimal deposits which project into the lumen of the open artery. They are often yellow-white in colour (Fig. 5.4). They are frequently irregular and are seen close to the bifurcations or branches of arteries. Atheroma may become complicated in that ulceration, haemorrhage, or overlying thrombosis and calcification may

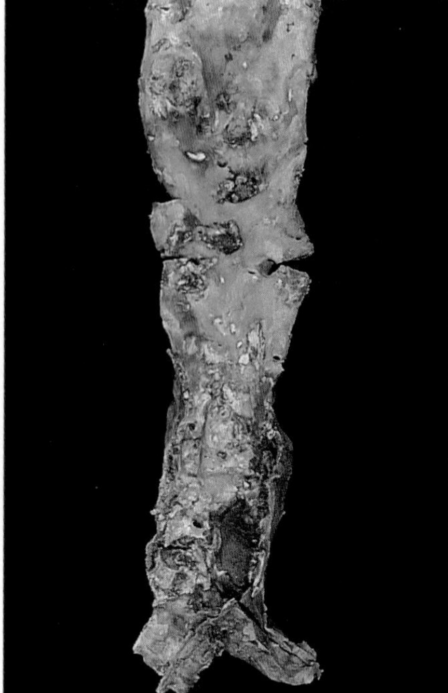

Fig. 5.4 Severe atheroma of the abdominal aorta.

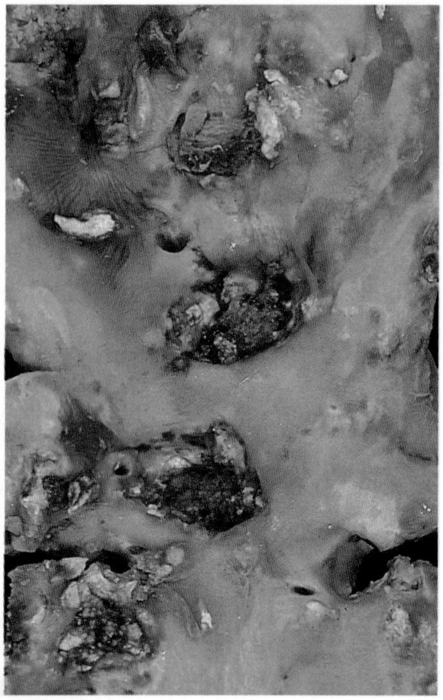

Fig. 5.5 Atheroma showing associated thrombus and occlusion of branches.

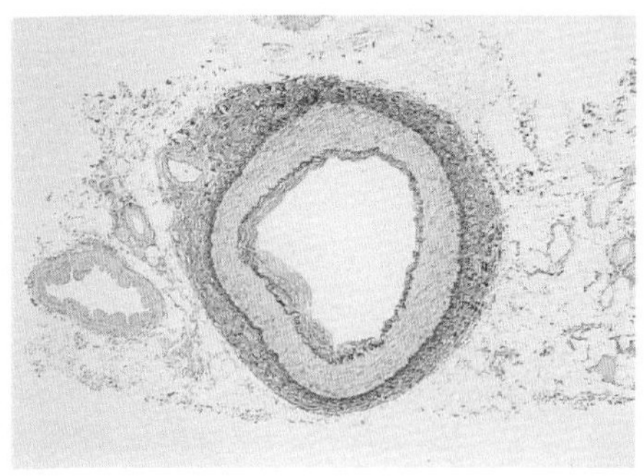

Fig. 5.6 Mild fibroelastic intimal hyperplasia in an artery.

occur (Fig. 5.5). The affected artery is thickened and nodular. Microscopically, a fatty streak consists of a small collection of macrophages, filled with lipid which lie beneath the endothelium in the intima. Early atherosclerosis shows only mild fibroelastic hyperplasia (Fig. 5.6). Established atherosclerosis consists of marked hyperplasia of intimal smooth muscle cells and fibroblasts. In fibrous plaques there is a marked increase in intimal elastic and collagen. In severe atheroma there is underlying fibrosis and atrophy of the underlying media. In the case of a muscular artery there is fibrosis and loss of smooth muscle and in the case of an elastic artery there is degeneration and breaking up of the elastic fibres of the vessel. In the softer type of plaques in association with the increased elastin and collagen there are extensive deposits of cholesterol and other lipids (Figs 5.7 and 5.8). Many of the fat deposits lie within macrophages. There is frequently a lymphocytic inflammatory response in the outer parts of the affected artery. Atheromatous plaques are frequently covered with endothelium, but ulceration is frequent and platelets are frequently adhered to the exposed subendothelial connective tissue. Calcification may be seen either within the intimal plaque itself or in the adjacent media. In complicated atheroma there may be splitting of the atheromatous plaque with haemorrhage into its substance and associated surface thrombosis. A summary of the features of an atheromatous plaque is shown in Fig. 5.9.

The cause of atherosclerosis

The occurrence of atherosclerosis in places with arterial pressure, and the sites of atherosclerosis suggests that the process relates to a response to shear stress and trauma. Established atherosclerosis with fatty deposits does not occur in veins which are subject to a much lower intraluminal pressure. Veins are, however, prone to fibrous intimal hyperplasia which may relate to episodes of previous thrombosis. Lipids appear very important in the cause of atheroma in that hypercholesterolaemia is a major risk factor for the disease. Elevated levels of lipoproteins are strongly

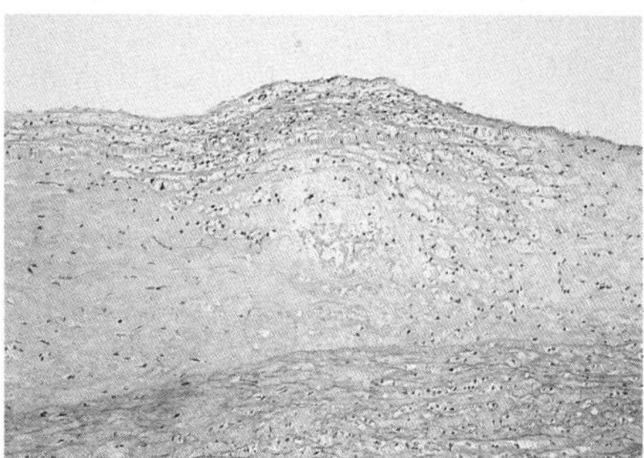

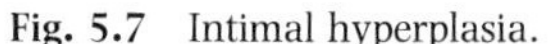

Fig. 5.7 Intimal hyperplasia.

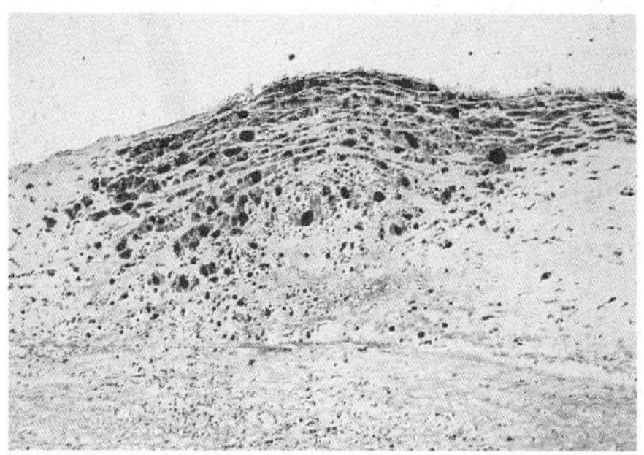

Fig. 5.8 Stains of Fig. 5.7 show lipid deposits (red).

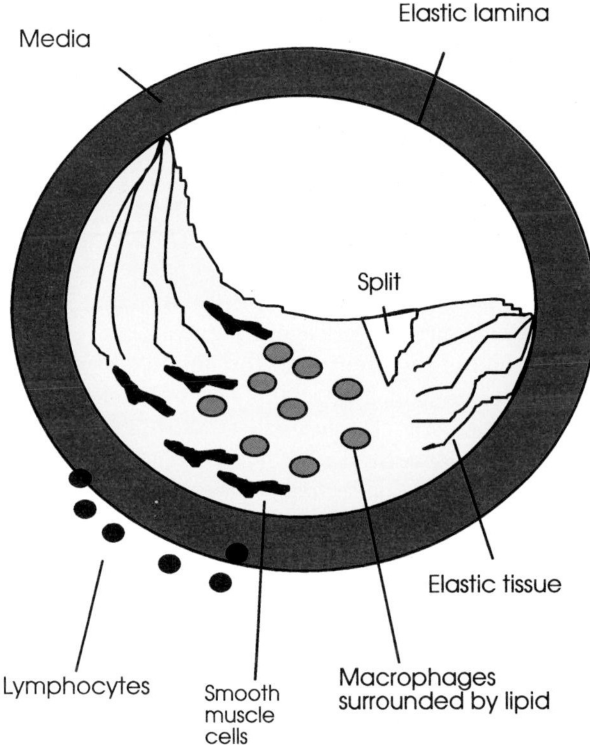

Fig. 5.9 Summary of the features of an atheromatous plaque.

associated with the development of atherosclerosis. In familial hypercholesterolaemia there is an abnormality of the low-density lipoprotein receptors. Low-density lipoprotein (LDL) is very important in the transport of cholesterol from the cells of the body to the liver (Fig. 5.10). With an abnormality of the LDL receptor there is loss of the normal negative feedback inhibition of cholesterol production by the liver. There is then an abnormally high production of cholesterol by the liver with a subsequent increase in the circulating plasma cholesterol levels.

As well as the deposition of cholesterol in the intima, endothelial damage is very important in the development of the intimal hyperplasia seen in atherosclerosis. In particular hypertension, possibly by direct stress, and cigarette smoking mediated by toxic agents is seen associated with endothelial damage. Diabetes, being a very important risk factor for atherosclerosis, may be contributing to the development of atherosclerosis due to the hypercholesterolaemia frequently present in association with this disorder.

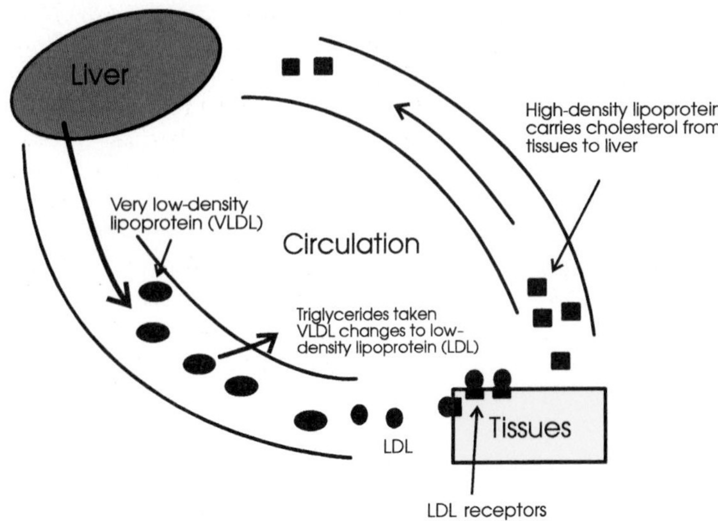

Fig. 5.10 Lipoprotein metabolism.

It has been shown that damaged endothelium, together with platelets adhering to the subendothelial connective tissue, release growth factors such as platelet-derived growth factor (PDGF). This growth factor causes proliferation of intimal smooth muscle cells and fibroblasts. There also appears to be a population of cells within the intima which share both smooth muscle and fibroblast characteristics. These cells migrate from the media of the artery into the intima and produce collagen and elastin. This results in frequent fibrosis and elastic tissue and elastic lamina reduplication seen in atherosclerosis. Intimal smooth muscle cells themselves are capable of producing platelet-derived growth factor. Smooth muscle cells also carry a receptor for PDGF. Activated macrophages are also relevant in the development of an atheromatous plaque in that they can produce PDGF and fibroblast growth factor (FGF). Other cytokines, such as tumour necrosis factor (TNF), are important in the development of atherosclerosis.

In essence, the development of atherosclerosis appears to be a response to injury.

ISCHAEMIC HEART DISEASE

Heart muscle is physiologically very similar to skeletal muscle. However, cardiac muscle has very little ability for anaerobic respiration and it has virtually no endogenous stores of energy in the form of glycogen. Although myocardium is capable of metabolizing a wide range of energy sources, it has a tendency to derive energy from free fatty acids. Cardiac muscle is therefore extremely aerobic, deriving high-energy phosphates by oxidation by metabolites in the mitochondria. Ischaemia, which is a compromised supply of blood, may occur due to increased demand by the myocardium or a reduction in blood flow due to occlusion of the coronary arteries. The most common cause for occlusive coronary artery disease is atherosclerosis.

The common complications of ischaemic heart disease are cardiac failure, infarction, angina, which may be either stable or unstable, and sudden death. Ischaemic heart disease is one of the most important causes of death in the Western world. The risk factors for ischaemic heart disease reflect the risk factors for atherosclerosis in that there is an increased incidence of hypercholesterolaemia, raised blood pressure, smoking, diabetes, and raised levels of the blood-clotting factors VII and VIII, and fibrinogen.

The myocardium cannot survive more than 40 minutes with an absent blood flow. If the cessation of blood flow continues any longer than this permanent and irreversible damage to the myocardium occurs, namely infarction. Myocardial function stops in the area of infarction and there is irreversible cell damage with death of the myocardium. Within six to eight hours, on microscopy there is visible necrosis of myofibres. It takes, however, approximately 24 hours before changes can be seen with the naked eye in the affected part of the myocardium. The earliest change is congestion and haemorrhage in the affected myocardium (Fig. 5.11). Within 3–4 days, there is migration of acute inflammatory cells into the area of infarction and part of the myocardium appears greenish or yellow in colour. Within 8–10 days, the affected myocardium becomes soft and weakened. The infarct then organizes and within 6–8 weeks there is laying down of collagen by fibroblasts. The hallmark of an old infarct is fibrosis.

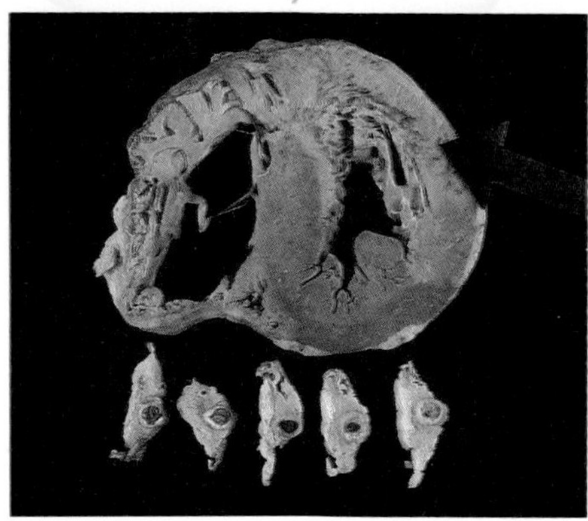

Fig. 5.11 An acute myocardial infarct (arrowed). The occluded coronary artery is dissected out below. This is occluded by thrombus.

The coronary arteries show a distinct regional supply to the myocardium and occlusion of any branches of coronary arteries tends to involve limited areas of myocardium only. In the normal coronary system there is very little in the way of collateral circulation. Infarcts may either involve the whole thickness of the myocardium or just part of the thickness, in particular just the area of the muscle beneath the endocardium, which lines the cavity of the ventricles (the subendocardium). Infarcts in the vast majority of cases involve the left ventricle of the heart; right-sided infarcts are extremely rare.

Complications of myocardial infarction are: sudden death (25 per cent); arrhythmias (75 per cent; the main reason for coronary care units); mural thrombus development on the endocardium (30 per cent); rupture of the myocardium (tends to occur on the 10th day when the infarct is at its weakest); cardiogenic shock; pericarditis; and left ventricular heart failure. Sudden death occurs in about 25 per cent of cases of myocardial infarction (Table 5.4).

Table 5.4 Complications of myocardial infarction

Sudden death
Arrhythmias
Mural thrombus with embolism
Pericarditis
Left ventricular failure
Congestive cardiac failure
Rupture of ventricle
Mitral incompetence due to papillary muscle rupture
Conduction defects
Ventricular aneurysm (either functional or caused by dilatation of a scar)

There is a wide variation in the distribution of occlusive disease of the coronary arteries due to atherosclerosis. The lesions tend to be near the begining of the vessel in the left side of the coronary circulation, and in the smaller distal region of the right coronary. A third of patients have disease of just one coronary artery, whilst 40 per cent of cases have disease of all three main coronary arteries.

The reason why a diseased coronary artery should suddenly thrombose is not clear, but factors such as fissuring, inflammation, and ulceration of the atheromatous plaque appear important. There is evidence that spasm of the coronary arteries may cause temporary occlusion.

ESSENTIAL HYPERTENSION

This is defined as an abnormally high blood pressure, and is usually said to be present when the systolic blood pressure is greater than 140–160 mmHg. It is also defined as an increased diastolic blood pressure of greater than 95 mmHg. Essential hypertension is defined as increased blood pressure of unknown cause. Hypertension may be secondary to renal disease such as renal artery stenosis or some tumours (Table 5.5). A continued raised blood pressure causes hypertrophy of the left ventricle and causes sclerosis of small arterioles in the kidney (arteriolosclerosis). Hypertensive patients also have a high risk of cerebral haemorrhage manifesting as a so-called stroke. Essential hypertension is frequently seen in patients in the fourth to fifth decade.

The most striking feature in the heart is hypertrophy of the left ventricle, up to twice its normal thickness of 1.5 centimetres in some cases. The kidneys in severe arteriolosclerosis show atrophy and marked granularity of the surface of the kidney beneath the capsule.

Table 5.5 Hypertension (raised blood pressure)

Primary (essential) 95% of cases (cause unknown)
Secondary (cause known)
Kidney disease
Renal artery occlusion or stenosis
Any chronic renal disease, including glomerulonephritis and pyelonephritis
Endocrine (hormonal)
Raised aldosterone (Conn's syndrome)
Raised corticosteroids (Cushing's syndrome)
Phaeochromocytoma (raised catecholamines)
Raised growth hormone (acromegaly)
Thyrotoxicosis
Aortic coarctation
Polyarteritis nodosa
Others
Neurogenic
Pregnancy pre-eclampsia

RHEUMATIC HEART DISEASE

Rheumatic heart disease develops as a consequence of a previous episode of rheumatic fever.

Rheumatic fever

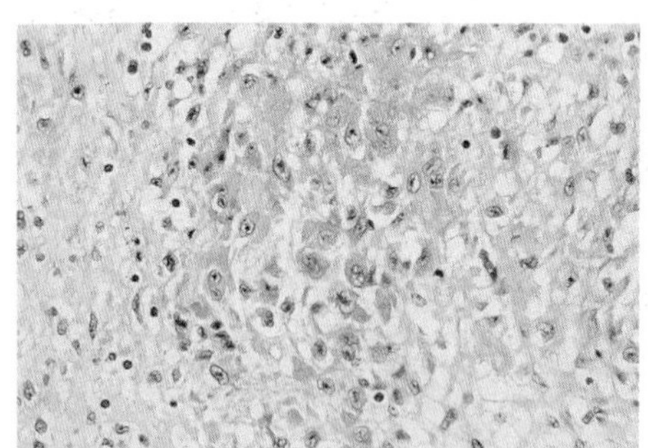

Fig. 5.12 Aschoff nodule consisting of a granulomatous response to immune complexes.

This is primarily a disease in children, usually below the age of six years of age, and due to an immunological response to a streptococcal infection. The infection is usually a group A beta-haemolytic streptococcal infection. The usual history is of a child presenting with a sore throat. One to two weeks later features of rheumatic fever develop. These are fever, skin rash, carditis, joint pains, and chorea (involuntary movements).

The disease is due to antibodies formed against the streptococcal infection that cross-react with the patient's own tissue antigens. Immune complexes are deposited at the sites of the cross-reaction. Granulomas (Aschoff nodules) may be seen (Fig. 5.12). These immune complexes are seen in the myocardium, heart valves, joints, and certain areas of the brain including the basal ganglia. The endocarditis that develops causes deposits of fibrin on valves, particularly on the left side of the heart. The disease then regresses and the patient recovers. However, there has been damage to the heart valves which then presents many decades later as rheumatic heart disease.

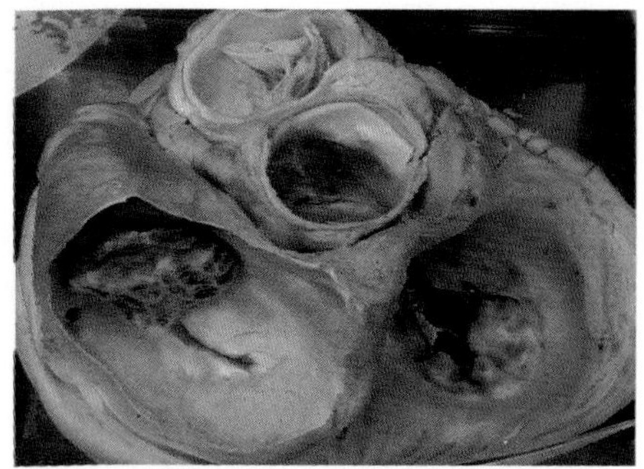

Fig. 5.13 The mitral valve of the heart (below left) showing marked fibrosis and narrowing of the opening (mitral stenosis). There is thrombus in the atrium.

Rheumatic heart disease is therefore a later complication of rheumatic fever. It affects the mitral and aortic valves. The hallmark of rheumatic fever in the mitral valve is mitral stenosis (Fig. 5.13). Aortic disease may also occur. The heart valves show marked fibrosis, remodelling of their architecture, and vascularization with chronic inflammation. Rheumatic heart disease greatly increases the risk of infective endocarditis.

RIGHT-SIDED HEART FAILURE

In severe and persistent left heart failure, extra load is put on the right ventricle and right heart failure may result. This results in increased pressure in systemic veins, with oedema in the tissues of dependent areas of the body such as the ankles. This is called *congestive* cardiac failure.

Extra load may be put on the right ventricle in the case of increased pressure in the pulmonary artery (pulmonary hypertension). This may be due to pulmonary vascular constriction with increased resistance to blood flow through the lung. This is often secondary to hypoxic lung disease such as chronic bronchitis. If right heart failure is due to lung disease, the term *cor pulmonale* is applied. Pulmomary hypertension may also be due to congenital heart disease (atrial or ventricular septal defects, patent ductus arteriosus) where blood can pass from the left side of the heart to the right, with increased blood flow through the lungs. Multiple small pulmonary emboli may obstruct the arterial circulation of the lungs.

The normal thickness of the right ventricle is only 0.4–0.5 centimetres, and right ventricular hypertrophy is the main feature seen in pulmonary hypertension. Another feature seen in pulmonary hypertension is the development of atherosclerosis within the pulmonary artery (Fig. 5.14).

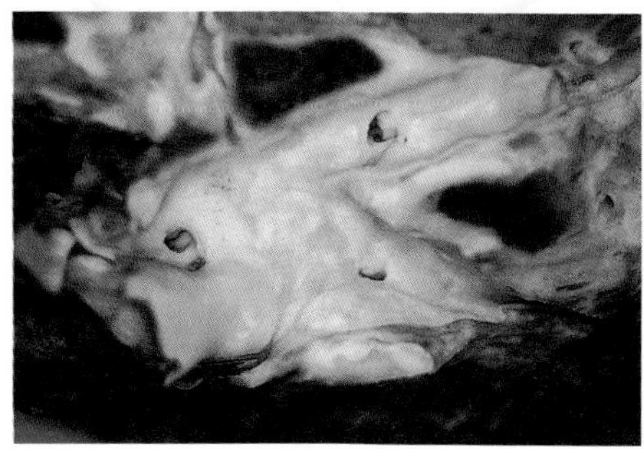

Fig. 5.14 Atheroma in the pulmonary artery in pulmonary hypertension.

DISEASES OF CARDIAC VALVES

Most valve pathology is seen on the left side of the heart in view of the high pressures seen at that side.

Aortic stenosis

This may be due to rheumatic heart disease or calcification. The latter is termed senile calcific sclerosis and is frequently seen in elderly females (Fig. 5.15). Aortic stenosis is a well-recognized cause of sudden death. Aortic stenosis may also occur with congenitally abnormal bicuspid valve.

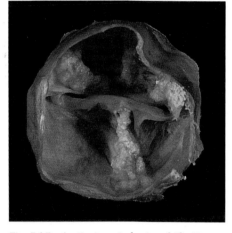

Fig. 5.15 Aortic stenosis due to calcification. The cusps are fused.

Aortic regurgitation

This may be due to rheumatic heart disease, with distortion of the valve cusps. It may also be due to widening of the aorta at the level of the aortic valve. It is commonly seen in syphilis or Marfan's syndrome. Infective endocarditis also can cause cusp damage and regurgitation.

Mitral stenosis

The most common cause of mitral stenosis is rheumatic heart disease, as described above.

Mitral regurgitation

Lesions intrinsic to the valve

This may follow rheumatic heart disease, infective endocarditis, or mucinous degeneration (particularly of the posterior cusp). Mucinous (myxoid) degeneration may occur in association with Marfan's syndrome or in isolation.

Lesions extrinsic to the valve

Increased diameter of the valve due to heart failure or ischaemic heart disease may cause valve leakage. Fibrosis or rupture due to infarction of a papillary muscle supporting the valve chordae tendinae may also cause valve incompetence.

INFECTIVE ENDOCARDITIS

Table 5.6 Sources of infective carditis

Dental surgery, including extractions
Infected intravenous fluids (drug addicts)
Cardiac surgery
Instrumentation, particularly of gastrointestinal and urinary tract
Skin infection
Chronic sepsis in extracardiac site

Table 5.7 Causes of infective endocarditis

Streptococcus viridans
Streptococcus bovis
Streptococcus faecalis
Staphylococcus aureus
Streptococcus pneumoniae
Gram-negative bacilli (*E. coli*)
Candida
Aspergillus
Other fungi
Rickettsiae (Q fever due to *Coxiella burnetti*)
Chlamydia

Infective endocarditis occurs when microorganisms colonize the endocardium within the heart. There are about 1500 cases a year in the United Kingdom, and before antibiotics the condition was uniformly fatal. It still has about a 30 per cent mortality. Endocarditis usually occurs in association with an abnormal heart valve on the left side of the heart. Artificial valves are also at risk of infection. The normal source of infection is the bloodstream, and a period of bacteraemia is therefore necessary before colonization of the heart valves by the infective organism can occur. Some organisms, such as *Staphylococcus aureus*, are capable of infecting normal valves, in view of the high virulence of this organism. This organism is well known to cause serious destructive acute endocarditis, and is associated with intravenous drug abuse. It is more common, however, for endocarditis to develop on previously abnormal valves. Valves may either be congenitally abnormal or have acquired abnormalities such as in rheumatic heart disease. The organisms that cause this form of endocarditis tend to be of low virulence and act as opportunistic organisms. Infective endocarditis is particularly relevant to dentists in view of the frequency of bacteraemia which is induced by dental manipulation or surgery, particularly extraction and scaling (Table 5.6). Many of the organisms that cause infective endocarditis are normally resident in the mouth, such as *Streptococci viridans*, *oralis*, *mitis*, and *sanguis*. This is why antibiotic cover of dental procedures is so important, particularly in patients with abnormal heart valves. However, it must be stated that dental procedures are a relatively uncommon cause of infective endocarditis, and dentists are blamed too frequently for causing this condition! In one study, only 15 per cent of cases could be related to a dental procedure within three months of the development of the endocarditis. Pre-existing dental sepsis could be found in 30 per cent of cases, although 16 per cent of cases were edentulous, and 20 per cent of cases had healthy teeth. Other portals of entry of bacteria are urological procedures such as prostate resection, gastrointestinal procedures, intravenous cannulae, and wound infection.

It has a very variable clinical presentation, making diagnosis very difficult. It may present as fever, heart failure, chest pain, or embolic phenomena such as paralysis, sudden blindness, or limb ischaemia. New heart murmurs may appear. Complications relate to valve destruction, spread of infection into the tissue surrounding the valve, and emboli from the fibrinous vegetations. The prognosis strongly relates to the causative organisms; *Staphylococcus aureus*, and fungal infections are associated with a poor prognosis. A list is given of the common microorganisms that cause infective endocarditis in Table 5.7.

The characteristic naked-eye appearance of endocarditis is that of vegetations which develop on the surfaces of the cusps of the valve. Vegetations consist mainly of thrombus, in association with colonies of bacteria and acute inflammatory cells (Fig. 5.16). There is frequently destruction of the underlying cusp architecture and this is the main reason for the failure of valves in infective endocarditis. Infective endocarditis usually causes valve regurgitation (Fig. 5.17). This can cause cardiac failure. Other complications of infective endocarditis are immune complex disease which can affect the kidneys. Also, there may be embolism of fragments of the vegetations to other organs such as the spleen, kidney, and brain. Complications may also result from treatment, including antibiotic sensitivity or penicillin allergy. Antibiotics are used as the main treatment after blood has been taken for culture. Penicillin and gentamicin are frequently used to cover most organisms; if *Staphylococcus aureus* is suspected then flucloxacillin is used. Clindamycin may be used in penicillin-sensitive patients. Surgical valve repair or replacement is performed if there is high risk of embolism, complications such as severe valve dysfunction, or poor response to medical treatment.

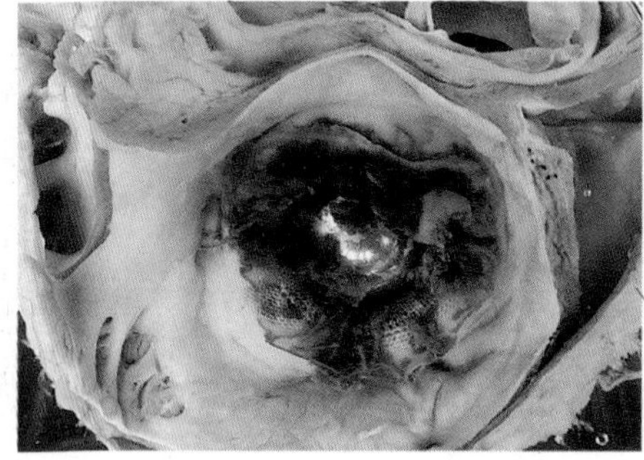

Fig. 5.16 Infective endocarditis on an artificial heart valve.

Preventative measures include reducing foci of infection by good dental hygiene, local antisepsis during dental treatment, and antibiotic cover during a surgical procedure. Amoxycillin, 3 g, 1 hour before the treatment is frequently used (600 mg clindamycin if there is penicillin sensitivity). If *Streptococcus faecalis* is suspected, then gentamicin may be added. Vancomycin can also be used if there are other risk factors.

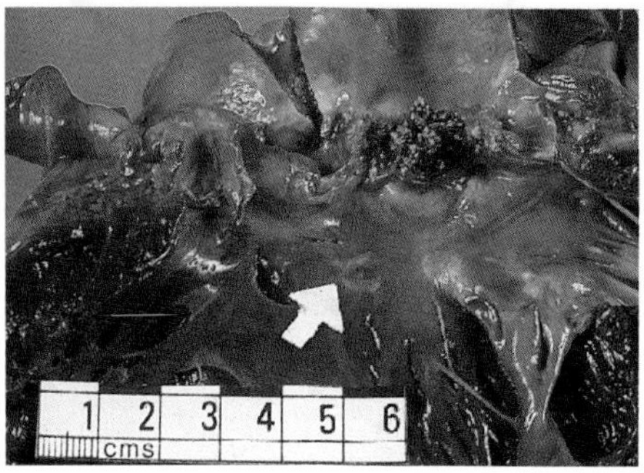

Fig. 5.17 Infective endocarditis on the aortic valve. There are large vegetations. A regurgitant 'jet' lesion consisting of fibrosis is arrowed.

MYOCARDITIS

Myocarditis is important in that it is a well-recognized cause of unexpected cardiac failure and death. Sudden death may in fact be a presenting feature of myocarditis. Myocarditis is most commonly of viral origin.

CARDIOMYOPATHY

The term cardiomyopathy really defines a disease process that affects the myocardium. It presents as a functional disorder of the heart muscle which generally causes heart failure. Cardiomyopathies are generally divided into three types: these are the dilated cardiomyopathies, the non-dilated cardiomyopathies, and restrictive cardiomyopathies.

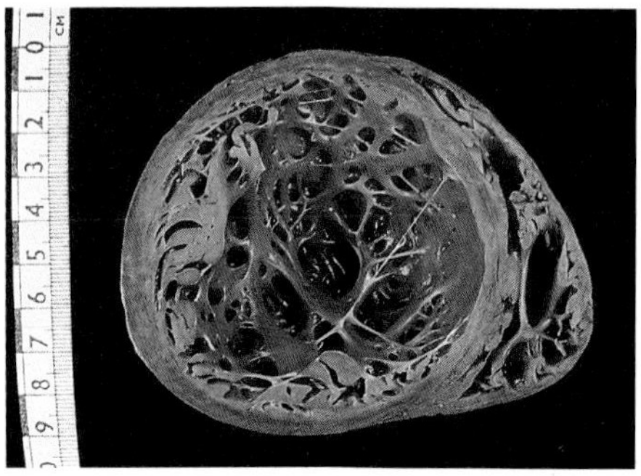

Fig. 5.18 A large dilated left ventricle due to ischaemic heart disease.

Dilated cardiomyopathy

This presents as cardiac failure. Pathologically there is marked dilatation of the ventricles with poor ventricular function. There is a wide range of causes. Ischaemic heart disease is the most common cause of dilated cardiomyopathy (Fig. 5.18). The next most common cause is probably a postviral myocarditis which goes on to cause a cardiomyopathy. There are many metabolic causes including excess alcohol intake and drug toxicity.

Non-dilated cardiomyopathy

The most important non-dilated cardiomyopathy is called hypertrophic cardiomyopathy. This is usually of familial type and presents as cardiac enlargement with no other apparent cause (Fig. 5.19). It is now known to be due to an abnormality in the genes for the myosin proteins of the myocardium. The usual clinical story is of a young person who presents with arrhythmias or sudden death who shows striking cardiac enlargement, particularly of the left ventricle and septum. There may also be obstruction of the aortic valve. Physiologically, there is a marked increase in sensitivity of the myocardium to sympathetic stimulation, in particular catecholamines.

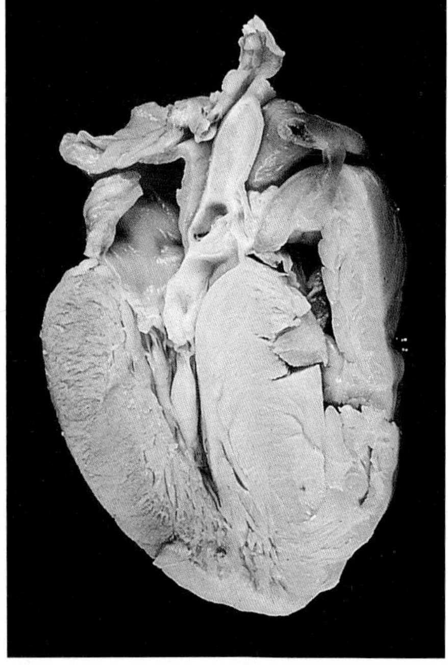

Fig. 5.19 Hypertrophic cardiomyopathy showing a marked thickening of the left ventricle.

Restrictive cardiomyopathies

This is when there is increased resistance to filling of the heart. One common type is due to cardiac amyloidosis in the elderly.

VASCULITIS

Inflammation of blood vessels, normally small arteries and capillaries, may occur, usually in association with immunologically mediated diseases such as autoimmune

Table 5.8 Classification of vasculitis

Associated with other disease or autoimmunity
Hypersensitivity (capillary) vasculitis
Henoch–Schönlein purpura
Drug-associated vasculitis
Associated with collagen vascular disease (systemic lupus erythematosus, rheumatoid arthritis)
Kawasaki's disease
Systemic
Polyarteritis nodosa
Wegener's granulomatosis
Takayasu's disease
Buerger's disease
Granulomatous (sarcoid, Crohn's disease)
Giant cell arteritis
Infection
Fungi
Rickettsiae
Hepatitis B
Infective endocarditis
Syphilis
Tuberculosis
Pseudomonas

disease. Inflammation may also be caused by injury due to infection, toxic agents, radiation, and physical trauma. There is associated damage to the vessel wall with occasional thrombosis. Causes are summarized in Table 5.8.

Hypersensitivity vasculitis may be caused by drugs such as antibiotics, and bacteria such as group B-haemolytic streptococci. The skin is a frequent site of involvement. Kawasaki's disease occurs in children and is also called the mucocutaneous syndrome. It may show the serious complication of coronary artery involvement. Polyarteritis nodosa (PAN) involves medium-sized arteries of the kidneys, heart, liver, and gastrointestinal tract. It may also involve the brain, muscle, and skin. There is an association with hepatitis B virus infection in up to 45 per cent of cases. The vasculitis leads to ischaemia in involved organs. Wegener's granulomatosis involves the upper respiratory tract, including the nose and nasal septum, the kidneys, brain, and skin. It occurs mainly in males, 40–50 years in age. Affected organs show vasculitis, necrosis, acute inflammation, and giant cells. Despite the name, granulomas are not prominent. It has a very poor outlook if untreated; the majority of patients respond to cyclophosphamide. Takayasu's arteritis involves large branches of the aorta in females from South-East Asia, causing obstruction to upper limb vessels in particular. Buerger's disease (thromboangitis obliterans) is a disease of male heavy cigarette smokers which causes obliteration of small arteries of the limbs. Amputation may be required if gangrene occurs. Giant cell arteritis, otherwise known as cranial arteritis, is a condition of the elderly which involves arteries of the head and neck. The most serious complication is when the ophthalmic arteries are involved, giving a high risk of blindness. The cause is unknown; up to 50 per cent of cases are associated with a connective tissue disorder called polymyalgia rheumatica. A vasculitis with giant cells destroying elastic tissue is seen. Biopsy of a temporal artery, which is easily accessible, will frequently confirm the diagnosis. Treatment is with corticosteroids.

AORTIC DISSECTION

This is the development of a split that originates in an aortic intimal tear and tracks down the aortic media (Fig. 5.20), frequently rupturing through the full thicknes of the wall. It occurs in association with hypertension and Marfan's syndrome, the latter associated with mucinous degeneration of the aorta.

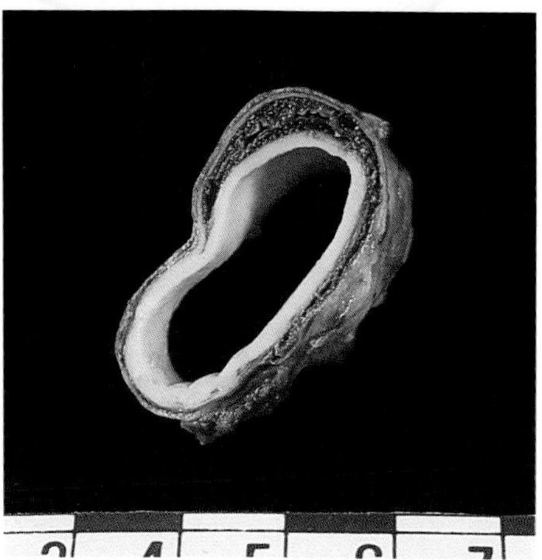

Fig. 5.20 A transverse section of an aortic dissection showing a split within the wall.

SUMMARY

Shock is reduced perfusion of tissues by the circulation. Types of shock are:

–hypovolaemic
–cardiogenic
–bacteraemic (septic)

Arteriosclerosis: the most important condition in this group is *atherosclerosis*. In summary, this is a proliferative condition that involves the intimal layer of arteries. The underlying cause appears to be endothelial injury. There is proliferation of smooth muscle cells within the intima with the production of collagen and elastin.

Risk factors for atherosclerosis are familial hyperlipidaemia, being male, hypertension, diabetes, smoking, and lesser factors such as diet, obesity, and lack of exercise. Complications of atherosclerosis include occlusion, thrombosis, and aneurysm development. Organs most affected by atherosclerosis are the heart, brain, and the extremities, particularly the lower limb. The abdominal aorta is most prone to aneurysm development.

Ischaemic heart disease: coronary arteries are particularly prone to atherosclerotic occlusion and thrombosis. Complications of ischaemic heart disease are cardiac failure, infarction, angina, and sudden death. Complications of infarction include arrhythmias (sometimes fatal), thrombosis, rupture, shock, and left heart failure.

Hypertension: this is defined as an abnormally increased blood pressure: the diastolic pressure is usually taken to be above 90 mmHg, a sustained systolic pressure above 149 mmHg. Almost all cases of hypertension, however, are of unknown cause (essential hypertension). The majority of causes of secondary hypertension are related to disease of the kidney. Endocrine causes are also a well-recognized cause of secondary hypertension. Complications of hypertension include hypertensive heart disease, and hypertensive renal disease characterized by nephrosclerosis.

Rheumatic heart disease: this is a consequence of rheumatic fever occurring many years earlier in childhood. Rheumatic fever is a post-streptococcal syndrome, characterized by fever, skin rash, carditis, joint pains, and chorea. There is, in a proportion of cases of rheumatic fever, long-lasting damage to the heart valves, which is progressive, and presents in later life with post-inflammatory scarring of the mitral and aortic valves. Typically, mitral stenosis occurs.

Other diseases of cardiac valves

Mitral regurgitation
–rheumatic heart disease
–infective endocarditis

–mucinous degeneration
–rupture of papillary muscle
–dilatation of valve ring

Aortic stenosis
–rheumatic heart disease
–calcification (senile or secondary to bicuspid aortic valve)

Aortic regurgitation
–rheumatic heart disease
–widening of aorta (syphilis or Marfan's syndrome)
–infective endocarditis

Infective endocarditis
Colonization of a heart valve with microorganisms. Usually occurs on the left side of the heart. It is almost always associated with bacteraemia with colonization of the heart valves by infective organisms. A common source of bacteraemia is the mouth, secondary to dental manipulation. A common cusative organism is *Streptococcus viridans*. However, there is a wide range of other organisms which cause infective endocarditis.

Cardiomyopathy
This defines a disease which intrinsically affects the myocardium. Cardiomyopathies are:

–dilated
–non-dilated (hypertrophic)
–restrictive

6 The respiratory tract

6 The respiratory tract

OVERALL respiratory disease is an important cause of illness and death in the population. In the first year of life up to 25 per cent of deaths are due to respiratory pathology, and in people over 75, respiratory disease accounts for a substantial cause of death. Almost 1 in 10 men who die in the United Kingdom die of lung cancer and although the rate in females is lower this is rapidly catching up.

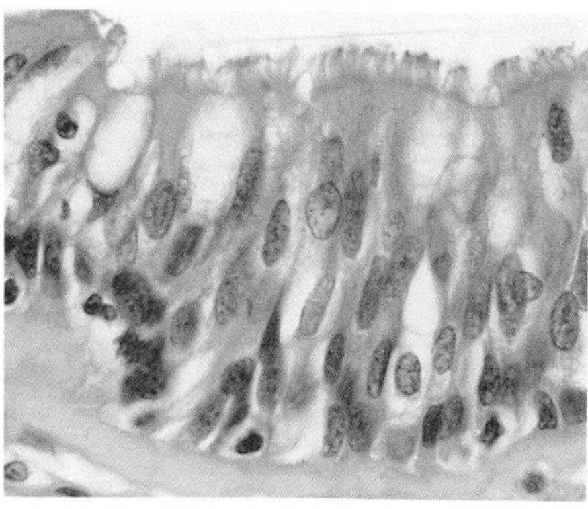
Fig. 6.1 Pseudo-columnar ciliated respiratory epithelium. Cilia are seen at the top.

The respiratory system can be divided into the upper and lower respiratory tracts. The upper respiratory tract consists of the nose, nasopharynx, and larynx. The lower respiratory tract consists of the trachea, bronchi, and bronchioles, and lung tissue distant to that including alveolar ducts and alveoli. The respiratory airways from the nasopharynx to the distant bronchioles are lined by pseudo-stratified columnar ciliated epithelium (Fig. 6.1). Alveoli are lined by predominantly a thin type 1 epithelium. There are occasional type 2 cells which are responsible for surfactant production, and also provide a reserve population of cells. The bronchi and bronchioles divide in a tree-like fractal pattern which provides the most efficient way of division and provide the maximum surface area for respiratory gas exchange within the limited space of the chest. Gas exchange only occurs in airways distal to terminal bronchioles, where alveoli start to form.

UPPER RESPIRATORY TRACT

Infections

The nasopharynx is susceptible to many virus infections, particularly those causing the common cold, which tend to be rhinoviruses. More specific virus infections include respiratory syncytial virus, parainfluenza viruses, and bacteria including *Haemophilus influenzae*. An increasing problem is inflammation of the upper respiratory tract due to allergies, for example to pollen in the case of hay fever (type I hypersensitivity) (see p. 000).

Inflammation

A manifestation of chronic inflammation which is commonly due to allergy is the development of nasal polyps (Fig. 6.2). These consist of large masses of oedematous mucosa which show an inflammatory infiltrate of lymphocytes and eosinophils, the latter indicative of type 1 hypersensitivity. Plasma cells are also seen. The paranasal sinuses may be similarly involved with the development of sinusitis. This is due to impaired drainage of the sinuses in most cases, but may also be due to direct spread from infective foci in adjacent tissues, particularly the teeth. The maxillary sinus is particularly prone to this phenomenon in view of the close proximity of the maxillary molar teeth, the roots of which project into the sinus. A rare complication of acute sinusitis is local spread upwards into the cranial cavity with the development of meningitis.

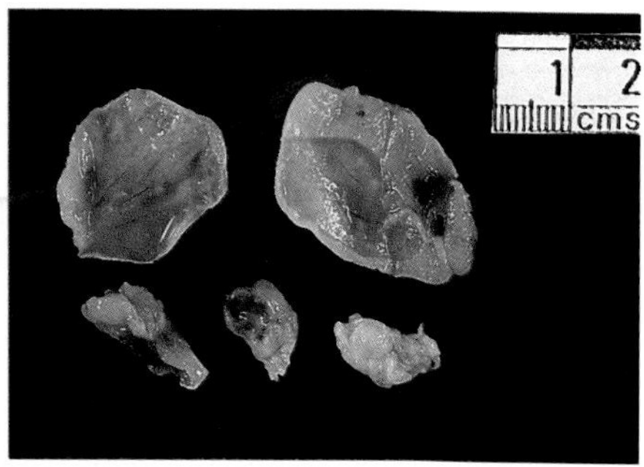

Fig. 6.2 Nasal polyps consisting of oedematous nasal mucosa.

Neoplasms

Common benign tumours of the nasopharynx include haemangioma, papillomas, and the rare juvenile angiofibroma. The angiofibroma is an entity which occurs within the distinct clinical situation of young males with a highly vascular tumour occurring in the upper lateral part of the nasopharynx. This tumour appears to be hormonally sensitive, responding to growth stimulation by androgens. Important malignant tumours of the nasopharynx are squamous cell carcinomas, and adenocarcinomas, the latter in many cases rising from salivary glands. Nasopharyngeal carcinoma, which represents a poorly differentiated form of squamous cell carcinoma, is often associated with a heavy lymphocytic inflammatory infiltrate (it is also known as a 'lymphoepithelioma'). Nasopharyngeal carcinoma is relatively common in the Chinese and South East Asians. It is related to infection with the Epstein–Barr virus.

The term 'lethal midline granuloma' is sometimes used for a destructive process that involves the nasal septum and face. It is a term which is best avoided as it includes a number of diseases. Many cases turn out to be T cell lymphomas.

LARYNX

Inflammatory pathology

Viral and bacterial infections of the larynx result in laryngitis. Laryngitis can also be due to chronic irritation to inhaled material, particularly cigarette smoke or secondary to surgical intubation. Laryngeal nodules commonly occur in cases where there is vocal abuse, particularly prolonged use of the voice in the case of singers. These lesions consist of congested and oedematous tissue covered with thickened squamous epithelium.

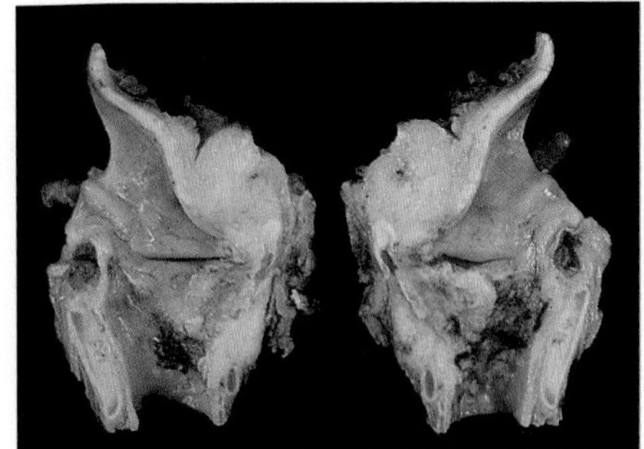

Fig. 6.3 A laryngeal carcinoma. The larynx has been opened up vertically to show an ulcerated tumour of the vocal cords.

Neoplasia

Laryngeal tumours are uncommon. An example of a benign laryngeal tumour is the viral papilloma which is associated with human papilloma virus infection. These are often multiple in children and can extend into more distal airways. The best known malignant tumour of the larynx is squamous cell carcinoma (Fig. 6.3) which is seen particularly in males over 50 years of age and is closely associated with cigarette smoking. Squamous cell carcinomas of the larynx are associated with adjacent mucosal dysplasia. Carcinoma-*in situ* appears to be the precursor lesion of invasive carcinoma.

NON-NEOPLASTIC LUNG DISEASE

The lungs have a very limited way of responding to an insult. Fibrosis tends to be the response to a wide range of insults, particularly infections or inflammatory disorders. In contrast to this, the lung shows a large diversity of tumours.

Infections

The lungs are normally sterile, a continuous escalator of mucociliary clearance providing very efficient host defence. Anything that interferes with this host defence predisposes the lung to infection.

Acute bronchitis

Most cases of acute bronchitis are viral in cause and in children are often associated with laryngitis. Viruses that are commonly implicated are the respiratory syncitial viruses and bacteria such as *Haemophilus influenzae* and *Streptococcus pneumoniae*. As will be described later, many cases of chronic bronchitis have episodes of acute bacterial infection causing acute bronchitis.

Bronchiolitis

This is generally limited to young children below 18 months of age. The respiratory syncitial virus is the most common cause of this condition. In adults, there is a condition called bronchiolitis obliterans which is either of unknown cause or associated with toxic gases, autoimmune disease such as rheumatoid arthritis, or chronic repeated infection. It is also seen in allergic lung disease and is characterized by obliteration of small airways, particularly bronchioles, by a proliferation of connective tissue.

Pneumonia

Pneumonia is defined as inflammation of the lungs and can be classified in two ways. It is commonly classified anatomically, but a more useful classification takes account of the causative organisms causing in the inflammation (Table 6.1).

Anatomical classsification: lobar pneumonia (Fig. 6.4)

This is defined as an inflammatory process which appears limited to a lobe of the lung. It is generally due to virulent organisms and tends to affect young adults. The pneumococcus (*Streptococcus pneumoniae*) is the commonest cause of this disease although *Klebsiella* is another well-recognized cause of lobar pneumonia. The clinical picture tends to be of a very acute illness and shows a tendency for rapid resolution.

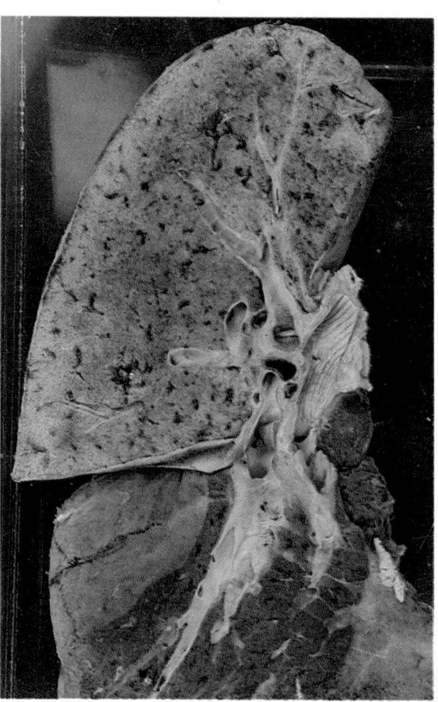

Fig. 6.4 The upper lobe of the lung (top) is white and consolidated with pneumonia. The lower lobe is normal.

Table 6.1 Causes of pneumonia

Acute pneumonia
Streptococcus pneumonia
Klebsiella pneumoniae
Haemophilus influenzae
Mycoplasma pneumoniae
Legionella pneumophila
Staphylococcus aureus
Chlamydia
Q fever
Influenza virus
Opportunistic
Gram-negative bacilli (*E. coli*, Pseudomonas)
Anaerobic infection
Aspergillus
Nocardia
Cryptococcus
Cytomegalovirus
Pneumocystis
Branhamella catarrhalis
Chronic pneumonia
Tuberculosis

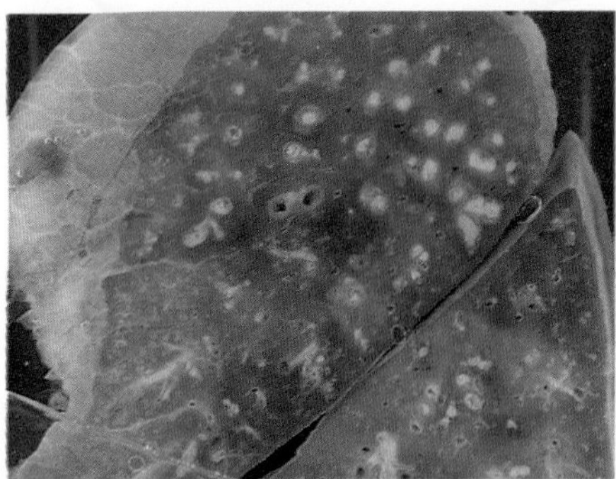
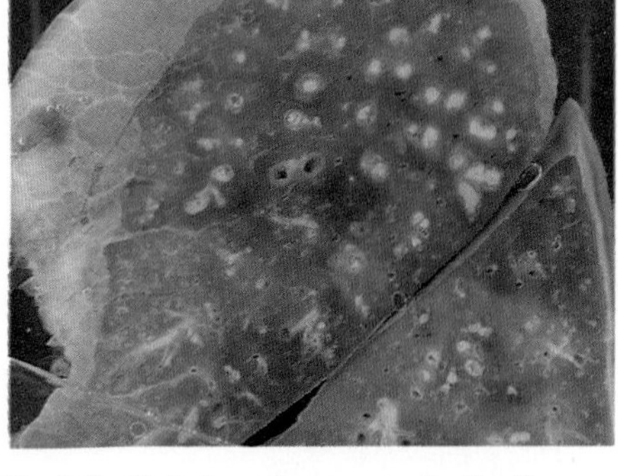

Fig. 6.5 Early bronchopneumonia. Small airways are filled with white pus.

Anatomical classification: bronchopneumonia (Fig. 6.5)

Bronchopneumonia is characterized by an inflammatory process that originates in bronchioles and tends to spread in a radial pattern into the surrounding lung parenchyma. It has a great tendency to involve basal lung segments and is primarily a disease of the elderly or in patients with immunosuppression or compromised respiratory function. The organisms causing bronchopneumonia tend to be opportunistic in the sense that they are of low virulence in normal situations and take advantage of reduced host defence. Gram-negative organisms are a common cause of bronchopneumonia. Staphylococcal pneumonia tends to form multiple abscesses.

Aspiration pneumonia

Aspiration pneumonia is particularly relevant to dentists in view of the continual hazard of inhalation of dental instruments. When a patient is in a vertical position any foreign objects that are inhaled tend to go down the right intermediate bronchus. Any such object that occludes the bronchus results in disruption of normal host defence, as described previously, and then predisposes the distal lung to infection. This may ultimately result in an abscess. Patients at high risk of aspiration are those with loss of protective reflexes to the airway, inability to cough, patients who are sedated or unconscious, and oesophageal obstruction.

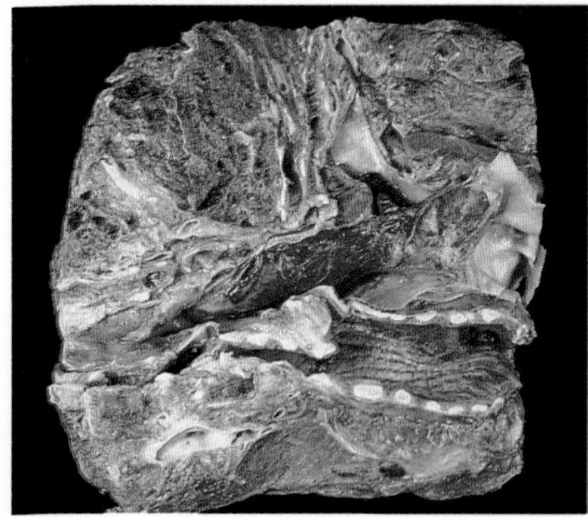

Fig. 6.6 A solid red pulmonary embolus is seen above the main bronchus in this lung.

Pulmonary embolus

Most pulmonary emboli are of thrombotic origin, arising particularly from the leg and pelvic veins. A pulmonary embolus is a common cause of sudden death. Deep vein thrombosis is usually secondary to immobilization and is extremely common in hospital patients, being seen in up to 10 per cent of admissions. A thrombus travels with the blood flow up the inferior vena cava and through the right side of the heart through the pulmonary valve and then lodges within a pulmonary arterial branch (Fig. 6.6). In view of the dual circulation of the lung, small pulmonary emboli often occur without symptoms. If there is any compromised cardiac function, however, a pulmonary infarct may result. This is seen as a well-circumscribed wedge-shaped area of lung congestion and oedema with disruption of the alveolar epithelium and extravasation of blood and plasma into alveolar spaces. An associated pleuritis occurs accounting for the typical pain frequently occurring with pulmonary embolism. A large pulmonary embolus often presents, however, with sudden death. This is due to complete occlusion of the circulation or cardiac arrythmias. Deep vein thrombosis in the leg can be prevented by anticoagulation and fibrinolytic drugs can be used to treat pulmonary embolism. Other forms of embolus include fat from bone trauma, air or tumour (see p. 000).

Pulmonary vascular disease

The most common distinct pulmonary vascular disease is pulmonary hypertension. This may be primary (of unknown cause), particularly in young females presenting with right heart failure and pleural effusions. Secondary pulmonary hypertension is commonly seen in association with hypoxia. This may be due to chronic obstructive airways disease or living at high altitude. Another cause of pulmonary hypertension of secondary type is congenital heart disease involving shunting of blood from the left to the right side of the heart. Examples include atrial or ventricular septal defects, or patent ductus arteriosis.

Pulmonary oedema

The causes of pulmonary oedema are either haemodynamic or microvascular.

Haemodynamic

In this form of oedema there is no abnormality of the lung. The primary cause of the oedema, which involves the outpouring of low-protein fluid into the alveoli spaces (transudate) is an imbalance between the forces pushing fluid into the alveolar spaces and the forces pulling fluid back into the circulation. The capillary pressure forms a force trying to push fluid into the alveolar spaces and is increased in cases of left heart failure. The forces trying to pull fluid back into the circulation are primarily due to colloid osmotic pressure of plasma proteins. Causes of left ventricular failure include myocardial infarction and ischaemic heart disease. Mitral stenosis is also a classic cause of pulmonary oedema. Conditions that result in a lowered colloid osmotic pressure of the plasma due to loss of protein include nephrotic syndrome of the kidney and protein-losing enteropathies. Haemodynamic pulmonary oedema is rapidly reversible with appropriate treatment.

Microvascular injury

This form of pulmonary oedema is also known as shock lung or adult respiratory distress syndrome. There is a wide diversity of causes (Table 6.2) which result in the production of microvascular injury in the lung. These include endotoxic shock due to predominantly Gram-negative infection, surgical shock, circulatory collapse due to, for instance, obstetric accident, and exposure to toxic gases including sulphur dioxide and continuous pure oxygen.

Other causes of microvascular injury include viruses such as influenza, drugs such as bleomycin and busulphan, and radiation. The disease presents clinically as an insidious progression of respiratory failure following the insult. There is progressive dyspnoea with respiratory failure which requires increasing amounts of inspired oxygen and high-pressure ventilation to maintain blood gases. The chest X-ray shows features of severe pulmonary oedema but there is no clinical evidence of heart failure. The primary problem seems to be an inability of the endothelium and epithelium of the lung to hold fluid out of alveoli. The pathology is characterized by an outpouring of high protein exudate into alveolar spaces together with a large number of inflammatory cells. There is an inappropriate activation of inflammatory mediators such as tumour necrosis factor. Other processes involved are neutrophil activation in the capillaries, platelet activation with endothelial damage, and epithelial damage. Radicals are also relevant, particularly those derived from oxygen (Fig. 6.7). The prognosis of the condition is very poor. The lungs become very poorly compliant due to an interruption of the normal surfactant production of the lung by type II pneumocytes.

Table 6.2 Causes of adult respiratory distress syndrome

Septic (endotoxic) shock
Trauma
Burns
Surgery, including abdominal and cardiac procedures
Pancreatitis
Viral infections
Oxygen toxicity
Inhalation of toxic agents
Fat embolism
Aspiration of gastric contents
Drugs (bleomycin, busulphan)
Radiation

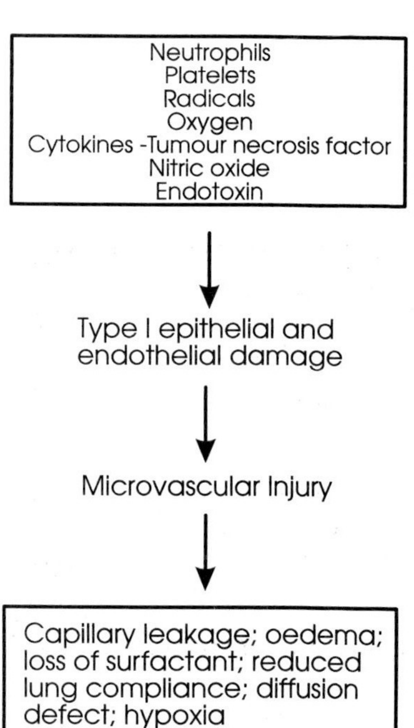

Fig. 6.7 Mechanisms causing adult respiratory distress syndrome.

Chronic obstructive airways disease

Chronic obstructive airways disease is a term that really encompasses two conditions, namely, chronic bronchitis and emphysema (Fig. 6.8). There tends to be an overlap between the two conditions in many patients.

Chronic bronchitis

Chronic bronchitis is defined clinically as an abnormal sputum production which occurs for more than three months a year for two years. The hallmark of chronic bronchitis is this excess sputum production. There appears to be a continued insult to the lung, in many cases smoking, although living in a damp or dusty climate is

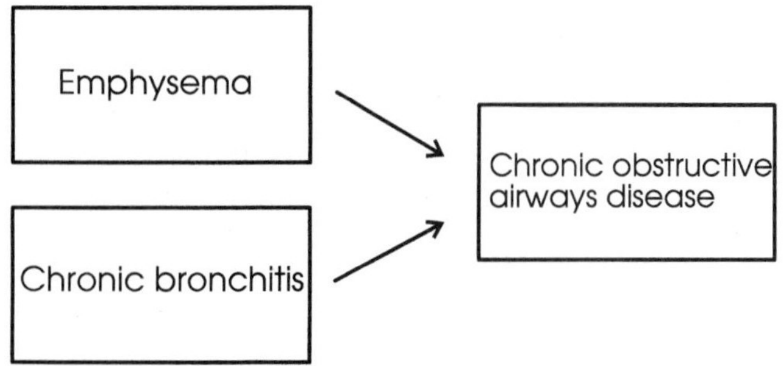

Fig. 6.8 Chronic obstructive airways disease.

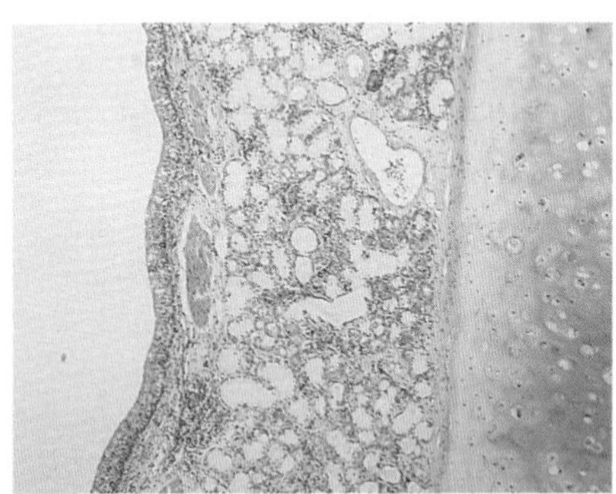

Fig. 6.9 Chronic bronchitis with marked hyperplasia of mucous glands replacing most of the tissue beneath the epithelium.

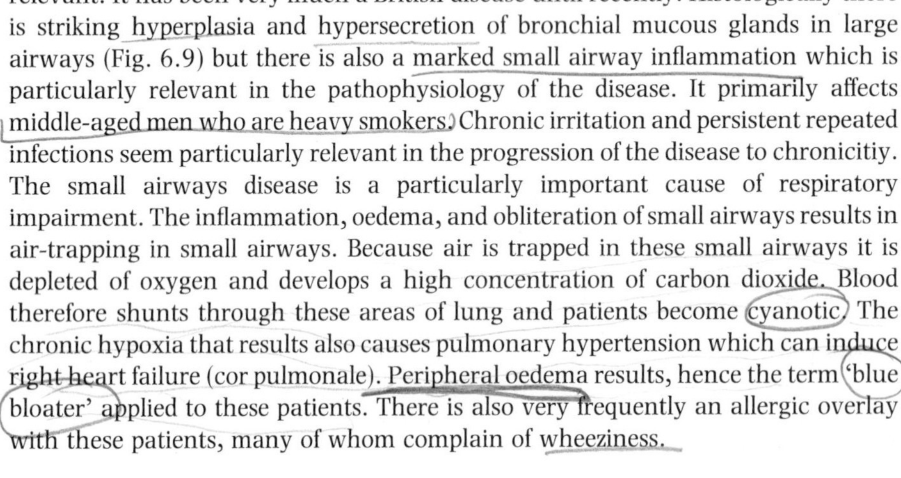

relevant. It has been very much a British disease until recently. Histologically there is striking hyperplasia and hypersecretion of bronchial mucous glands in large airways (Fig. 6.9) but there is also a marked small airway inflammation which is particularly relevant in the pathophysiology of the disease. It primarily affects middle-aged men who are heavy smokers. Chronic irritation and persistent repeated infections seem particularly relevant in the progression of the disease to chronicitiy. The small airways disease is a particularly important cause of respiratory impairment. The inflammation, oedema, and obliteration of small airways results in air-trapping in small airways. Because air is trapped in these small airways it is depleted of oxygen and develops a high concentration of carbon dioxide. Blood therefore shunts through these areas of lung and patients become cyanotic. The chronic hypoxia that results also causes pulmonary hypertension which can induce right heart failure (cor pulmonale). Peripheral oedema results, hence the term 'blue bloater' applied to these patients. There is also very frequently an allergic overlay with these patients, many of whom complain of wheeziness.

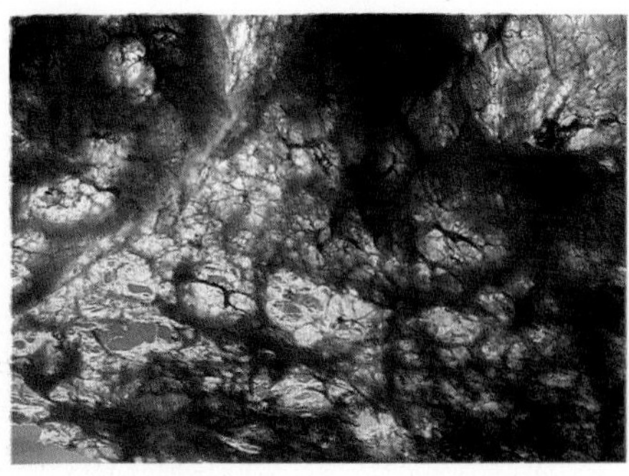

Fig. 6.10 Emphysema.

Emphysema

In contrast to chronic bronchitis this is best defined pathologically by direct examination of lung tissue. However, with modern techniques such as computer tomographic scanning, the disease can be defined in life. Emphysema is a permanent enlargement of alveolar spaces distal to the terminal bronchiole (Fig. 6.10). It is associated with destruction of lung tissue. As mentioned previously there is a common association with chronic bronchitis. A number of different types of emphysema are recognized.

Centrilobular emphysema

This is characterized by destruction of lung tissue in the centre of lung lobules, particularly surrounding bronchioles. It is frequently associated with dust exposure, for example coal.

Panlobular emphysema

This involves all air spaces in the lung lobules distal to the terminal bronchioles. The lung can often be converted into a soft sponge-like structure in view of the severe destruction seen with this disease. If emphysematous spaces become greater than 1 cm then the term *bulla* is used. The underlying mechanism of the development of emphysema is an imbalance between mechanisms protecting the lung from endogenous elastases and processes trying to destroy the lung tissue which are primarily proteolytic enzymes derived from neutrophils. Anything that decreases the resistance of the lung to proteases, such as alpha-1-antitripsin deficiency, or conditions that increase the exposure to endogenous elastases, such as smoking, result in emphysema.

Asthma

This condition is not normally included within the spectrum of chronic obstructive airways disease. It is a clinical definition with the presence of increased airway irritability and reversible small airway obstruction due to smooth muscle contraction. There are a number of different types of asthma, the most common being atopic asthma associated with allergy. There is also a clinical condition where asthma occurs with no history of allergy, and asthma is described in association with exposure to chemicals and drugs. Finally, patients may become sensitive to fungal antigens such as *Aspergillus*.

Atopic asthma

This is increasing in frequency probably due to exposure to environmental antigens. It is associated in particular with dust, pollen, food, and exposure to certain animal antigens. House dust mites are particularly implicated. There is frequently a family history of atopy, with eczema commonly seen. The small airway smooth muscle contraction is mediated by type 1 hypersensitivity (immediate hypersensitivity) which results in airway obstruction which presents as wheezing and increased respiratory rate and breathlessness. The wheeziness is intermittent in character, often occurring several minutes to hours after the initial exposure to the antigen. The pathogenesis of allergic asthma involves the binding of specific (immunoglobulin E) IgE to mast cells which then become sensitive to a particular antigen. Almost all IgE is bound to cells such as mast cells and basophils. On exposure to the antigen, the mast cells degranulate and release histamine, and other inflammatory mediators such as platelet-activating factor and eosinophil chemotactic factor. Eosinophils are attracted to the bronchial wall and are characteristically seen at histology. The small airway obstruction causes distal over-inflation of the lung and there is also an excessive production of mucus with plugging of bronchioles and bronchi. There is also marked disruption of the bronchiolar epithelium which is shed into the lumen. In chronic asthma there is frequently striking mucous gland hypertrophy, smooth muscle hyperplasia, and thickening of the basement membrane.

Bronchiectasis

This is defined as a permanent enlargement of bronchi and bronchioles, frequently due to destruction, fibrosis, and chronic inflammation in the surrounding lung (Fig. 6.11). It occurs as a secondary effect of bronchial obstruction and secondary infection results which tends to potentiate the situation. It is associated with tuberculosis, and in view of this is less frequently seen these days.

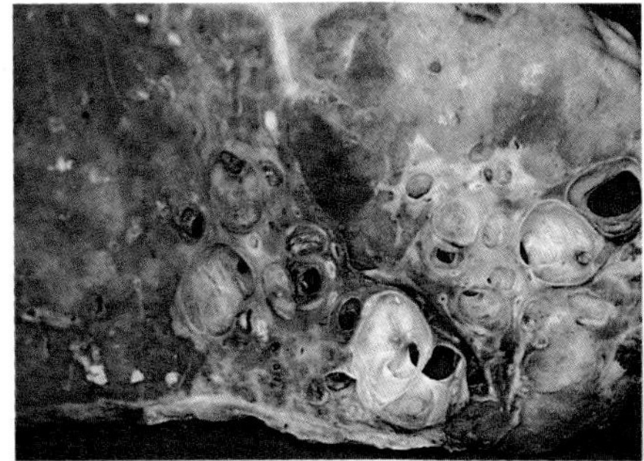

Fig. 6.11 Bronchiectasis associated with cystic fibrosis.

Bronchiectasis is also associated with defects of ciliary function with impairment of host defence. There is a condition called Kartagener's syndrome where cilia are immobile due to a structural abnormality. In view of this ciliary clearance problem there is chronic infection in the distal parts of the lung with development of severe bronchiectasis. Bronchiectasis may also follow occlusion of airways due to tumours or foreign bodies and it is typically seen in cystic fibrosis (see p. 000). It is usually classified as being of cylindrical or saccular type. Clinical features are those of chronic sepsis, with production of purulent sputum. The production of sputum tends to reflect which part of the lung is affected; bronchiectasis tends to involve lower lobes and repositioning patients may accentuate the production of sputum. Complications of bronchiectasis includes those of chronic sepsis, in particular amyloid. Also pneumonia may surpervene with pus escaping into the pleural cavity to cause an empyema and subsequent septicaemia. There may be escape of infective material into the circulation with septic emboli to the kidney and brain. Histologically, as well as severe chronic inflammation and fibrosis, characteristically there is a striking loss of elastic tissue in the bronchi which probably contributes to the loss of strength and dilatation of these airways.

Tuberculosis

This is the most common infective disease in the world. It is caused by the bacillus *Mycobacterium tuberculosis hominis* and *M. tuberculosis bovis*. We will focus primarily on *M. Tuberculosis hominis*.

The bacillus is a strict aerobe and infects primarily macrophages, living as an intracellular organism. It is very resistant to drying and can survive many weeks to months in the environment outside of a host. It has a thick waxy coat which is difficult to stain. A Zeihl–Neelson stain is used to visualize the bacillus. The true incidence is difficult to determine because:

1. Most people who get the disease have no symptoms.
2. All infected people remain at risk of active disease.
3. The reporting of cases is incomplete.

The disease flourishes in poor social and nutritional conditions.

Tuberculosis is intrinsically a *virulent* disease. A 'cord' factor in the waxy coat gives the bacterium its virulence. There are many other species of mycobacteria in the environment which do not cause disease—they are not virulent and are not pathogenic.

Immunology

People with tuberculosis do not develop a significant antibody respose against the organism, that is, the humoral B cell mediated immune system does not play much of a role. Because tuberculosis is an intracellular organism, the *cell-mediated immune system* is important in controlling the infection. The response seen is that of helper T cell-activated macrophages forming aggregates around foci of infection. These macrophages have increased killing ability. They show a switch from phagocytic activity to secretion; on microscopy they appear large and resemble epithelial cells, hence they are named epithelioid cells. These aggregates of macrophages are called epithelioid cell granulomas.

The emergence of *hypersensitivity* to the tubercule bacillus plays a very important role in the tissue damage seen in the disease. Sensitivity to tuberculosis develops about two to four weeks after infection by the organism. This can be measured by skin hypersensitivity (tuberculin test, Heaf test) where a small amount of protein derived from killed tuberculosis is implanted into the skin. In an infected person, a red swollen area will develop in three to four days. This reactivity remains for life. This is probably due to persistence of a few live tuberculous bacteria which maintain an antigenic stimulus to the immune system.

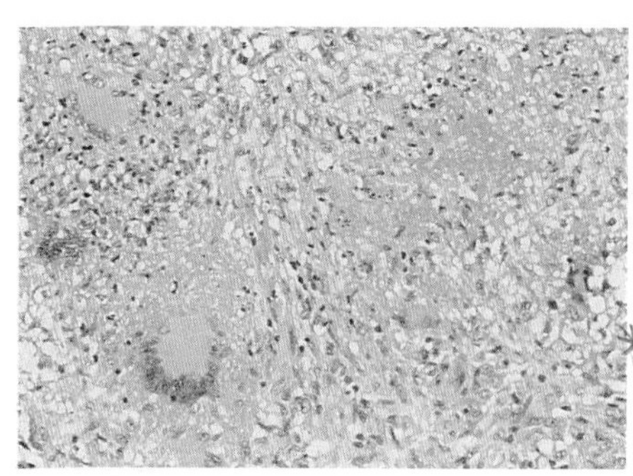

Fig. 6.12 Necrotizing tuberculous granulomas.

In an infected person, the onset of hypersensitivity heralds an important change in the behaviour of the host to the mycobacteria. At first, there is only a phagocytic response from macrophages and neutrophils. The mycobacteria act as a non-specific irritant. When hypersensitivity develops, an epithelioid cell granulomatous response develops. Because so many active cytokines and macrophage products are around, there is frequently central necrosis (Fig. 6.12). *Granulomas and necrosis are features of tuberculosis.*

This granulomatous reaction can cause a lot of tissue destruction, but it is the price paid for having a greatly increased killing ability and resistance to infection by tuberculosis.

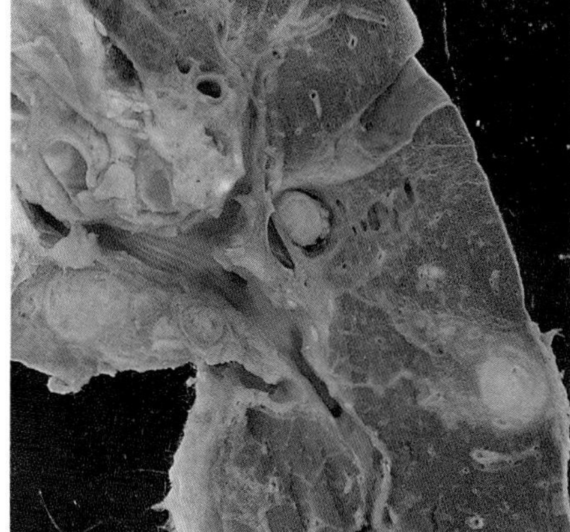

Fig. 6.13 Primary tuberculosis with a Ghon focus (right lower) and involved lymph node (centre) forming a Ghon complex.

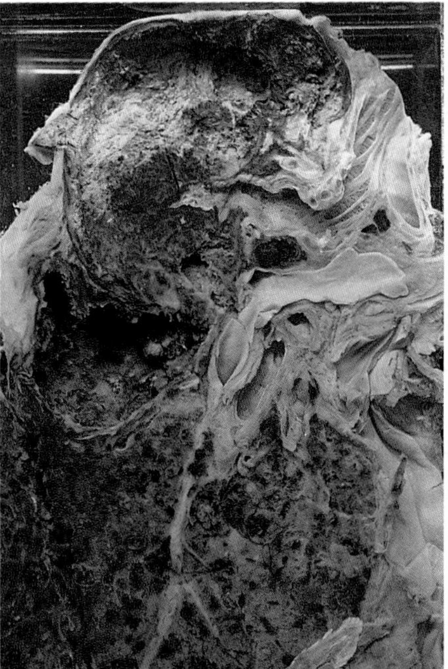

Fig. 6.14 Secondary tuberculosis with lung fibrosis and destruction of the upper lobe.

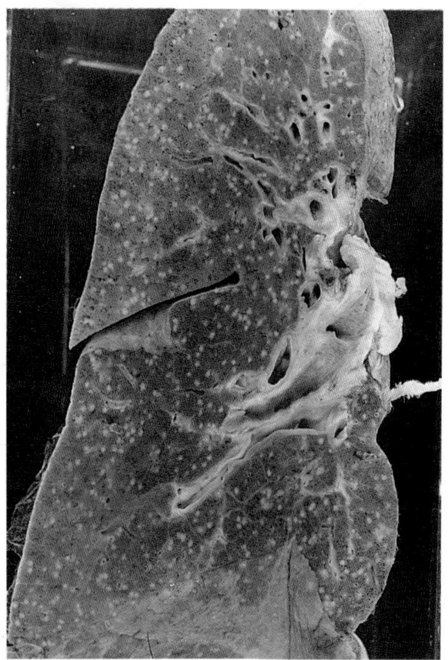

Fig. 6.15 Miliary tuberculosis (looks like millet seed).

Primary tuberculosis

This is when an individual is infected with tuberculosis with no previous history of infection by this organism. This usually starts as an infection in the lower part of the upper lobe or the upper part of the lower lobe of a lung (there is more ventilation by air as compared to perfusion by blood in the upper lobes; it is the opposite way round in the lower lobes). Tuberculosis is, of course, *aerobic*. This area of infection is called a Ghon focus. When the local lymph nodes are involved as well, this is called a Ghon complex (Fig. 6.13). In most cases, as stated above, the infection does not progress, and the lesion eventually shrinks down and frequently becomes calcified. However, an important concept is that although the infection is *controlled* it is not completely *eradicated*.

In a few situations, particularly in children, the infection is not self-limiting. In these cases, the infection spreads into adjacent lung tissue and, via the bloodstream, distant sites, including the meninges.

If the infection is acquired by another route, such as the gastrointestinal tract, there is a similar immunological reaction to that seen in the lungs, with the involvement of local mesenteric lymph nodes in this case. In most cases of primary tuberculosis, the person does not have any symptoms. The disease is detected by screening chest X-ray or skin tests.

Secondary tuberculosis

This is tuberculosis occurring in a previously sensitized individual—someone who has had the infection before. The tuberculosis organisms may be derived from the outside (exogenous) or from re-activation of the previous infection (endogenous).

This occurs in the apex or posterior regions of the upper lobes. On histology, there is a florid necrotizing granulomatous reaction. There may be extensive lung destruction (Fig. 6.14). A number of consequences may develop:

1. The infection may 'arrest' and calcify.
2. There may be spread to other parts of the lungs.

3. There may be extensive spread to other organs of the body (miliary tuberculosis).
4. An isolated organ, such as the kidney, adrenals, bone or brain, may become involved with tuberculosis.

In both primary and secondary tuberculosis, widespread infection of the lungs may occur, with the development of miliary tuberculosis (Fig. 6.15).

Interstitial lung disease

The interstitium of the lung is the tissue within the septa of the alveoli and tissues surrounding airways and blood vessels. The normal interstitium, the space between basement membranes of the alveolar epithelium and endothelium, normally contains a small number of fibroblasts, smooth muscle cell, lymphatics, and occasional lymphocytes and plasma cells. The characteristic feature of interstitial lung disease of the lung independent of cause, tends to be increased fibrous tissue within the interstitial space. In severe interstitial lung disease there is collagen which is laid down between the blood vessels and alveolar epithelium thereby causing severe gas diffusion defects. Fibrotic lungs also show a reduced compliance and marked restriction in lung function, with reduced vital capacity. Interstitial lung disease can be classified into cases where the cause of interstitial disease is known and cases where the cause of the fibrosis is not apparent (Table 6.3).

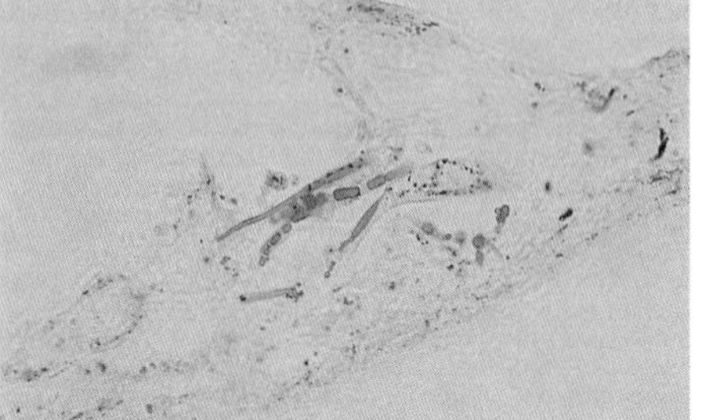

Fig. 6.16 Asbestos bodies in a lung.

Cause of interstitial lung disease known

Pneumoconioses

This is defined as a lung disease due to inhalation of dust, either organic or inorganic. Typical examples involve exposure to coal dust, silica, asbestos (Fig. 6.16), and mineral dusts such as iron or talc.

Extrinsic allergic alveolitis

This develops when a patient is sensitive to an inorganic dust such as material from a pet bird or animal. It may also occur with sensitization to fungal spores, in the case of

Table 6.3 Causes of lung fibrosis

Dust exposure (pneumoconiosis)
Inorganic particles (coal, asbestos, silica)
Organic dusts (fungi, foreign proteins from animals/birds causing extrinsic allergic alveolitis)
Toxic gas (sulphur and nitrogen dioxide)
Drugs and toxic agents
Busulphan
Bleomycin
Cyclophosphamide
Penicillamine
Paraquat
Radiation
Post-inflammatory
Pneumonia
Adult respiratory distress syndrome (shock lung)
Immunological disorders and others
Sarcoidosis, rheumatoid arthritis or other autoimmune disease, in particular scleroderma
Cryptogenic fibrosing alveolitis (no apparent associated cause)

'farmers lung'. It is a manifestation of immune hypersensitivity, involving immune complex (type 3) and delayed hypersensitivity (type 4).

Infection

The result of pneumonia may be interstitial lung disease. Viral infections in particular occasionally result in interstitial lung fibrosis.

Drugs and toxins

Toxins, such as paraquat and drugs, typically bleomycin and busulphan, may cause lung fibrosis. Radiation may also result in fibrosis within the interstitium.

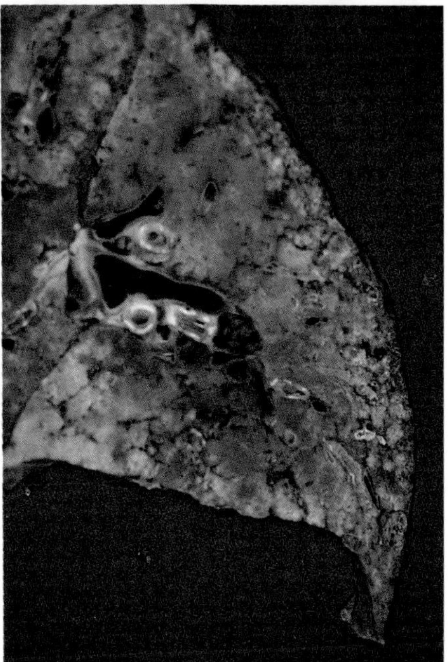

Fig. 6.17 Cryptogenic fibrosing alveolitis. There is subpleural fibrosis in the bottom right part of the lung.

Cause of interstitial lung disease unknown

Sarcoidosis

This is defined as a condition where there is granulomatous inflammation in many organs of the body, with no apparent cause. In particular, mycobacteria are not found. The non-caseating granulomata frequently resolve leaving fibrosis. Sarcoidosis can involve the oral cavity.

Cryptogenic fibrosing alveolitis

This is a condition where there is severe chronic inflammation and resulting inflammation in the interstitium of the lung which may be associated with autoimmune disease, such as rheumatoid arthritis or scleroderma, or may show no association with any other clinical syndrome (Fig. 6.17).

Rare causes

There are a number of other causes of lung fibrosis which are of unknown aetiology, such as excess iron deposition (haemosiderosis), and a proliferation of Langerhans cells called histiocytosis X.

Other non-neoplastic lung disease

Wegener's granulomatosis

This rare disease is mentioned because it may have oral manifestations. It is of unknown cause, but immunological mechanisms are important. It may present in the mouth with a hyperplastic gingivitis or with upper respiratory inflammation and necrosis. It most frequently involves the lung and kidneys. In the lung there are areas of necrosis associated with neutrophils, vasculitis, and giant cells; despite the name, granulomas are not prominent. In the kidney a glomerulonephritis may be present. Antineutrophil cytoplasmic antibodes (ANCA) are present in the majority of patients. The disease responds well to the cytotoxic drug cyclophosphamide.

NEOPLASTIC LUNG DISEASE

Ninety-five per cent of lung tumours are malignant and the majority are of epithelial origin, that is, carcinomas. Most of these carcinomas arise from the bronchus. Rare benign tumours are the bronchial adenoma, carcinoid (an endocrine tumour), and hamartoma. An important point is that the lung is a common site of metastatic tumour.

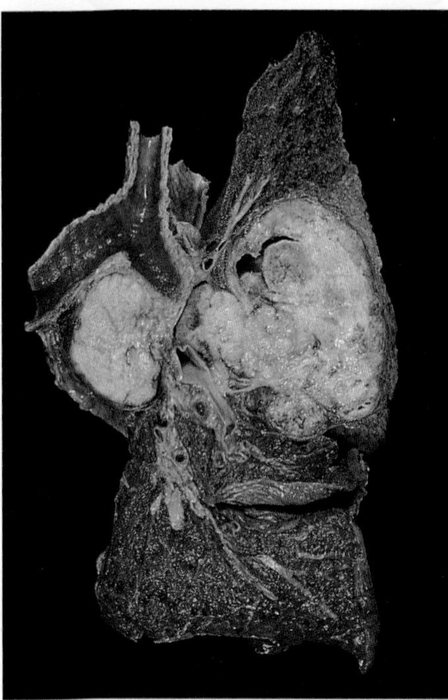

Fig. 6.18 A central carcinoma with metastases to lymph nodes.

Carcinoma of lung

Carcinoma is the most common cancer in men and the second most common cancer in women after breat carcinoma. It was a rare disease before the industrial revolution, and its increased incidence mirrors that of the increased incidence of smoking in the population. It is an urban disease and is predominantly seen in males, although the incidence in females is increasing. It primarily occurs in men over 50 years of age who have a history of smoking or dust exposure, in particular asbestos or radioactive material. A major problem with lung carcinoma is that clinically it is a late-presenting disease; by the time people present with symptoms the tumour is already very advanced. Patients may present with haemoptysis, cough, or weight loss. Pain is usually a late symptom. There are frequently secondary effects such as obstruction of the lung due to the tumour.

Most carcinomas of the lung arise from bronchi and therefore are central in position (Fig. 6.18). However, other forms of carcinoma occur in the lung parenchyma with no relation to bronchi, and are termed peripheral. There are four histological types of lung carcinoma listed below:

1. Squamous cell carcinoma (50 per cent) (Fig. 6.19).
2. Small cell undifferentiated carcinoma (30 per cent) (Fig. 6.20).
3. Adenocarcinoma (10 per cent).
4. Large cell undifferentiated carcinoma (10 per cent).

Squamous cell carcinoma, adenocarcinoma, and large cell undifferentiated carcinoma tend to have a similar, rather low-grade clinical behaviour in that they tend to grow slowly. Small cell carcinoma, often called 'oat' cell carcinoma in view of its histological appearance, is a very malignant tumour, in contrast to the other three tumours listed above.

The normal lung does not have squamous epithelium within in, and squamous cell carcinoma arises from squamous metaplasia of bronchial respiratory epithelium. Dysplasia then supervenes forming initial carcinoma-*in situ* and then invasive carcinoma.

Small cell carcinoma appears to be a very malignant form of endocrine cell tumour and arises from normal endocrine cells found in the lung. Many adenocarcinomas appear to rise from glandular elements in the lung, particularly bronchial glands and occasionally alveolar epithelium.

Large cell carcinomas in most cases appear to be squamous cell carcinomas or adenocarcinomas that are so poorly differentiated that their type cannot be determined using normal techniques such as light microscopy.

Generally, the prognosis of lung cancer, particular small cell carcinoma is very poor. In view of the very high growth rate of small cell carcinoma, chemotherapy

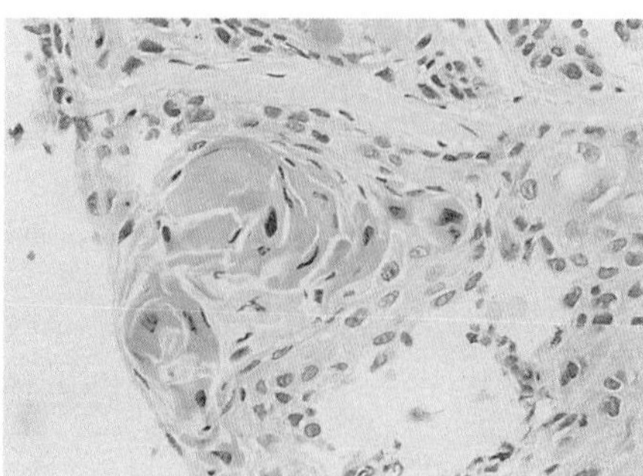

Fig. 6.19 Keratinizing squamous cell carcinoma.

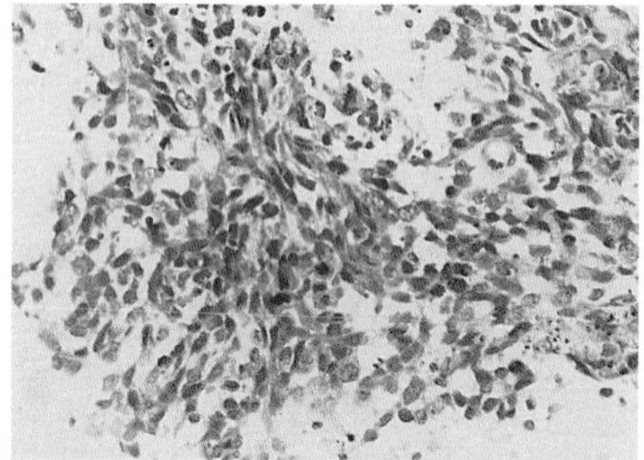

Fig. 6.20 How small cell carcinoma got its name. The cells are small and dark staining.

and radiotherapy is often used. It is also important to remember that the lung is a common site of metastasis of carcinomas from other sites in the body (Fig. 6.21).

The stage of the disease has a great influence on the prognosis. The system used in staging lung cancer is shown in Table 6.4, together with the two-year survival rates in Table 6.5.

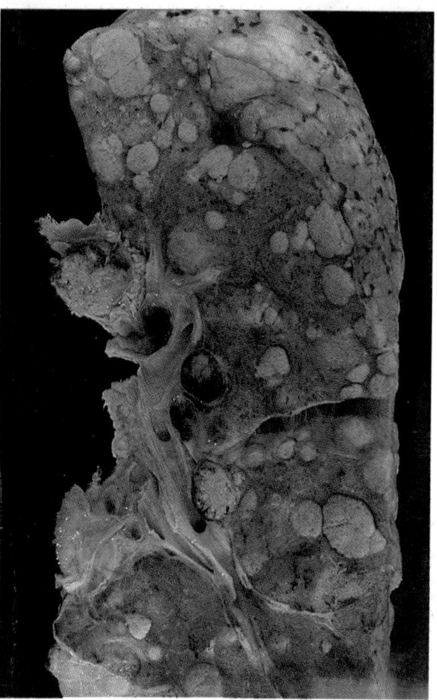

Fig. 6.21 Lung metastases.

Table 6.4 Staging of lung cancer

Stage 1–Less than 3 cm diameter (T1), no nodal involvement in same lung (N0), or, greater than 3 cm in diameter 2 cm distal to carina (T2) and no nodes involved (N0)

Stage 2–T1 or greater than 3 cm, with nodes involved in same lung (T2, N1)

Stage 3–Pleural or mediastinal involvement, with/without nodes involved in hilum of same lung (N0 or N1) or any T with nodes involved in opposite side (N2)

Stage 4—Any T, any N, distant metastases (M1)

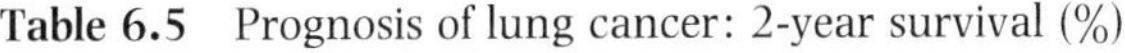

Table 6.5 Prognosis of lung cancer: 2-year survival (%)

Stage	Squamous cell carcinoma	Adenocarcinoma	Large cell	Small cell carcinoma
1	47	46	43	6
2	40	14	13	5
3	11	8	13	2

SUMMARY

Upper respiratory tract

Nasopharynx: this is particularly susceptible to viral infections. Inflammatory disorders include hay fever, a type I hypersensitivity to inhaled antigens; nasal polyps are an associated complication.

Neoplasms of the nasopharynx may be benign (haemangioma, papillomas and angiofibroma. Malignant tumours of the nasopharynx that arise are squamous cell carcinoma (nasopharyngeal carcinoma) and lymphoma.

Larynx

Inflammatory pathology

–viral and bacteria infection
–laryngeal nodules

Benign tumours: benign squamous papillomas are the most common benign tumours of the larynx. They are associated with human papillomavirus. The most common malignant tumour of the larynx is squamous cell carcinoma.

Lung

Lung disease can be divided into non-neoplastic and neoplastic types.

Infections

–acute bronchitis
–chronic bronchitis

–bronchiolitis
–pneumonia (may be classified by anatomical involvement, either lobar or bronchopneumonia, or may be classified according to the causative organism)

Pulmonary embolism: most pulmonary emboli are thrombi, arising particularly in deep leg veins and the pelvis. A common cause of sudden death. Very common in immobilized patients.

Pulmonary hypertension: this may be primary, or secondary to chronic hypoxia.

Pulmonary oedema: this may be haemodynamic (due to cardiac failure or due to microvascular injury (so-called shock lung or adult respiratory distress syndrome).

Chronic obstructive airways disease: this encompasses two disease processes, chronic bronchitis (defined clinically as excessive sputum production) and emphysema (defined as enlargement of air spaces due to destruction of lung substance). Chronic bronchitis is also associated with inflammation and constriction of small bronchioles.

Asthma: this is a condition where there is increased irritability of bronchioles causing airway obstruction. It occurs in episodes and is reversible. Mechanisms involve immediate hypersensitivity to inhaled antigens.

Bronchiectasis: this is a permanent enlargement of bronchi and bronchioles secondary to chronic inflammation.

Interstitial lung disease: the lung has a limited way of responding to an insult, and interstitial lung disease manifests itself as fibrosis in the connective tissue between the alveolar epithelium and the blood vessels of the lung. It may be due to known causes, such as inhaled dust or infection, or unknown causes, such as immunologically mediated disease, that is, sarcoidosis or connective tissue disorders.

Lung tumours: most lung tumours are malignant and are carcinomas. Lung carcinoma is the most common cancer in men and the second most common cancer in women. It is strongly associated with smoking. There are four main types: squamous cell carcinoma, small cell undifferentiated carcinoma, adenocarcinoma, large cell undifferentiated carcinoma.

7 The gastrointestinal system

7 The gastrointestinal system

MOUTH

The mouth, as with any other structure that is subject to continuous wear and tear, is lined by squamous epithelium. The basic structure of the epithelium is similar in the oesophagus and the skin, although the latter, in contrast, shows overt keratinization. The oral mucosa is generally non-keratinized. If there are signs of chronic irritation there may be hyperplasia of the epithelium which may manifest itself clinically as leukoplakia. This whiteness is due to the keratinization that occurs in this situation. Important tumours of the mouth that are seen in surgical pathology are listed below.

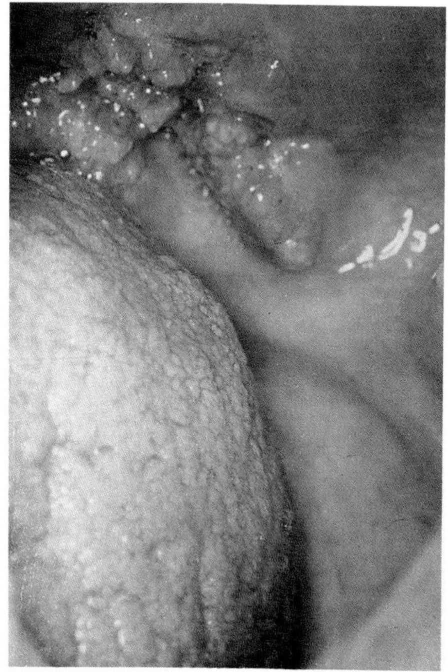

Fig. 7.1 Oral squamous cell carcinoma.

Benign tumours

- Papilloma.
- Benign tumours of minor salivary glands.
- Fibroma (epulis).

Malignant tumours

Squamous cell carcinoma (Fig. 7.1)

This tends to occur on the lateral border of the tongue and on the floor of the mouth, occurring in about 4 per 100 000 of the population in the United Kingdom. The lip is also a frequent primary site. It is associated with alcohol, tobacco smoking or chewing, and Betel nut chewing (see p. 000). It is also associated with lichen planus, systemic lupus erythematosus, human papilloma virus infection, and immunosuppression. It is a disease of the elderly. They are most frequently well-differentiated tumours. Oral cancer shows extensive local spread, and metastasizes to local lymph nodes late in the disease.

The overall 5-year survival rate for oral cancer is about 40 per cent. Poor prognostic factors are a tumour greater than 4 cm diameter, greater than 0.5 cm invasion into the soft tissue, lymph node metastases, and a poorly differentiated tumour. The TNM classification (devised by the International Union Against Cancer: IUCC) is shown in Table 7.1.

Adenocarcinoma (frequently arising in minor salivary glands)

Malignant melanoma

This arises from melanocytes present in the oral mucosa.

Tumours may also arise from the structures associated with the teeth:

- Odontome (a tooth malformation).
- Ameloblastoma (arises from odontogenic epithelium; it may be benign or malignant).

Table 7.1 The staging of oral cancer

T0	No primary tumour seen
T1	2 cm or less diameter (stage I if N0, III if N1)
T2	2–4 cm diameter (stage II if N0, III if N1)
T3	Larger than 4 cm (stage III if N0, III if N1)
T4	Involved deep tissue and bone (stage IV if N0 or N1, M0)
N0	No node metastases
N1	Mobile enlarged nodes on side of tumour
N2	Mobile enlarged nodes on opposite side or bilaterally (stage IV, any T)
N3	Fixed enlarged nodes (stage IV, any T)
M0	No distant metastases
M1	Distant metastases (as soon as any distant metastases, stage IV, any T or N)

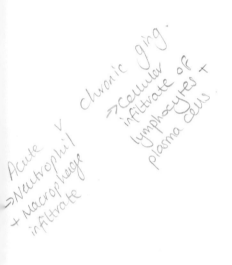

- Cementoma (contains cementum; cementomas are closely related to an osteoma, a benign bone tumour).

Inflammatory diseases of the mouth

Gingivitis

Inflammatory reactions, which are a non-specific response to injury or infection, are commonly seen in the mouth. Gingivitis may be either acute or chronic, and which is normally caused by anaerobic bacteria such as *Borrelia vincentii* and so-called fusiform bacilli. A dentist will see gingivitis every day of his or her practice and it represents an inflammatory reaction to bacterial plaque present on the teeth. As in inflammation in any other site of the body, acute inflammation is characterized by a neutrophil and macrophage infiltrate. Chronic gingivitis is characterized elsewhere by a cellular infiltrate of lymphocytes and plasma cells. Inflammation may track down to the tooth apex and form an abscess or radicular cyst.

Ulcers

The cause of many mouth ulcers is unknown, as in the case of aphthous ulcers. Ulcers may be due to known viruses, such as herpes simplex, or may be associated with other systemic disease, the most important being Crohn's disease. Another important infection of the mouth, seen particularly in association with immunodeficiency is *Candida*, a yeast.

PHARYNX

Pharyngitis due to viruses is far more common than bacterial pharyngitis. Most viruses are in the adenovirus group. The tonsils are a frequent site of acute inflammation, particularly in children. The most common tumour of the pharynx is nasopharyngeal carcinoma which is generally a poorly differentiated squamous carcinoma, and is associated with Epstein–Barr virus infection.

SALIVARY GLANDS

Inflammatory Disorders

Acute and chronic inflammatory disorders of the salivary gland are usually associated with duct obstruction, frequently due to a stone. Infection ascends the ducts and involves the salivary gland lobules. Mucoceles (mucous cysts) are associated with obstruction of the ducts of minor salivary glands.

Sjögren's syndrome

This is an autoimmune disease which may involve the salivary glands in isolation, or occur as a secondary phenomenon in association with other autoimmune disease such as rheumatoid arthritis. Circulating antibodies to the salivary epithelium may occur. Frequently antibodies to antigens such as nuclear proteins (called Ro and La, or SS-A and SS-B, respectively), and IgG (rheumatoid factor) are found. The disease most frequently affects late middle-aged females.

There is a lymphocytic destruction of the salivary gland tissue with reduction in the production of saliva. The process is most evident in the major salivary glands, causing a dry mouth (xerostoma), but the inflammation also involves minor salivary glands and the lacrimal glands of the eye (causing dry eyes, xerophthalmia). The combination of dry eyes and dry mouth is called the sicca syndrome. Sicca syndrome is also seen in association with rheumatoid arthritis, systemic lupus erythematosus, and scleroderma.

Sjögren's syndrome is associated with other immunological diseases such as primary biliary cirrhosis of the liver, Hashimoto's thyroiditis, and arthritis.

Tumours

The salivary glands are a rich source of tumours of a wide variety. Benign tumours tend to involve both the epithelium and myoepithelium, whilst malignant tumours involve just the epithelium. The most common types of tumours are listed below.

Benign

Pleomorphic adenoma—this is generally a benign tumour growing commonly in the parotid gland. It has a very variable appearance in different parts of the tumour (Fig. 7.2).

Monomorphic adenoma—this shows a very similar appearance throughout the tumour.

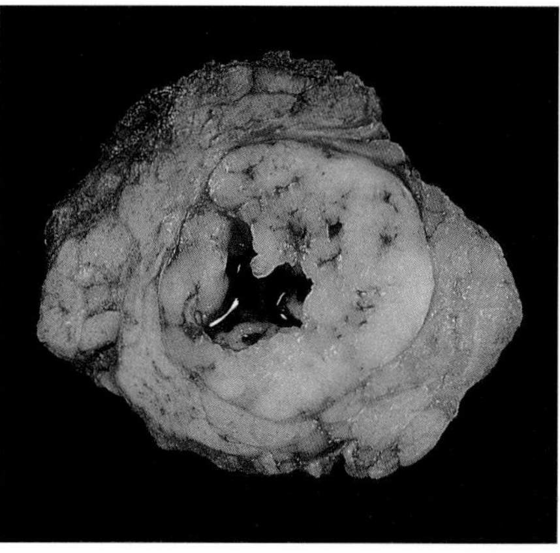

Fig. 7.2 Pleomorphic adenoma of the parotid.

Adenolymphoma (Warthin's tumour)—this is a tumour arising from salivary gland epithelium and is associated with lymphoid tissue. Despite its inappropriate name, it is benign.

Malignant

Mucoepidermoid carcinoma—this is a rare malignant tumour showing mixed mucinous and squamous differentiation.

Adenoid cystic carcinoma—this is a rare tumour and tends not to metastasize, but shows extensive local invasive activity. It typically invades along nerves, an unusual route of tumour spread.

Adenocarcinoma

Low- and high-grade adenocarcinomas may occur in salivary glands.

OESOPHAGUS

As with the mouth, the oesophageal mucosa is of squamous type, but without the distinct outer keratinized layer as seen in the skin. In many ways, the oesophagus is prone to similar disorders to the mouth and pharynx.

Oesophagitis

This is usually classified as detailed below.

Reflux oesophagitis

Inflammation of the oesophagus is most frequently due to the reflux of gastric acid secretions through the gastro-oesophageal junction. This may occur with hiatus hernia where the functional gastro-oesophageal junction is herniated into the thorax through a widened diaphragmatic hiatus or opening. There is frequently heavy acute-on-chronic inflammation with ulceration. The squamous epithelium of the oesophagus responds by turning into metaplastic mucinous epithelium, termed Barrett's oesophagus.

Infective oesophagitis

In immunocompromised patients there may be infection such as *Candida*, causing oesophagitis. *Klebsiella* is described as causing oesophagitis, and viruses such as herpes may induce inflammation.

Chemical (corrosive)

Reflux oesophagitis can be regarded as a form of chemical inflammation in that gastric acid acts as a corrosive agent. Ingestion of corrosive agents, such as strong alkali, causes a severe erosive oesophagitis which may result in a fibrotic stricture.

If oesophagitis persists there may be a fibrosis, the hallmark of chronic inflammation, which may cause a stricture with chronic oesophageal obstruction.

Vascular disorders

The most important vascular abnormality of the oesophagus are acquired varices (enlarged veins) in the lower oesophagus (Fig. 7.3). There are potential communications between the portal venous system draining the gastrointestinal tract and systemic veins in the lower oesophagus. When there is raised blood pressure in the portal system due to, for example, liver cirrhosis from chronic alcohol abuse, these communications or *anastomoses* open up and enlarge. These veins are very thin and are easily damaged, and can cause life-threatening haemorrhage into the stomach.

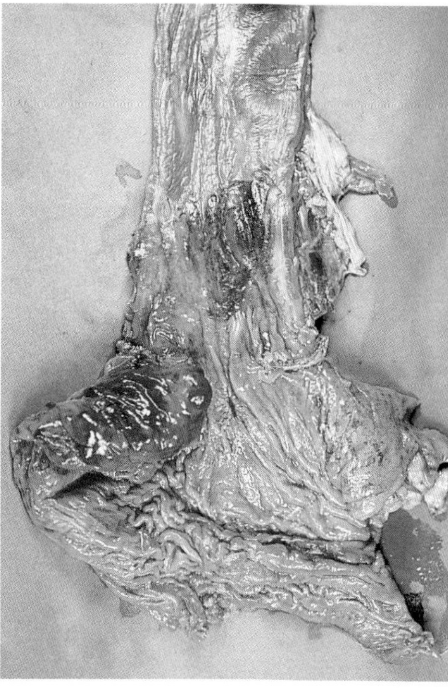

Fig. 7.3 Oesophageal varices in the mid-part of the specimen. There are linear ulcers over the varices.

Systemic disorders

With the autoimmune disease *systemic sclerosis* there may be oesophageal involvement manifesting as fibrosis.

Tumours

Leiomyoma

This is the most common benign tumour in the eosophagus and arises from the smooth muscle of the oesophageal wall. It is usually of no clinical significance and is found incidently.

Other tumours that can be found at this site are neurofibromas, lipomas, and haemangiomas.

Carcinoma

The most common malignant epithelial tumour of the oesophagus, as with the mouth and pharynx, is squamous cell carcinoma. Throughout the world, there is tremendous variation in the incidence of this tumour, the highest incidence being in countries such as the Middle East and China. In the United Kingdom the tumour has an incidence of 5–10 per 100 000. There is strong evidence that oesophageal carcinoma is associated with environmental factors in the diet, particularly alcohol and organic chemicals such as nitrosamines. There is also an association with certain viruses, particularly human papilloma virus (HBV). Most squamous cell carcinomas of the oesophagus arise in the lower oesophagus (Fig. 7.4). The most common presenting clinical symptom is difficulty in swallowing (dysphagia).

The second most common type of oesophageal carcinoma is adenocarcinoma. This type of carcinoma is strongly associated with Barrett's oesophagus due to reflux oesophagitis.

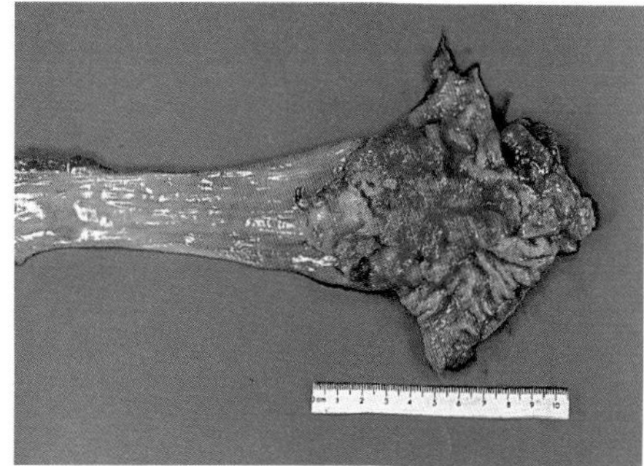

Fig. 7.4 Carcinoma of the lower oesophagus.

STOMACH

The stomach is a reservoir that converts an intermittent flow from the oesophagus into a continuous flow into the duodenum. It is a highly acid environment with a mucosa that is specialized and resistant to digestive enzymes. The stomach is divided into two areas. The proximal area of the stomach is called the body which has specialized acid-secreting mucosa. The distal part of the stomach is known as the antrum, and has non-specialized mucus-secreting epithelium. It is here that the hormone-secreting gastrin cells are found. Gastrin stimulates acid secretion in the specialized mucosa of the gastric body.

One congenital or developmental abnormality of the stomach is infantile hypertrophic pyloric stenosis. In this condition there is a marked thickening of the muscle around the pylorus, the outflow from the stomach. This is a well-recognized cause of gastric outflow obstruction in babies.

Table 7.2 Classification of gastritis

A—Autoimmune (pernicious anaemia)
B—Bacterial (*Helicobacter*)
C—Chemical (bile, corrosives, drugs)

Gastritis (Table 7.2)

Autoimmune gastritis

This is associated with vitamin B_{12} deficiency due to loss of cells which produce intrinsic factor. This occurs in pernicious anaemia. A heavy destructive chronic inflammatory infiltrate of lymphocytes and plasma cells is seen. There is frequently a change of gastric epithelium type into small intestinal epithelium, known as metaplasia. There is a high incidence of gastric cancer in these patients.

Bacterial gastritis

Helicobacter pylori is a common bacterial infection of the stomach that is associated with acute and chronic gastritis. It appears that this organism is commonly carried in the mouth. It can survive gastric acidity by producing an alkaline ammonia metabolite from the metabolism of urea by ureases.

Less common bacteria that can cause gastritis are *Salmonella*, *Yersinia*, *Candida*, and viruses such as herpes.

Chemical gastritis

This may be due to drugs, the most common being non steroidal anti-inflammatory drugs. These include aspirin and drugs that are frequently used for treatment of rheumatoid arthritis and as analgesics. There may be a range of pathology seen in this type of gastritis, from multiple small gastric erosions to overt ulceration. Gastritis may also be due to the influx of bile and duodenal secretions into the stomach. Spicy irritant food can also cause gastritis.

Other causes

Gastritis is rarely associated with dietary allergy, parasites, or inflammatory disorders such as Crohn's disease. Gastritis is also seen as a response to stress.

Gastric ulceration

Gastric or peptic ulceration is essentially due to an imbalance between factors trying to damage the gastric mucosa and defences which protect the gastric mucosa from such digestion. The strongest associated factor which appears to precipitate gastric ulceration is the presence of gastric acidity. Drugs that reduce gastric aciditiy such as cimetidine, which is a histamine H_2 receptor blocker, or the more recently released acid secreting-cell inhibitor omeprazole, are effective healers of chronic peptic ulcers. In gastric ulcers, however, there is frequently reduced gastric acid secretion, and ulceration appears to be due to reduced mucosal resistance. Other factors that are associated with gastric ulcers are infection with the bacterium *Helicobacter pylori* as mentioned above, non-steroidal anti-inflammatory drugs, and smoking. Gastric and duodenal ulcers are more common in males than females. Ulcers may be acute, in that they only involve the superficial parts of the mucosa or they may be chronic in that they penetrate through the mucosa to involve the underlying submucosa and muscle wall beneath. Gastric ulceration is frequently associated with bleeding due to erosion into blood vessels in the base of the ulcer (Fig. 7.5). Perforation through the muscle wall may also occur (Fig. 7.6), and severe fibrosis and malignant change may develop. Through the endoscope, gastric ulcers are usually solitary, show a flat edge with a punched-out appearance, and show inflammatory slough in the base. An ulcer is defined as a loss of epithelium, and the central part of a peptic ulcer is composed of degenerate and inflamed granulation tissue.

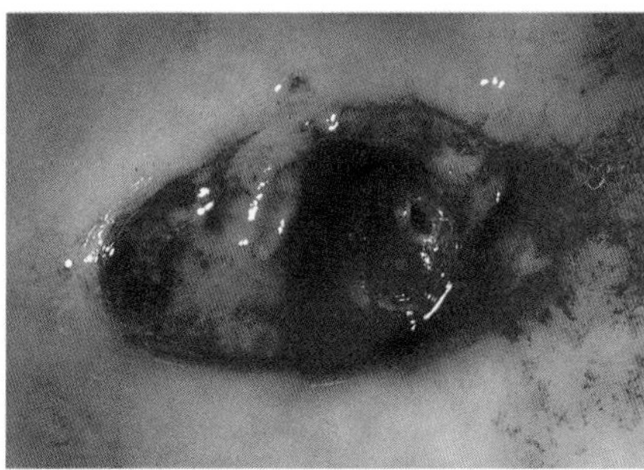

Fig. 7.5 Gastric ulcer showing a prominent central projecting artery which has bled.

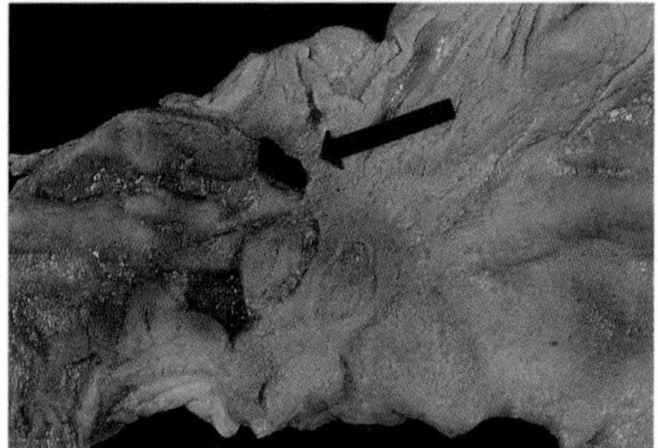

Fig. 7.6 A perforated gastric ulcer (arrow) with a further non-perforated chronic ulcer below.

Benign tumours

As with the oesophagus, the most common benign tumour of the stomach is the leiomyoma which arises in the muscle wall. These often protrude into the lumen of the stomach and are associated with focal ulceration and haemorrhage. A benign tumour of the stomach mucosa is the adenoma. Adenomas, by definition, show epithelial dysplasia, and are strongly associated with malignant change.

Malignant tumours

The majority of cancers of the stomach are adenocarcinomas. Dietary factors have been implicated in explaining the high incidence of gastric ulcers in some populations, particularly Japan, Chile, Russia, and Finland. Patients with chronic gastritis, gastric atrophy, previous gastrectomy, and loss of gastric acidity in, for instance pernicious anaemia, have a high incidence of carcinoma. In contrast to benign ulcers, a malignant ulcer has typically a raised rolled edge and shows invasive activity into the muscle wall. The tumours usually occur on the lesser curve. Gastric carcinoma is, unfortunately, a late-presenting disease and at presentation frequently shows extensive metastatic disease, particularly in local lymph nodes and the liver (Fig. 7.7).

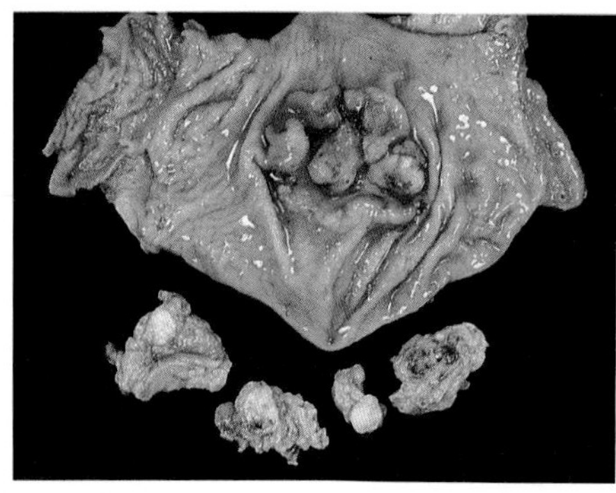

Fig. 7.7 Gastric carcinoma with metastases to lymph nodes (bottom).

With population screening, gastric cancer in the mucosa can be discovered before it involves the gastric muscle wall (early gastric cancer) and it is then potentially curable.

Gastric lymphoma is a well-recognized lymphoid malignancy of the stomach. The stomach has normally its own population of lymphoid cells, termed mucosal-associated lymphoid tissue (MALT). In view of the normal 'homing' ability of lymphocytes in the stomach to re-circulate between local lymph nodes and the stomach, the lymphomas that arise in this tissue generally remain localized in the stomach for a long period of time, and therefore have a good prognosis, particularly with surgical removal. Some lymphomas appear to be associated with chronic immunological stimulation by *Helicobacter* infection.

DUODENUM

The most important pathology of the duodenum seen in surgical pathology is the duodenal ulcer. This is a form of peptic ulcer with similar characteristics as gastric ulcers. Anterior duodenal ulcers have a strong tendency to perforate, in view of the absence of any anatomical structures over that surface of the duodenum. Posterior duodenal ulcers tend to erode into the deep wall of the duodenum and bleed from gastric arteries. Duodenal ulcers, in contrast to gastric ulcers, are associated with high acid secretion from the stomach. Multiple and persistent duodenal ulcers are associated with a gastrin-secreting carcinoid of the pancreas islets in the *Zollinger–Ellison syndrome*. Gastrin stimulates the production of acid by the body mucosa of the stomach, and although this syndrome is rare, it illustrates in the form of a biological 'experiment' the importance of gastric acidity in the development of duodenal ulceration. This syndrome is also of interest in that gastrin is produced from a pancreatic islet cell tumour when normal islets do not contain gastrin. This shows that, in tumours, genes can be activated that are normally inactive.

SMALL INTESTINE

Congenital abnormalities

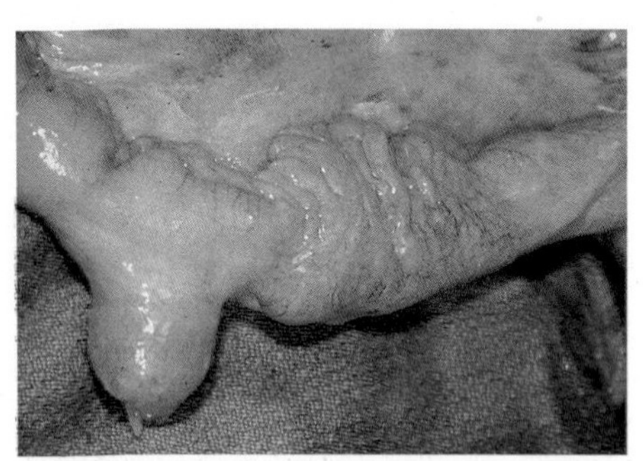

Fig. 7.8 A Meckel's diverticulum.

Diverticulae of the small intestine may be multiple, as in the case of multiple diverticulosis where the diverticuli are arranged along the mesenteric border of the bowel. Another form of congenital abnormality of the small bowel is the Meckel's diverticulum (Fig. 7.8) which is an embryonic remant associated with the umbilical cord. This has a tendency to be lined with gastric acid producing mucosa and may ulcerate. The Meckel's diverticulum is usually found approximately 50 cm from the caecum. Inflammation of Meckel's diverticulum can imitate appendicitis.

Malabsorption

In view of the absorptive function of the small bowel, many inflammatory disorders of the small intestine are manifested as problems in nutrition. Recognized causes of this are listed below.

Coeliac disease—this occurs as an allergic or immune response against dietary gluten. The immune response causes loss of villi, which are responsible for the normally high surface area of the small bowel (Figs 7.9 and 7.10). The presence of cell-mediated immunity is supported by the large numbers of lymphocytes seen in the surface epithelium of the mucosa. Antibodies to gliadin, which is part of gluten, can be found in the circulation. Coeliac disease is associated with a blistering skin disorder called dermatitis herpetiformis. There is also an increased incidence of T cell lymphoma of the small intestine.

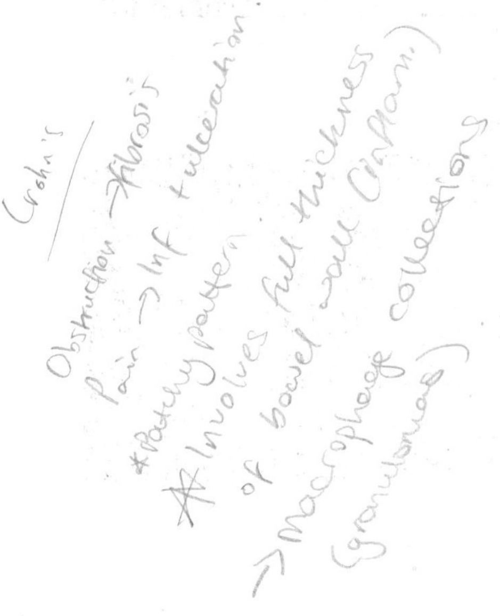

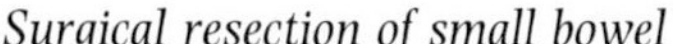

Surgical resection of small bowel

Excision of a large length of small bowel reduces the surface area of the intestine and is therefore associated with malabsorption.

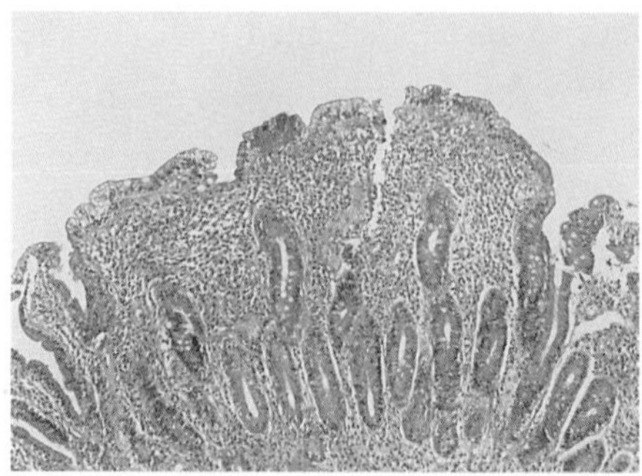

Fig. 7.9 Coeliac disease with villous atrophy.

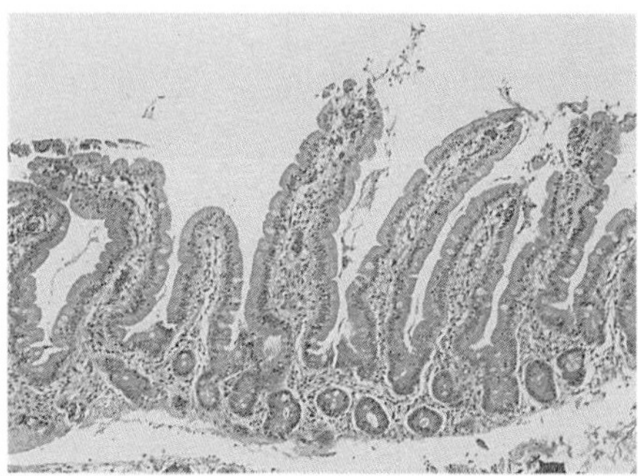

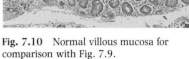

Fig. 7.10 Normal villous mucosa for comparison with Fig. 7.9.

Impaired digestion

Surgery to the stomach, liver, or pancreas can interfere with intestinal absorption. Occasionally the mucosa may be deficient in an enzyme such as disaccharidase which may produce intolerance to some food, resulting in malabsorption.

Intestinal damage

Radiation and ischaemia impair intestinal function. Whipple's disease, parasites (for example, *Giardia*), and infections such as tropical sprue caused probably by abnormal bacterial overgrowth in the small intestine cause damage to mucosal villi.

Inflammatory disorders

Common infections of the small bowel are listed in Table 7.3.

Table 7.3 Common infections of the small intestine

Salmonella
Dysentery
Shigella
Cholera
Campylobacter
E. coli (enterotoxic: half of cases of 'travellers' diarrhoea')
Staphylococcal
Tuberculosis
Whipple's disease
Viruses (Norwalk type)
Fungi
Parasites (*Giardia*)
Entamoeba histolytica
Cryptosporidium parvum

Crohn's disease

This is an inflammatory bowel disease of unknown cause which can involve any part of the gastrointestinal tract, from the mouth to the anus. It is most frequently seen in the small bowel and colon. It is a chronic and persistent disease which frequently presents with obstruction due to the associated fibrosis, or pain due to inflammation and ulceration (Figs 7.11 and 7.12). It occurs most frequently in the 15–30 year age group. The disease has a typically *patchy* pattern of distribution, lesions 'skipping' from place to place in the bowel. Involved areas of small bowel show acute-on-chronic inflammation of the mucosa with ulceration. Fissuring ulcers penetrate into the muscle wall and inflammation is seen involving the full thickness of the bowel wall. The resulting fibrosis causes stricturing of the bowel which narrows the lumen and can cause obstruction. Microscopically, there is also patchy acute-on-chronic inflammation which extends through the full thickness of the bowel wall. A characteristic feature is frequent collections of macrophages termed granulomas. No microorganisms have been found as a cause of Crohn's disease, although a form of tuberculosis has been suspected. Crohn's disease is frequently associated with malabsorption, in view of the excessive ulceration. It also is classically a disease that causes fistula. A fistula is a communication between two epithelial-lined cavities, or an epithelial-lined cavity and the skin. A fistula can occur between the small bowel and any other adjacent structure such as the bladder or other loops of bowel, either small or large.

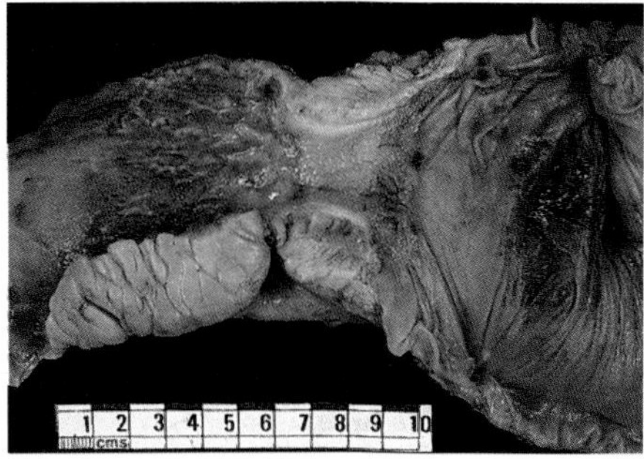

Fig. 7.11 Crohn's disease showing ulceration and stricture of the colon.

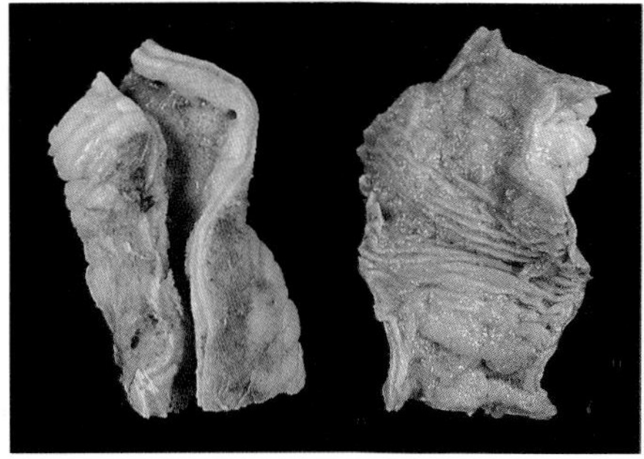

Fig. 7.12 Crohn's disease showing fibrosis and narrowing of small bowel (left specimen). Less involved bowel on the right.

Tumours

Despite the high surface area of the small bowel, tumours of the small intestine are rare. Adenocarcinomas and endocrine tumours (carcinoids), are described. Lymphomas also occur, particularly in coeliac disease.

Peutz-Jegher's syndrome comprises of multiple benign tumours of the small bowel associated with pigmentation around the mouth (circumoral pigmentation). The polyps are composed of branching smooth muscle with overlying mucosal tissue.

LARGE INTESTINE

Appendix

The most common surgical pathology of the appendix is appendicitis (Fig. 7.13). The underlying cause of appendicitis is not known, although obstruction of the appendix lumen seems to be a common factor. Appendicitis is a very common cause

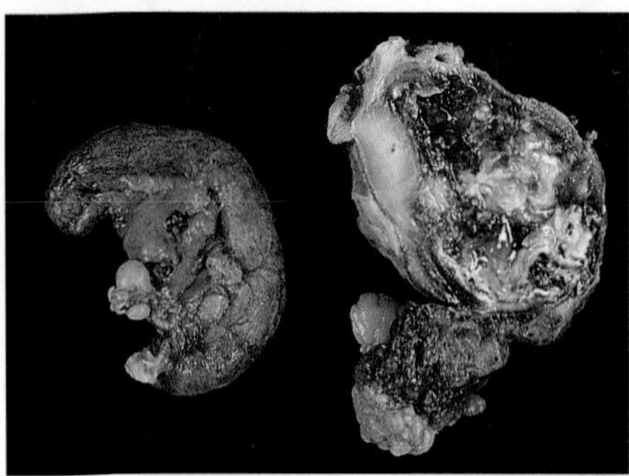

Fig. 7.13 A moderately inflamed (left) appendicitis and a severely inflamed appendicitis (right), the latter with an abscess.

of the 'acute surgical abdomen'. Appendicitis may be associated with peritonitis, perforation, and abscess formation.

Diverticulosis

Diverticulosis or diverticular disease is due to increased pressure in the large bowel due to a low-fibre diet. The diverticulae frequently occur in the sigmoid colon, which is in the distal region of the bowel. They develop as herniations of mucosa through natural weaknesses in the bowel wall where blood vessels penetrate through the muscle to supply the mucosa (Fig. 7.14). Complications of diverticulosis are diverticulitis with acute inflammation or abscesses developing in association with the diverticulae. Also severe haemorrhage may occur and diverticulitis may progress to overt perforation of the bowel. Bowel involved with diverticular disease shows striking muscle hypertrophy and diverticulae can be seen with the naked eye protruding from the outer surface of the bowel, close to the mesentery.

Ischaemic bowel disease

This is due to a compromised blood supply to the large bowel, commonly due to atherosclerosis. Overt infarction may occur (Fig. 7.15). The bowel may show features which resemble inflammatory bowel disease, in that there is mucosal ulceration, acute and chronic inflammation, and bowel fibrosis. The most commonly involved area with ischaemic colitis is the splenic flexure, which is a 'watershed' area between the two blood supplies of the superior mesenteric artery and the inferior mesenteric artery. Radiation colitis, which is basically ischaemia due to damaged blood vessels, is associated with radiotherapy.

Inflammatory bowel disease

Ulcerative colitis

This is an inflammatory bowel disease of unknown aetiology which is characterized by acute-on-chronic inflammation which begins in the rectum and progresses proximally in a continuous fashion and may eventually involve the whole colon (Fig. 7.16). The disease characteristically does not involve the small bowel and this is an important feature that differentiates the disease from Crohn's disease. On histology, the inflammation is characteristically limited to the mucosa and is continuous and diffuse. There is often striking remodelling of the architecture of the mucosa, with notable glandular atrophy. The cause of the disease is unknown, but the mucosal limitation of the inflammation suggests a factor in the lumen which induces the disease. There is probably an immunologically mediated process

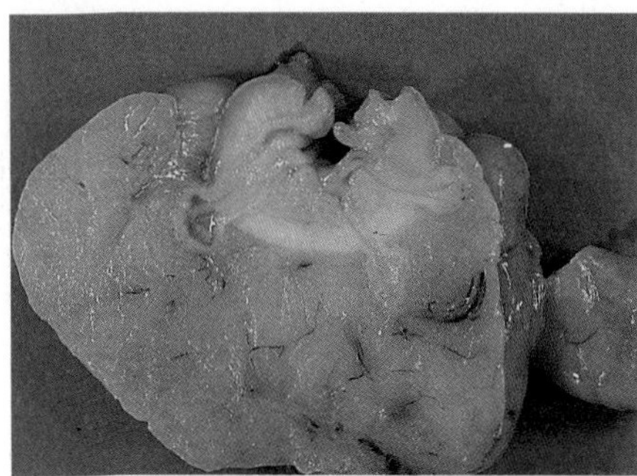

Fig. 7.14 Three diverticulae are present.

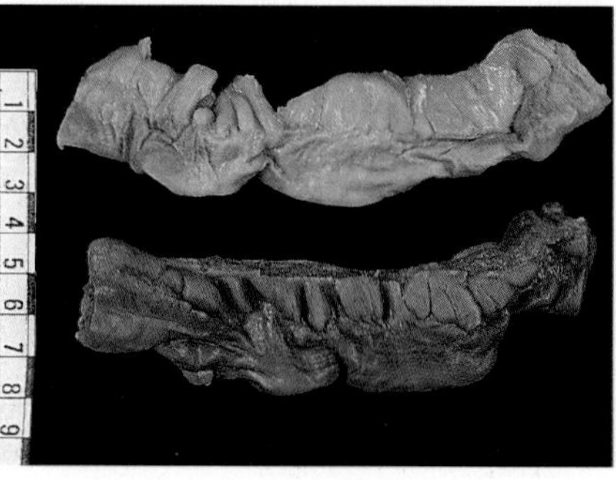

Fig. 7.15 Infarcted bowel which is black (lower specimen). Normal bowel upper specimen.

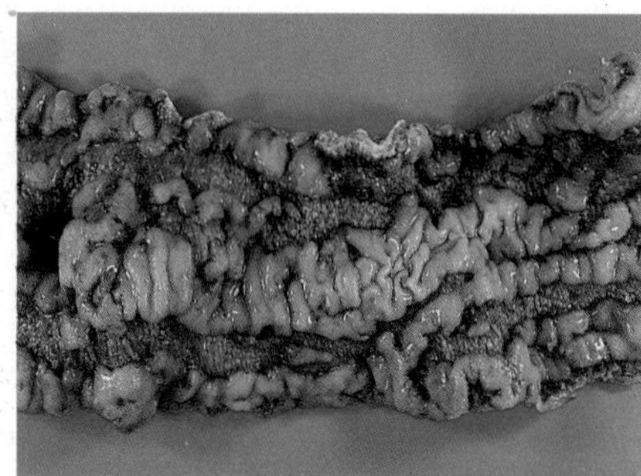

Fig. 7.16 Ulcerative colitis with severe mucosal inflammation and distortion of architecture.

Table 7.4 A comparison of ulcerative colitis and Crohn's disease

Ulcerative colitis	Crohn's disease
Affects the colon only	Any part of the intestines
Diffuse, continuous	Patchy, skip lesions
Particularly distal colon	Particularly small intestine
No scarring	Typically scarring
Superficial mucosal disease	Full thickness of colon wall
No fistulae	Typically fistulae form
No granulomas	Granulomas typical
Disease outside colon is rare	Disease outside colon more common

occurring as well. Complications of ulcerative colitis include haemorrhage, perforation, and occasionally malignant change. Ulcerative colitis is also associated with disease processes outside the colon, particularly in the liver and skin. There may also be eye and joint involvement.

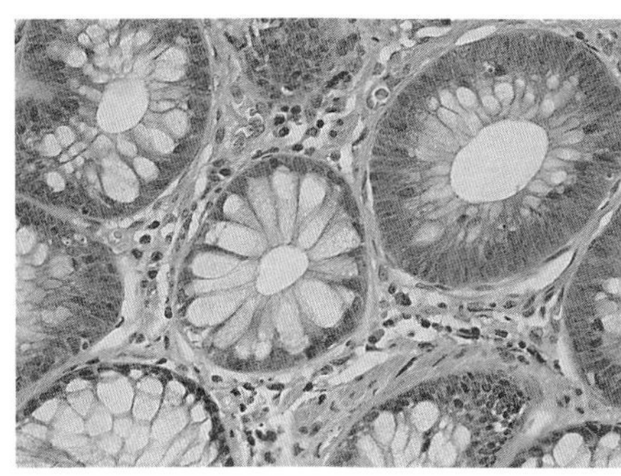

Fig. 7.17 A dysplastic gland with thick blue epithelium, top right, is compared to a normal gland centrally.

Crohn's disease

This is described in the section on the small intestine. A comparison of ulcerative colitis and Crohn's disease in the colon is given in Table 7.4.

Tumours

Benign tumours

A polyp is a nodule which projects above the surface of the mucosa. Most arise within the epithelium and the various common types are listed below:

Metaplastic polyps—these represent localized hyperplastic proliferations of surface epithelium. They have no malignant potential.

Adenomas—these differ from metaplastic polyps in that they show atypical epithelial proliferation. The term applied to the histological appearances of abnormal proliferation of epithelium, with nuclear abnormalities and architectural disturbance with dysplasia. (Fig. 7.17). There are two types of adenoma, one that shows a predominantly glandular or tubular form and the other, which is less frequent, showing papillary projections of epithelium termed a villous adenoma (Fig 7.18). A large proportion of adenomas are of a mixed pattern. They frequently have a well-formed stalk which enables surgical excision (Figs 7.19 and 7.20). The importance of adenomas is their pre-malignant potential in that almost all bowel carcinomas are

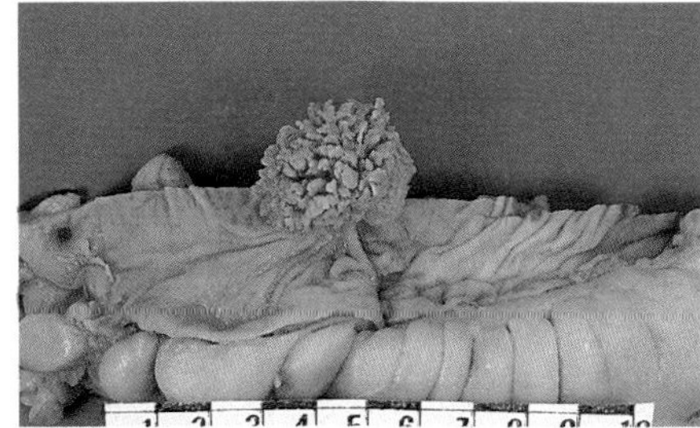

Fig. 7.18 A villous adenoma.

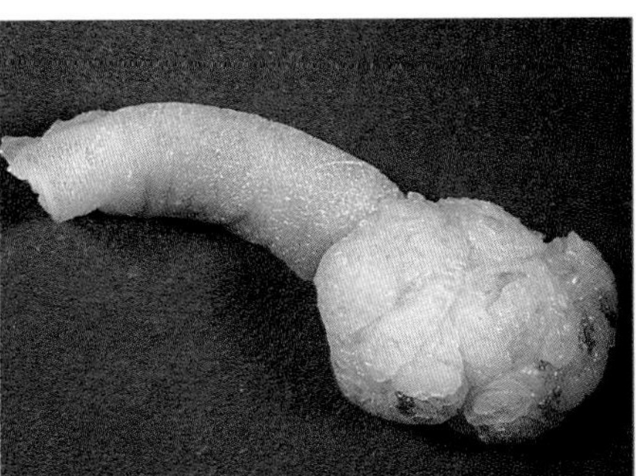

Fig. 7.19 A tubular adenoma with a well-formed stalk.

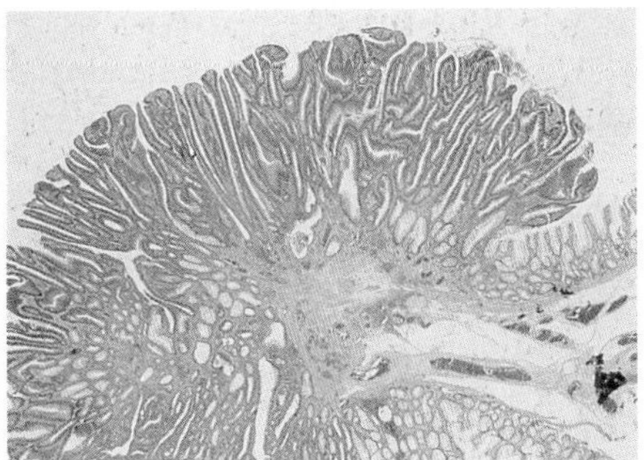

Fig. 7.20 Histology of an adenoma.

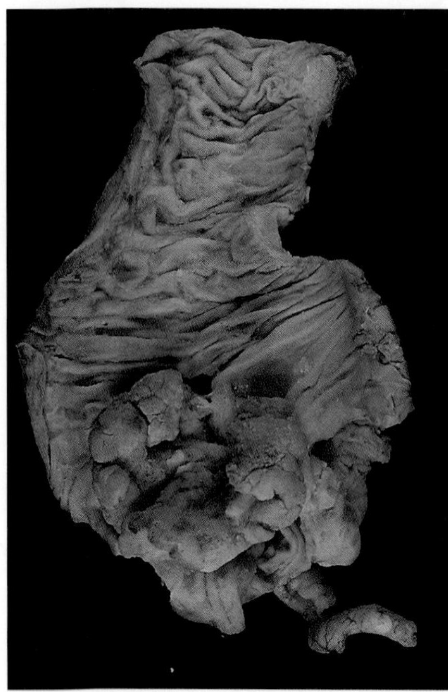

Fig. 7.21 Carcinoma of the caecum.

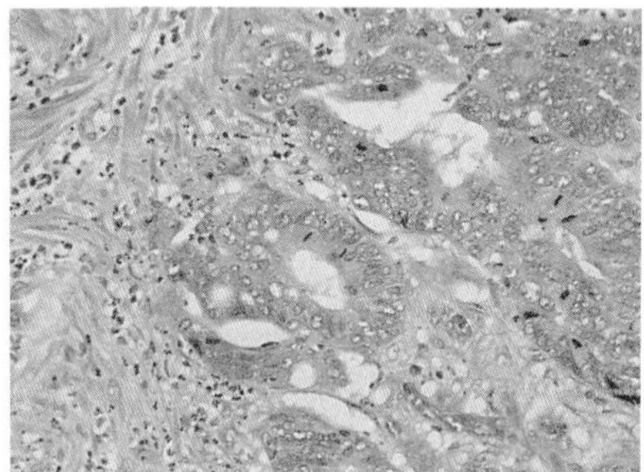

Fig. 7.22 Invasive adenocarcinoma.

derived from adenomas. A progression can be demonstrated in the development of carcinoma starting from benign adenomas which acquire increasingly severe dysplasia. A point is reached when the dysplasia is severe enough to warrant the description of carcinoma-*in situ*. This then eventually progresses to overt invasion through the basement membrane with the development of invasive carcinoma.

Juvenile polyps

These are a form of hamartoma in that they are formed from elements of the lamina propria forming a mass. They are most frequently solitary and may detach and be passed spontaneously.

Malignant tumours

Carcinoma

Carcinoma of the colon and the rectum is a very common tumour. The underlying cause has a strong environmental factor in that it is a Western disease and is seen in people with low dietary fibre. About 25 000 people die a year from colon cancer in the United Kingdom. Other factors implicated in the development of colon cancer are bile acids. It is possible that certain bacteria can degrade bile acids to form carcinogens. Approximately half of all large bowel cancers occur in the rectum. Approximately a third occur in the sigmoid colon. They may present as chronic anaemia due to rectal bleeding or obstruction. They are seen as ulcerated tumours with a raised rolled edge which may project into the lumen and cause obstruction (Fig. 7.21). Microscopically, the majority of these tumours are adenocarcinomas (Fig. 7.22), most frequently showing well-formed glands with or without mucin production. Colon cancer is surgically staged using the Dukes system, named after a pathologist who worked at St Mark's Hospital in London. This is a very useful staging system which closely correlates with overall prognosis of the tumour. It is summarized below and in Fig. 7.23:

Stage A –the tumour has not penetrated the bowel wall

Stage B –the tumour has penetrated the bowel wall to involve serosal tissues

Stage C –the tumour involves lymph nodes draining the colon

Colon cancer has a tendency to show distant spread, particularly to the liver. The five-year survival rate of a stage A Dukes carcinoma is at least 90 per cent. The survival rate of a stage B Dukes carcinoma is 70 per cent, and stage C is 35 per cent.

Other tumours

Endocrine cell tumours. These are derived from the endocrine cells normally found in the bowel. They are predominantly benign and present as so-called slow growing carcinoid tumours.

The anal canal is a site of squamous cell carcinoma.

Lymphomas

As with the stomach, these appear to be derived from the mucosal associated lymphoid tissue of the colon. Lymphomas are much less common in the colon than in the small bowel.

Infarcts

The gastrointestinal tract generally has a very good blood supply with many vascular anastomoses. However, obstruction of large arteries of the bowel can cause necrosis of tissue due to loss of blood supply. The most frequent area of the bowel to be subject to infarcts is the small intestine. Infarcts may be associated with severe atheroma of the inferior mesenteric artery, or be associated with emboli, usually of thrombotic nature. Infarcts may also be associated with inflammation of blood vessels resulting in thrombosis. They are characteristically seen with the naked eye as areas of discoloration of the bowel (Fig. 7.15), with softening and as a late complication perforation. Infarction may also be due to compression of the bowel due to herniation into a structure such as the inguinal canal.

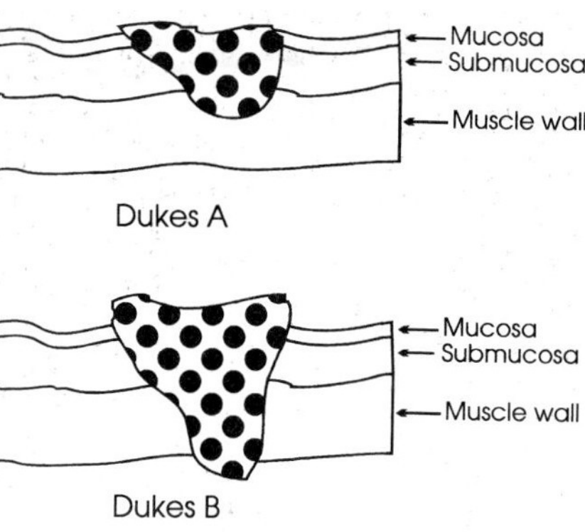

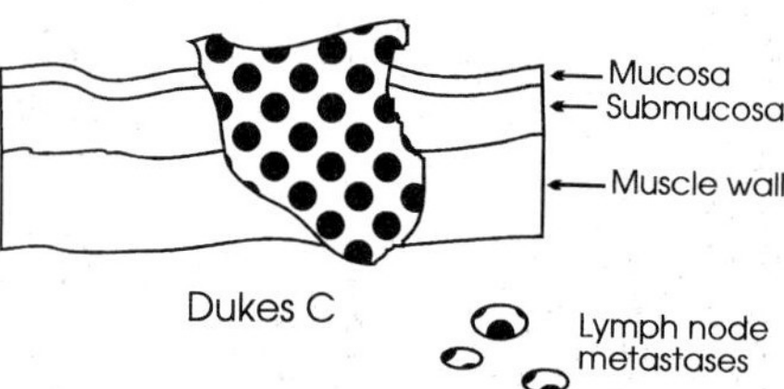

Fig. 7.23 The Dukes classification of colon and rectal carcinoma.

SUMMARY

The mouth

Inflammatory disorders: important inflammatory disorders of the mouth include gingivitis, lichen planus, and lupus erythematosus. Common tumours of the mouth are:

–*Benign*: papilloma, fibroma
–*Malignant*: squamous cell carcinoma

Salivary glands

Inflammatory disorders: common inflammatory disorders of the salivary glands usually relate to duct obstruction and infection and manifest as acute or chronic sialadenitis.

Tumours: there is a wide range of salivary gland tumours. Common types are:

–pleomorphic adenoma
–adenolymphoma
–monomorphic adenoma
–mucoepidermoid carcinoma
–adenoid cystic carcinoma

Oesophagus

Common conditions of the oesophagus are:

–reflux oesophagitis
–oesophageal varices due to portal hypertension secondary to liver failure
–tumours, in particular, squamous cell carcinoma and adenocarcinoma

Stomach

Inflammatory disorders: gastritis may be *autoimmune*, *bacterial* (*Helicobacter*), or *chemical*.

Peptic ulceration: gastric ulcers are due to a reduced host defence against gastric acid and enzymes which protect the gastric mucosa from self-digestion. Acid secretion in gastric ulceration is low. In contrast, duodenal ulceration is associated with increased acid secretion. Both gastric and duodenal ulcers are associated with infection with *Helicobacter pylori*.

Gastric tumours (benign):

–leiomyoma
–hyperplastic polyp
–adenoma

Gastric tumours (malignant):

–adenocarcinoma
–lymphoma

Small intestine

Congenital abnormalities: the most common congenital abnormality of the small intestine is a Meckel's diverticulum.

Malabsorption—causes include:

–coeliac disease
–surgical resection
–impaired digestion
–intestinal damage

Inflammatory disorders:

–infective
–idiopathic
–inflammatory—Crohn's disease

Tumours: these are uncommon, the carcinoid being the most frequently recognized. Adenocarcinoma and lymphoma also occur.

Large intestine

Pathology involving the large intestine includes:

–acute appendicitis
–diverticulosis (diverticulitis)
–ischaemic colitis
–inflammatory bowel disease (ulcerative colitis and Crohn's disease)

Benign tumours:

–hyperplastic polyps
–juvenile polyps
–Peutz–Jegher polyps

Malignant tumours:

–adenocarcinoma (clinically staged using the Dukes classification)
A: tumour confined to the bowel wall
B: tumour penetrates the bowel wall
C: lymph node metastases

8 The liver and pancreas

8 The liver and pancreas

LIVER

The liver is the largest organ of the body weighing an average of about 1500 grams. On light microscopy the liver can be divided anatomically into lobules which consist of stacked units of the liver which are delineated by portal tracts which contain the portal vein, bile duct, and hepatic artery. The portal vein and hepatic artery branch in a repetitive pattern and drain along hepatocyte plates towards the central vein in the centre of the lobule. The bile ducts begin as small channels or canaliculi between the hepatocyte plates which then join up to form large ducts. The hepatocytes closest to the portal vein are exposed to the highest concentrations of metabolites and blood. The hepatocytes in the centre of the lobules receive blood that has already passed through the sinusoids and is depleted of oxygen. The hepatocytes around the central vein are relatively hypoxic. These cells are most susceptible to injury due to low blood flow to the liver. This functional way of looking at the liver is reflected in the acinar method, where the liver is divided into zones. Zone 1 is the liver adjacent to portal tracts, Zone 3 is closest to the central vein, and Zone 2 is between these two zones.

The liver has a very wide function, both being an exocrine gland that produces bile and also an organ that has a wide metabolic activity. It is also involved in the breakdown of haemoglobin to produce bilirubin pigments. The liver produces many proteins such as albumin, clotting factors involving the blood coagulation system, and complement components. It is also involved in carbohydrate and lipid metabolism. Other functions include detoxification and processing of metabolites from the gastrointestinal tract. Clinical features of liver failure reflect this metabolic activity of the liver. Abnormalities in bilirubin metabolism result in jaundice, the yellow discoloration of the skin seen in liver failure. Reduced protein secretion causes oedema, with reduced colloid osmotic pressure due to low protein levels in the plasma. There is, therefore, less absorption of fluid from extracellular areas through the post-capillary venules. Problems in blood-clotting factor production cause coagulation disorders. Failure to metabolize toxins cause cerebral and renal problems. Reduced metabolism of some hormones also manifest as hormonal abnormalities. For instance, excess oestrogens which are not metabolized by the liver may cause enlargement of the breasts in men, known as gynaecomastia. Excessive oestrogens also cause testicular atrophy.

Pathological causes of jaundice

Jaundice is a yellow discoloration of the skin or eyes by bile pigment, in particular bilirubin. Jaundice is usually a general symptom of underlying liver disease. In the case of increased production of bilirubin or reduced clearance of bilirubin from the circulation, the type of bile in the circulation is mainly unconjugated. This means that the bile pigments are not linked to proteins produced by the liver. Conjugated bilirubin is increased in biliary obstruction; the bile that has been conjugated in the liver cells effectively 'refluxes' back into the circulation. There are a wide number of causes of jaundice. They can be summarized as follows.

Haemolytic

Increased production of bile pigments due to increased breakdown of red blood cells. The liver has considerable metabolic reserve and jaundice only occurs with a high rate of haemolysis. The bilirubin in the circulation in this type of jaundice is unconjugated. Organizing blood clot in a haematoma may also produce enough haemoglobin breakdown products to result in haemolytic jaundice.

Hepatocellular

Disordered liver function with reduced metabolism of bile pigments from the circulation. Causes are:

Congenital

Gilbert's syndrome: a relatively common condition where there is mild impairment of bile conjugation.

Dubin–Johnson syndrome: a problem with excretion of bile into the bile canaliculi between the hepatocytes.

Criggler–Najjar syndrome: a frequently fatal disease of infants where there is an enzyme deficiency leading to an inability to secrete bile. This condition emphasizes the importance of normal bile metabolism.

Chronic liver disease

Chronic liver disease may be induced by drugs, toxins, autoimmune disease or viruses (particularly the hepatitis viruses B and C). There is reduced uptake of bile pigments by liver cells.

Viral hepatitis

This subject is covered below; damage to hepatocytes prevents the uptake of bilirubin, interferes with bile conjugation, and disturbs the bile canaliculi.

Liver cell necrosis

This is most frequently caused by viral hepatitis, particularly type B. It may also occur with drugs, toxins, shock, cardiac failure, and septicaemia. In the case of toxic chemicals, the pattern of necrosis depends on the causative agent. Chemicals such as chlorinated hydrocarbons, for example carbon tetrachloride, the anaesthetic halothane, and paracetamol produce necrosis around the central vein (*centrilobular necrosis*). The diuretic frusemide can cause *mid-zonal* necrosis, and phosphorus can cause necrosis around the portal tracts (*periportal necrosis*).

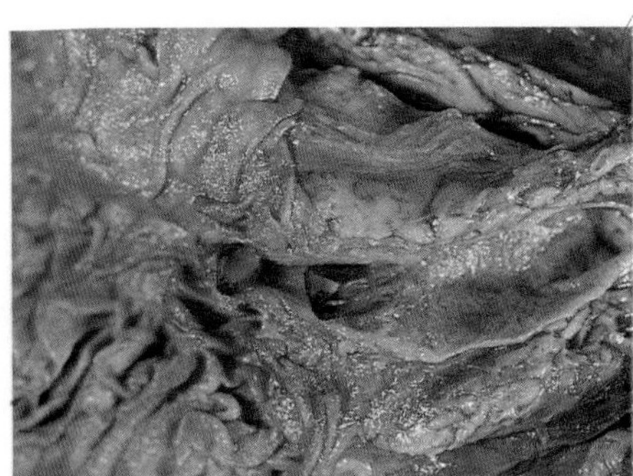

Fig. 8.1 Gallstones in the common bile duct causing obstruction.

Bile duct obstruction

This is reduced secretion of bile from the liver due to obstruction, either within the liver substance (intrahepatic) or within the major bile ducts (extrahepatic).

Extrahepatic

Obstruction may be due to a gallstone (Fig. 8.1), fibrosis of the bile duct due to chronic inflammation, pancreatic carcinoma, or chronic pancreatitis.

Intrahepatic

This is frequently associated with chronic liver disease. It also occurs in cystic fibrosis.

The clinical features of jaundice differ depending on the underlying cause. Typically, jaundice due to obstruction of bile ducts causes pale stools because of loss of bile pigments in the gut with an associated darkening of the urine. This is because of increased secretion of conjugated bile pigments into the circulation which are secreted into the urine. The increased level of bile acids in the circulation also causes a very typical itching of the skin. In addition, there may be increased lipids in the circulation causing the deposition of fat within the skin. Because of the reduced bile production into the gastrointestinal tract there is reduced absorption of fat and particular fat-soluble vitamins such as vitamins A, D, and K. It is very important to tell the difference between jaundice due to intrinsic liver disease, which is primarily treated medically, and jaundice due to obstruction of large bile ducts, which is amenable to surgical treatments. Surgery on patients whose liver function is already compromised by liver damage will make the situation worse.

Cirrhosis

Cirrhosis is defined as a diffuse fibrosis of the liver with nodular regeneration. It is a condition where there has been chronic liver injury with liver cell regeneration and associated fibrosis. The fibrosis occurs when there is severe disruption of the normal underlying liver architecture. It is the end-result of a wide range of underlying causes. It is really a reflection of the limited way the liver reacts to injury. A cirrhotic liver is typically small, firm, and shows numerous nodules on the cut surface (Fig. 8.2). There is disruption of the normal underlying liver cell architecture. It can be classified by the size of the nodules; micronodular cirrhosis is when the nodules are generally less than 0.3 cm in diameter, reflecting the general size of a liver lobule. Macronodular cirrhosis is when nodules are generally bigger than 0.3 cm in diameter. Micronodular cirrhosis is the most common type and can progress to form macronodular cirrhosis. Because of the bridging fibrosis that occurs with cirrhosis between portal tracks and central veins, blood can enter the liver and leave by the hepatic veins without coming into contact with hepatocytes. Liver failure will then result. Due to obstruction of portal veins there may be increased blood pressure within the portal vein giving portal hypertension. Cirrhotic livers are also at high risk of developing liver cell carcinoma (hepatocellular carcinoma). Portal hypertension results in an increase in the size of normal communications between the portal veins and systemic veins. Large varices may develop at these sites. The most important site is the lower oesophagus where these varices may become dangerously enlarged and rupture causing catastrophic gastrointestinal haemorrhage. The causes of cirrhosis are listed in Table 8.1. In summary, any form of chronic liver injury may result in liver cirrhosis.

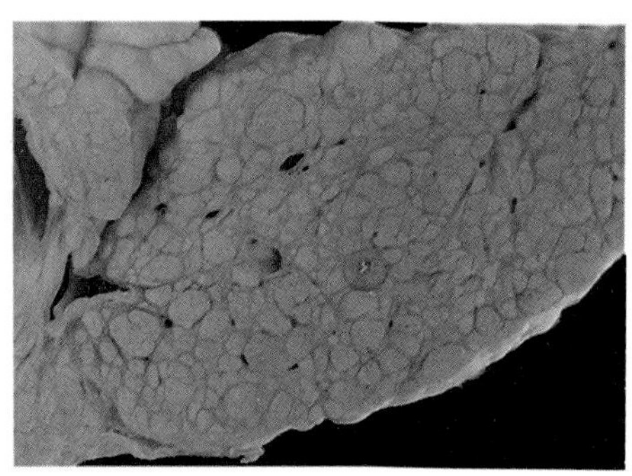

Fig. 8.2 A cirrhotic liver.

It is important to always remember that drugs are an important cause of liver injury (Table 8.2).

Liver disease is generally divided into acute and chronic hepatitis. Chronic hepatitis is defined clinically as a disease that persists longer than six months. It is also a useful pathological classification and this will be covered below.

Acute hepatitis

This is seen pathologically as active liver cell destruction or necrosis. A typical feature is degeneration of hepatocytes with individual cell necrosis (apoptosis). This is a form of active cell death, often immunological in origin. Biochemically, there is frequently release of enzymes, which are normally kept within the liver cells, into the circulation. Causes of acute liver cell injury include viral hepatitis, toxins, such as

Table 8.1 Causes of cirrhosis

- Alcoholic liver disease
- Chronic Hepatitis, either post-viral or autoimmune
- Primary biliary cirrhosis: an autoimmune attack on small bile ducts
- Secondary biliary cirrhosis due to obstruction
- Cystic fibrosis
- Metabolic disorders; galactosaemia, tyrosinaemia, haemochromatosis, Wilson's disease, alpha-1-antitrypsin deficiency
- Vascular disease: veno-occlusive disease, hepatic vein thrombosis (Budd–Chiari syndrome)
- Drugs: long-term cytotoxic therapy, e.g. methotrexate

Table 8.2 Drug-related liver injury

Liver injury	Drug
Fatty change	Alcohol, steroids, tetracycline, phenytoin
Massive necrosis	Paracetamol
Chronic hepatitis	Methyldopa
Cirrhosis	Methotrexate
Cholestasis	Chlorpromazine, anabolic steroids
Fatty change with hepatitis	Amiodarone
Hepatic vein thrombosis (Budd–Chiari syndrome)	Contraceptive pill
Adenoma	Contraceptive pill
Angiosarcoma	Thorotrast, polyvinyl monomer

alcohol or drugs, or obstruction to the bile ducts. Ischaemia tends to cause liver cell destruction around portal veins.

Viral hepatitis

There are at least five viruses which specifically attack the liver. They cause acute hepatitis, and in some cases are associated with chronic hepatitis. Hepatitis A and E spread by the faecal–oral route. Hepatitis B, C, and D spread via blood and other body fluids. These viruses are summarized below.

Hepatitis A

This is a single-stranded RNA enterovirus, 27–29 nm diameter, which spreads from the gastrointestinal tract in a faecal–oral method. It is generally a very mild disease with a very low incidence of chronic problems. It has a short incubation period of about a month and children in particular are susceptible. It appears in epidemics in situations with poor social conditions, and it has a world-wide distribution. In contrast to hepatitis B, no carrier state occurs. Clinically, jaundice is a frequent presenting feature with liver pain and loss of appetite, but it may have no symptoms, particularly in the elderly. In almost all cases there is recovery with no lasting damage. Pathologically, there is liver cell destruction caused by cytotoxic T cell destruction of infected hepatocytes.

Recent infection can be diagnosed by detecting IgM antibodies to the virus which persist in the serum for about 10 weeks. IgG antibodies to the virus appear later and persist for many years giving long-term immunity from further infection. The liver enzyme alanine transaminase (ALT) 'leaks' from the liver during acute infection, and levels are raised in the serum.

Hepatitis B

This is of much more importance, in particular to health care workers having a large amount of blood exposure, in particular dentists. This is a highly infectious virus of double-stranded DNA type, 42 nm diameter, which spreads by the transmission of blood products, in particular by needle injury and sexual transmission. There is about a 30 per cent risk of infection from a needlestick injury of infected blood. The virus has an outer envelope of surface antigen (HBsAg), and an internal core (HBcAg) surrounding the DNA. The 'e' antigen (HBeAg) is secreted into the serum during active infection.

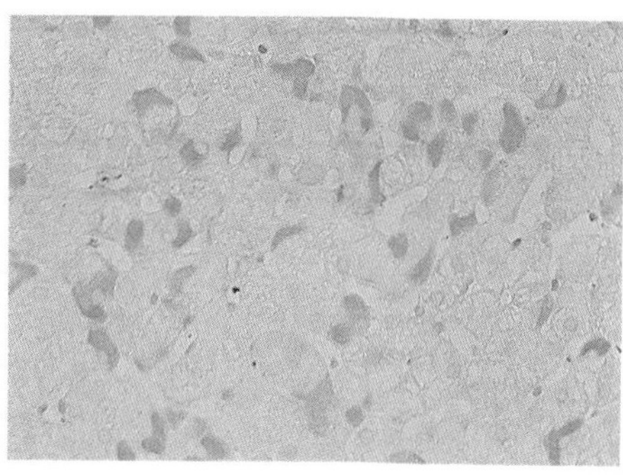

Fig. 8.3 An orcein stain shows brown hepatitis surface antigen-positive cells in the liver.

Hepatitis B has a longer incubation period than hepatitis A, in some situations up to six months. Infection of the virus may be asymptomatic or may cause acute hepatitis. It also has a high incidence of chronic liver cell injury and a carrier state may occur. The incidence of hepatitis B varies dramatically in different countries. In the United Kingdom, the incidence is around 0.5 per cent. However, in certain countries, particularly Africa and South East Asia, the incidence of infection may approach 30 per cent. In these situations there is frequently infection of a child from the mother at birth. The chronic liver disease that occurs in hepatitis B is due to continued stimulation of the host immune system. There is continued attack of the liver by T lymphocytes with subsequent liver cell fibrosis and cirrhosis.

In acute infection, the following appear in the serum in sequence: surface antigen (HBsAg), envelope antigen (HSeAg), and then the antibodies to the core antigen (HBcAg), envelope, and then the surface antigens. Acute infection can be determined by the detection in the serum of surface antigen which is produced in excess by the virus for a short period of time. HBsAg is a component of the surface capsule of the virus particle and can be identified by histological stains (Fig. 8.3). Raised IgM levels to the core antigen, a component of the capsule around the DNA and polymerase of the virus, also indicate recent infection. The presence of envelope antigen in the serum indicates a person who is a carrier and highly infective. If antibodies to the envelope antigen are present, this indicates a low risk of infectivity. Only a small proportion of people infected with hepatitis B virus go on to become chronic carriers. There is a significant risk of chronic liver disease (approximately 2–5 per cent) and eventual cirrhosis with hepatitis B infection.

Immunoglobulin can be given to cover a person who may have been exposed to the virus. There are now very effective vaccines available for the hepatitis B virus.

Hepatitis C

This used to be called non-A/non-B hepatitis and as with hepatitis B spreads by transmission of blood products. It is less infective than hepatitis B with only a 3 per cent risk of infection from a needlestick injury of infected blood. It is a single-stranded RNA virus with a relatively short incubation period of approximately one to two months and is now appearing to be a very common cause of chronic liver cell injury in Europe. Clinical symptoms may be very vague, even in a case of chronic underlying liver injury. Acute infection produces only mild symptoms, but chronic liver disease will develop in up to 50–80 per cent of patients. The virus structure has been predicted using molecular biological techniques; the virus itself has not been isolated to date. Infection with the hepatitis C virus can be determined by detecting serum antibodies to non-structural proteins of the virus.

The rate of infection in the United Kingdom is around 1 in 2000. The only effective treatment at present is alpha-interferon.

Delta agent

This is a small specialized RNA virus which needs an underlying hepatitis B infection before the delta agent can replicate. It is effectively a defective RNA virus. Its surface coat is provided by the hepatitis B virus. It is responsible for many acute exacerbations of disease in the case of a chronic hepatitis B infection.

Hepatitis E

This is transmitted in a faecal–oral route in a similar way to hepatitis A virus. The virus has an incubation period of about a month. It is a single-stranded RNA virus and is usually a mild illness with little risk of chronic liver disease. It is particularly common in Africa, India, and Central Asia.

Alcohol-induced liver disease

In view of the high incidence of excessive alcohol intake in the community, the subject warrants discussion under a separate heading. Alcohol is metabolized to acetaldehyde and acetate by the enzyme alcohol dehydrogenase and to a smaller amount by the microsomal ethanol oxidizing system (MEOS) in the smooth endoplasmic reticulum. Hydrogen ions are produced by alcohol dehydrogenase. In chronic high levels of alcohol intake, there is an increase in the MEOS system. Excess alcohol intake leads acutely to fatty change in the liver because the oxidation of fatty acids is inhibited. There is also increased cholesterol production by hepatocytes. Part of the change may also be due to nutritional deficiency. The change is entirely reversible and as long as the excessive alcohol intake does not persist no chronic liver injury results. Other effects include increased lipid in the circulation and decreased glucose production from protein (gluconeogenesis), the latter making alcoholics prone to hypoglycaemia.

If excessive alcohol intake continues, alcoholic hepatitis develops, with acute liver cell damage and necrosis of hepatocytes. There is also associated inflammation, particularly of neutrophils. It is probable that toxic metabolites of alcohol are responsible for the damage. There may also be an immunological component to the chronic liver cell injury.

Fibrosis may also result in chronic liver injury and this appears to be responsible for the onset of cirrhosis. Alcohol is one of the most common causes of cirrhosis. The fibrosis seen in alcoholic liver disease surrounds individual hepatocytes and central veins in a very typical pattern. There is also scarring around the central vein. The fibrosis in any form of chronic liver injury derives from collagen produced by the perisinusoidal cells. These are otherwise known as the fat-containing cells of Ito. Under the action of cytokines they are capable of transformation into connective tissues cells that can produce extracellular matrix such as collagen and laminin.

Chronic liver disease

In contrast to acute liver disease this is defined clinically as liver disease that persists for longer than six months. Pathologically, it is characterized by a chronic inflammatory infiltrate within the liver, composed of predominantly lymphocytes and plasma cells. There also may be active destruction of hepatocytes by lymphocytes. This is then known as 'piecemeal' necrosis. Chronic liver disease may be induced by drugs, viruses or may relate to autoimmune disease. Some chronic liver disease is due to an inborn error of metabolism, in particular Wilson's disease, alpha-1-antitrypsin deficiency, and haemochromatosis.

Liver tumours

Benign tumours

These are frequently an incidental finding. The most common types of benign tumours are: adenoma, angioma, hamartoma, and focal nodular hyperplasia.

Malignant tumours

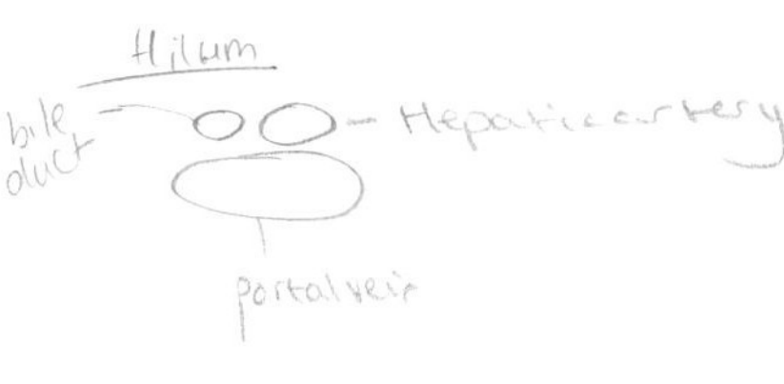

Hepatocellular carcinoma (hepatoma) is the most common cancer in the world with respect to its association with chronic hepatitis induced by hepatitis B infection. Hepatocellular carcinoma almost always occurs on a background of established cirrhosis. Other agents that are known to predispose to hepatocellular carcinoma are carcinogens such as toxins produced by *Aspergillus* fungus known as aflatoxins. These typically grow on peanuts. Many forms of cirrhosis, however, predispose to hepatocellular carcinoma. The next most common primary tumour of the liver is carcinoma of the bile ducts known as cholangiocarcinoma. This is an adenocarcinoma which develops in the bile duct epithelium. It typically occurs at the hilum or root of the liver. A rare but well-recognized connective tissue tumour of the liver is the angiosarcoma. This is particularly important because of its close association with exposure to vinyl chloride monomer. It is also associated with previous exposure to a thorium-containing X-ray contrast medium known as Thorotrast.

Metastases

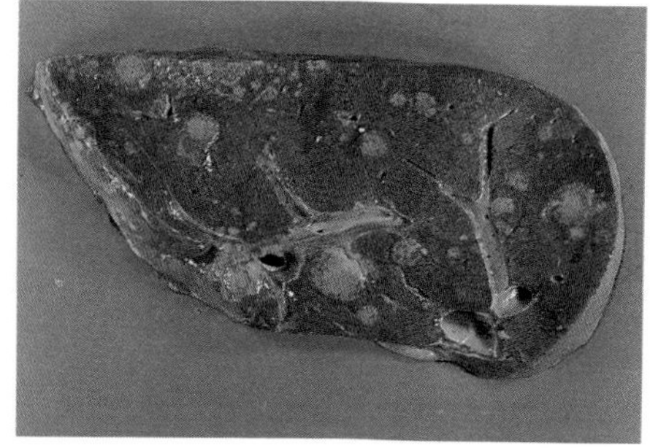

Fig. 8.4 Extensive liver metastases from a colon carcinoma.

It is important to remember that the liver is a very frequent site of metastasis from primary tumours, particularly in the gastrointestinal tract (Fig. 8.4). Other common primary sites include the breast and lung. They are most typically multiple and may be scattered throughout the liver cell substance. The liver involved with metastases may be extremely nodular and enlarged.

GALL BLADDER

The gall bladder is a sac aproximately 8 cm in length which is connected to the common bile duct by the cystic duct. It is effectively a blind-ending sac which is involved in storage and concentration of bile. By the nature of its ductal supply the gall bladder can be removed without any interruption into the flow of bile into the common bile duct. Cholecystectomy is the second most common operation performed in this country and it is usually carried out for chronic cholecystitis and gallstones.

Gallstones

Gallstones are very frequent in the population and are formed by the crystallization of substances derived from the bile. There are three main types of gallstones:

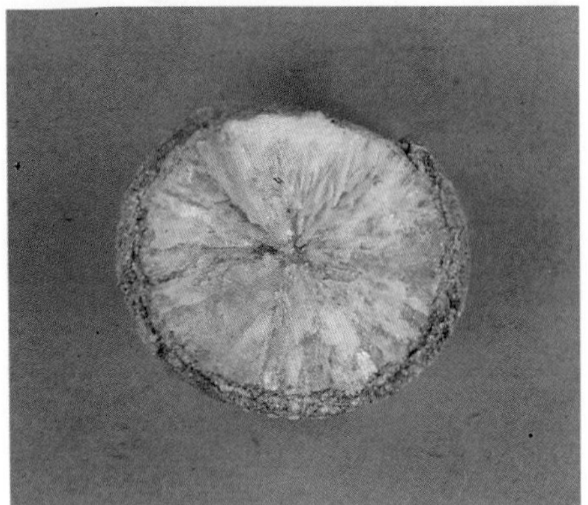

Fig. 8.5 A cholesterol gallstone.

cholesterol, bile pigment, and mixed gallstones. Bile is effectively a supersaturated solution composed of cholesterol, bile acids, and emulsifying lipids, predominantly lecithin. Mucin is also produced by the lining columnar epithelium of the gall bladder and bile ducts. There is a complex relationship between these three main elements of bile. If there is an imbalance in these elements, particularly due to abnormal lipid metabolism, an increase in bile acids or pigment, or bile stasis with infection, then there is an increased likelihood of stone formation.

Cholesterol stones

These are typically solitary, yellow, and range from 1 to 5 cm in diameter. On the cut surface they show a very crystal-like appearance with radiating crystals of cholesterol (Fig. 8.5). They are formed from cholesterol crystals bound together with mucin. They are particularly associated with obesity, hyperlipidaemia, diabetes, being female, and a high calorie diet.

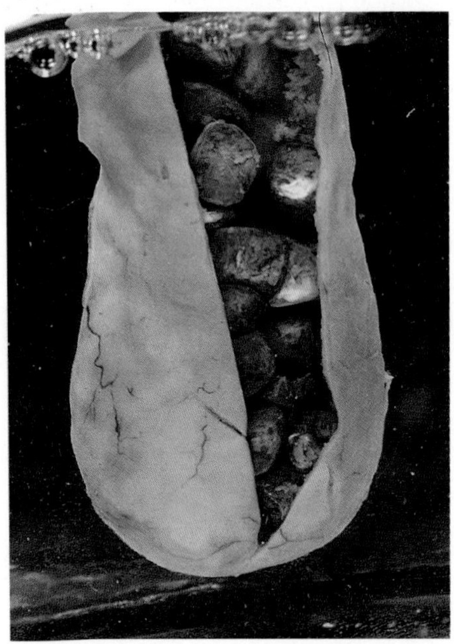

Fig. 8.6 Mixed gallstones in a chronically inflamed gallbladder.

Bile pigment stones

These are particularly frequent in association with haemolysis, where there is increased breakdown of red cells due to haemolytic anaemia. There is also an increased incidence of pigment stones in association with biliary infection, and alcoholic liver cirrhosis. Pigment stones tend to be more or less the same size, implying that they all began forming at the same time. Bile pigment stones are a polymer of bile pigments and are fairly insoluble.

Mixed gallstones

These are the most frequent type and are seen as large numbers of faceted gallstones of various sizes from 0.5 cm up to 1–2 cm (Fig. 8.6). They have a mixture of bile pigments with cholesterol or calcium towards the centre of the stones (Fig. 8.7).

Complications of gallstones

In many cases gallstones, cause no symptoms and have been observed in up to 20 per cent of the population of older age groups. However, a gallstone may obstruct the cystic duct at the outflow of the gall bladder causing distension of the gall bladder. The gall bladder may distend with mucin or, if it becomes infected, pus. This will form a mucocele or empyema, respectively. A gallstone may pass through the cystic duct and enter the common bile duct and may cause obstruction (Fig. 8.1). This may cause obstructive jaundice or, more seriously, pancreatitis. Gallstones are frequently associated with acute and chronic inflammation of the gall bladder (cholecystitis). Carcinoma of the gall bladder is invariably associated with gallstones, although this is a very rare form of carcinoma.

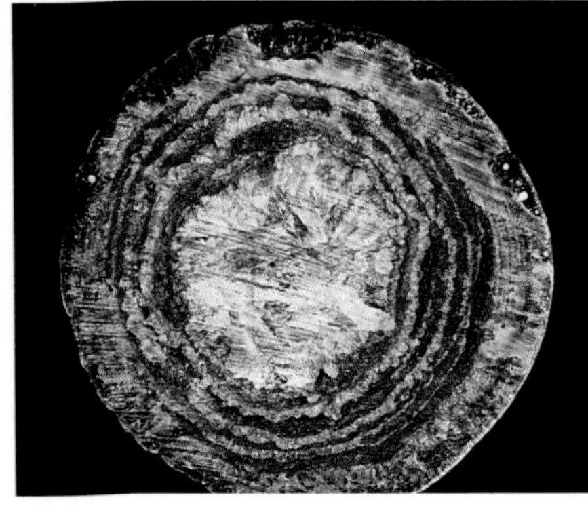

Fig. 8.7 A cut surface of a mixed gallstone.

PANCREAS

The pancreas weighs about 75 grams and lies behind the peritoneum. In view of its deep position it is not possible to palpate it clinically. Also, in view of its position many pathological processes of the pancreas do not present until quite late with involvement of adjacent structures such as the duodenum and stomach. It is effectively two glands in one, having an exocrine component which secretes digestive enzymes and bicarbonate and an endocrine component consisting of the islets of Langerhans. There are four main types of cells within the islets of

Langerhans: beta cells containing insulin, representing 17 per cent of the cells in the islets; alpha cells containing glycogen, representing 20 per cent of the cells; delta cells containing somatostatin, representing 8 per cent of the cells; and pancreatic polypeptide containing cells, representing 2 per cent of the cells of the islets.

Table 8.3 Causes of acute pancreatitis

Gallstones
Pancreatic duct obstruction
Alcoholism
Trauma
Ischaemic shock
Viral infections (mumps, hepatitis)
Hyperlipidaemia
Hypercalcaemia
Hypothermia
Drugs (sulphonamides, thiazide diuretics, azathioprine)

Acute pancreatitis (Table 8.3)

The pancreas contains a high concentration of inactive enzymes that only become active when they are secreted into the gastrointestinal tract. One of the dangers of inflammation of the pancreas is activation of the enzymes which then causes destruction of the pancreatic tissue. Acute pancreatitis is generally due to some form of obstruction to the duct due to gallstones or a tumour. Other factors which initiate acute pancreatitis include trauma, hypothermia, hypoglycaemia, some viral infections which include mumps, reduced circulation as in shock, and some toxins, particularly alcohol. In acute pancreatitis there is extensive leakage of active pancreatic enzymes into the surrounding tissue. Fat necrosis is often a prominent feature of pancreatitis (Fig. 8.8). Also, many toxins may be released into the circulation which may initiate shock.

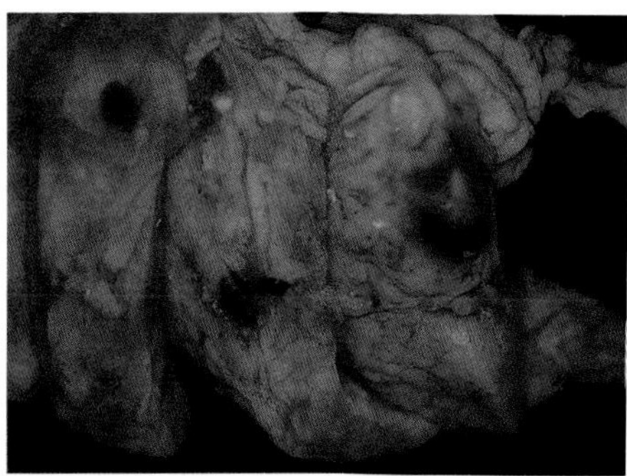

Fig. 8.8 Acute pancreatitis showing areas of haemorrhage and yellow focal fat necrosis.

Chronic pancreatitis

Chronic pancreatitis may occur after repeated episodes of acute inflammation of the pancreas. It is particularly associated with chronic alcohol ingestion. Pancreatitis also occurs in cystic fibrosis in which there is typically severe atrophy of the exocrine pancreas due to chronic duct destruction.

Pancreatic tumours

Exocrine pancreas

The most important tumour of the exocrine pancreas is carcinoma. It is almost always ductal adenocarcinoma and in view of its usual late presentation, the prognosis is very poor. Obstructive jaundice is a frequent presenting feature of pancreatic carcinoma.

Endocrine pancreas

There are a number of tumours that arise from the endocrine cells in the islets of Langerhans. Seventy per cent of these tumours are derived from the beta cells that produce insulin and are termed insulinomas. Twenty per cent of endocrine tumours of the pancreas secrete gastrin, termed gastrinomas (normal islets of Langerhans do not contain gastrin).

Failure of beta-cell function results in diabetes mellitus.

SUMMARY

Jaundice, the yellow skin discoloration, is a general symptom of underlying liver disease. Causes fall into three main groups:

1. Haemolytic.
2. Hepatocellular.
3. Bile duct obstruction.

Cirrhosis: this is defined as a diffuse fibrosis of the liver with nodular regeneration. It is a response to chronic liver cell injury. Causes of cirrhosis include:

–alcohol
–chronic hepatitis (viral, drug induced or autoimmune)
–biliary cirrhosis (primary or secondary)
–metabolic disorders
–vascular disease

Hepatitis: most infective hepatitis is of viral origin. There are at least five viruses which specifically involve the liver. Important viruses are hepatitis A, B, C, and D.

Alcohol-induced liver disease: this is a very important cause of chronic liver failure. Manifestations of alcohol liver disease include acute hepatitis, chronic hepatitis, and cirrhosis.

Liver tumours

Benign tumours: these are rare, the most common being an adenoma.

Malignant tumours: primary liver cancer (hepatocellular carcinoma) is closely associated with cirrhosis due to chronic hepatitis. The next most common primary liver tumour is cholangiocarcinoma. The liver is, of course, an important site of metastatic tumour.

Gall bladder: the most common pathology of the gall bladder is chronic cholecystitis secondary to gallstones.

Pancreas

Pancreatitis: this may be acute, secondary to, for example, alcohol or viral infection, or chronic, frequently secondary to chronic alcohol ingestion.

Pancreatic tumours

Exocrine pancreas: adenocarcinoma of the pancreas is a well-recognized primary tumour at this site. Obstructive jaundice is a frequent presenting symptom.

Endocrine pancreas: tumours may arise from the islets of Langerhans. Most secrete insulin, termed insulinomas.

9 The urinary and male genital tract

9 The urinary and male genital tract

KIDNEYS

The kidneys each weigh 120–150 grams and receive about 25 per cent of the cardiac output, which is disproportionate to their size. The majority of the renal blood flow is to the renal cortex, the site of the renal glomeruli.

The kidneys have a central role in controlling biochemical and metabolic functions in the body. In particular, they are involved in removing unwanted metabolic and biochemical waste products. They also regulate fluid balance and the levels of electrolytes in the circulation. In addition, the kidneys monitor and control the levels of hydrogen ions, carbonate, sodium, and potassium. Functionally, the kidneys act as a filter in which fluid filtrates into tubules from glomeruli and then the fluid is then processed to form urine. Blood is filtered through the basic functional unit of the kidney which is the nephron. Each kidney contains approximately one million nephrons. A nephron consists of a glomerulus where filtration occurs, a Bowman's capsule which collects the transudate, a proximal convoluted tubule, loop of Henle, a distal convoluted tubule, and a collecting duct. Blood flows through glomerular capillaries from the afferent arteriole to the efferent arteriole. Due to capillary pressure, fluid transudes through endothelial pores, endothelial and epithelial basement membrane, and spaces in between the surface epithelium of the glomeruli into the Bowman space. The basement membrane represents the main barrier to fluid passing from the capillary to the Bowman space. A frequent manifestation of abnormalities of the basement membrane is excessive protein loss into the urine known as proteinuria. If there is severe damage to the glomeruli, red cells can escape into the urine and this is known as haematuria. In the proximal convoluted tubule the majority of the sodium in the filtrate is reabsorbed together with amino acids, potassium, phosphate, and glucose. The loop of Henle is involved in water conservation. The distal convoluted tubule is involved in sodium concentration control and this part of the tubule is sensitive to antidiuretic hormone. In the presence of antidiuretic hormone there is marked resorption of water from the distal convoluted tubule. Each distal convoluted tubule finds its way back to its parent glomerulus and at the point of contact there is a specialized region of the tubule called the macula densa. There is also a specialized part of the afferent arteriole and at this point the so-called juxtaglomerular apparatus forms. This is involved in the control of blood pressure and blood flow to the kidneys. Renin is in the afferent arteriole at this point and this is released if there is reduced blood flow into the kidneys. It is also released if there is a reduced concentration of sodium in the distal convoluted tubule. The kidneys also function as an endocrine organ in that they produce prostaglandins which are involved in salt regulation, erythropoietin which is involved in the control of red cell production by the bone marrow, and 1,25-dihydroxycholecalciferol (1,25 dihydroxyvitamin D_3). This is involved in calcium metabolism increasing calcium absorption from the gut and phosphate resorption from the renal tubules. Renal failure occurs when there is inability of the kidneys to deal with waste products produced by the body.

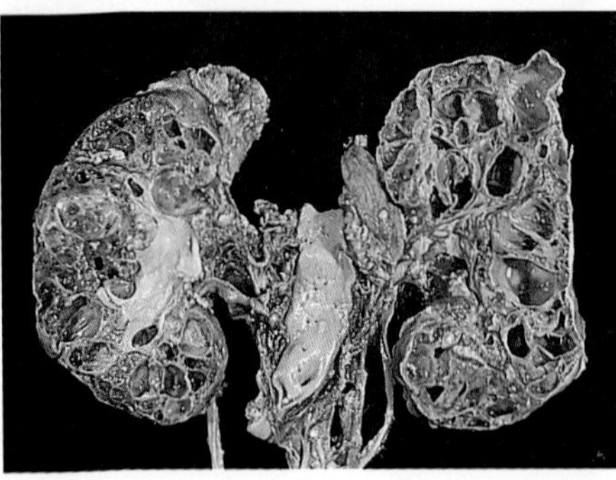

Fig. 9.1 This polycystic kidney disease showing replacement of both kidneys by multiple cysts of varying sizes.

Congenital abnormalities

Congenital abnormalities of the kidneys are relatively common. Agenesis of one kidney occurs in about 1 in 1000 people and displacement to another site occurs occasionally. There are a number of congenital disorders where there is obstruction at various levels in the renal tubules. These manifest themselves as cystic diseases. There are:

–infantile polycystic disease
–adult polycystic disease
–uraemic medullary cystic disease
–medullary sponge kidney

Adult polycystic disease is an important cause of chronic renal failure and has an autosomal dominant pattern of hereditary transmission. It presents in late middle age with renal failure and hypertension, the kidneys being enlarged and replaced by numerous cysts (Fig. 9.1). There is an increased incidence of death from cardiovascular causes. The condition has been linked to chromosome 6, and is associated with a gene called PKD-1. The cysts appear to be due to abnormal proliferations of renal tubules causing obstruction.

Cystic disorders

There are also a number of conditions where cysts are acquired during adult life. Simple renal cysts are very common and represent single obstructed nephrons which fill with urine to form large cysts. Cysts may also be acquired due to scarring. Also, kidneys which are left *in situ* with renal dialysis frequently develop multiple cysts.

Clinico-pathological correlation

The type of renal disease and the site of pathology can be predicted by clinical features, biochemical investigations, and examination of the urine. Some examples of findings and their significance are given in Table 9.1.

The diseases of the kidney can be related to the site of pathology, and are described below:

Glomerular disease

Diseases of the glomeruli are the most common reason for chronic renal failure. These patients are frequently assessed for renal transplantation. Diseases of the glomeruli are usually classified as primary (without any associated disease), or secondary (with another disease present).

Primary: generally immunological, for example, antiglomerular basement membrane antibody, immune complex disease.

Secondary: autoimmune disease, immune complex (infective endocarditis), metabolic (diabetes mellitus, amyloid), vascular disease (polyarteritis nodosa).

As can be seen, the majority of diseases of the glomeruli are of immunological origin. This damage by immunological mechanisms either involves antibodies against the basement membrane of the glomeruli or involves the deposition of immune complexes within the glomeruli. Glomeruli respond by either showing a *diffuse* pattern of disease where the pathology involves all the glomeruli, or a *focal* pattern where only a proportion of the glomeruli are involved. Looking at the glomeruli themselves the changes may either be total (*global*) affecting the whole

Table 9.1 Features of renal disease

Proteinuria	–increased permeability of the glomerular basement membrane
Uraemia	–renal failure
Haematuria	–severe glomerular injury, tumours, trauma
Urinary casts	–glomerulonephritis, nephrotic syndrome, pyelonephritis, acute tubular necrosis
Red cell casts	–glomerlonephritis
Hypertension	–renal ischaemia, polycystic disease
Oliguria, anuria	–renal failure, acute tubular necrosis, urinary tract obstruction, shock, dehydration
Polyuria	–excess fluid intake, diabetes mellitus (osmotic cause; reduced reabsorption from the renal tubules), diabetes incipidus (impaired concentration of urine)
Renal colic	–calculus, blood clot, ureteric tumour
Oedema	–nephrotic syndrome
Dysuria	–urinary tract infection

glomerulus or they may be partial (*segmental*) affecting only a small part of the glomerulus. The term *membranous* is involved when the basement membrane shows marked thickening. There may also be proliferation of cells within the glomeruli known as *proliferative glomerulonephritis*. This proliferation may either involve *epithelial* cells or the cells involved in the scaffold of the glomerulus, the so-called *mesangium*. Finally, there may be a crescentic or eccentric proliferation of epithelial cells within the Bowman's capsule. These terms used above are used to classify different types of glomerulonephritis. Several types of glomerulonephritis are described below.

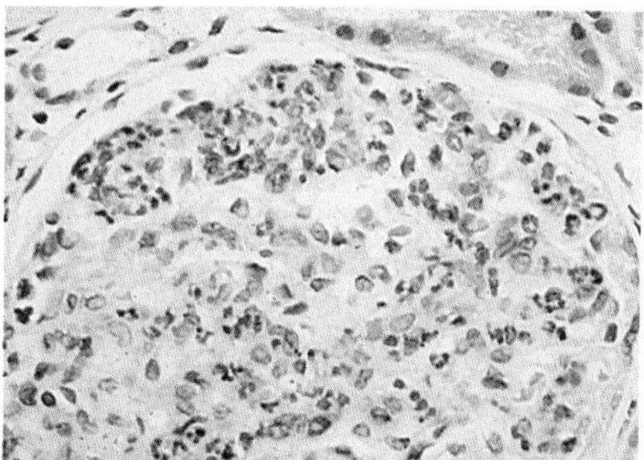

Fig. 9.2 Post-streptococcal glomerulonephritis showing increased numbers of cells in the glomeruli associated with neutrophils.

Post-streptococcal proliferative glomerulonephritis

Immune-complexes are deposited on the basement membrane of glomeruli, and is associated with recent infection by group A, beta-haemolytic streptococci (the same organism that can cause rheumatic fever). These immune complexes stimulate the production of complement via the classic pathway, and neutrophils are attracted to the glomeruli by complement byproducts (Figs 9.2 and 9.3).

Rapidly progressive (crescentic) glomerulonephritis

There is striking proliferation of epithelial cells and associated connective tissue around the inside of the Bowman's capsule, which compresses the glomeruli. The cause is usually unknown, but it may be seen with Goodpasture's syndrome (a good example of an autoimmune disease where there are circulating antibodies to glomerular basement membrane components). It may also be seen with systemic lupus erythematosus, and infective endocarditis.

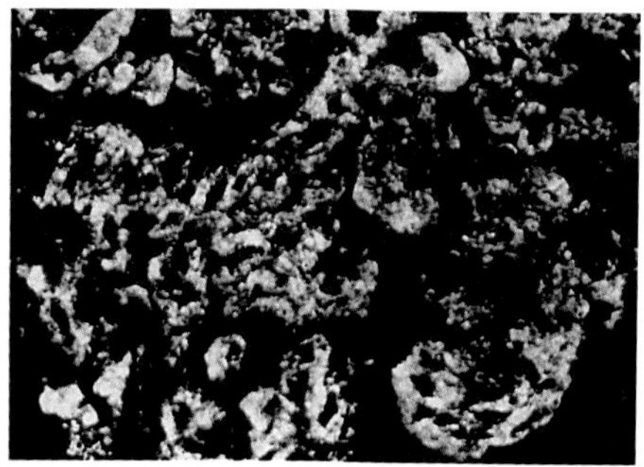

Fig. 9.3 Immunofluorescence of the glomeruli shows deposits of immune complexes in post-streptococcal glomerulonephritis.

Focal glomerulonephritis

This is secondary to other disease in a lot of cases. Examples include:

–infective endocarditis
–polyarteritis nodosa
–systemic lupus erythematosus

Membranous glomerulonephritis

Although the basement membranes in glomeruli are thicker in this disease, they are more 'leaky' and allow large molecules such as proteins to pass into the renal tubules. Causes include chronic infection, and drugs such as penicillamine and gold. Infections that can cause this include syphilis, hepatitis B, leprosy, schistosomiasis, and malaria. Immunological disorders such as rheumatoid disease, systemic lupus erythematosus, sarcoidosis, Sjögren's syndrome, some malignant tumours, transplantation, and bullous pemphigoid are also associated with membranous glomerulonephritis.

Membrano-proliferative glomerulonephritis

This may be seen with systemic lupus erythematosus. There is thickening of the glomerular basement membrane with associated proliferation of the epithelial and mesangial cells of the glomeruli. Other conditions where it may be seen are infective endocarditis, liver disease, cancer in other sites, and polyarteritis nodosa.

Vascular disease

Renal infarcts are relatively frequent because of the kidneys' vulnerable position to exposure to arterial emboli. Common sources of emboli causing renal infarcts are the heart, in particular infective endocarditis and mural thrombi overlying myocardial infarcts.

A complication of essential hypertension is accelerated arteriolosclerosis. This is characterized by intimal hyperplasia of arterioles in the renal cortex. There are also similar intimal changes in larger interlobular arteries. Atrophy and scarring of the renal cortex occurs. Hypertension is an important cause of renal failure.

There may be involvement of the kidney in vasculitic diseases. Examples include polyarteritis nodosa.

Minimal-change

There is a type of glomerulonephritis where there is no abnormality seen on light microscopy, but there is a marked basement membrane abnormality with leakage of plasma protein into the renal tubules causing protein loss in the urine, a low plasma protein, and oedema (nephrotic syndrome). It is seen mainly in children.

Tubulo-interstitial disease

Disorders of the renal tubules

Acute tubular necrosis

Acute tubular necrosis is a condition where there is damage to the epithelial cells forming the renal tubules. There are two main situations that cause acute tubular necrosis: reduced blood supply (ischaemia); and exposure to toxins. The renal tubules generally have a good regenerative capability.

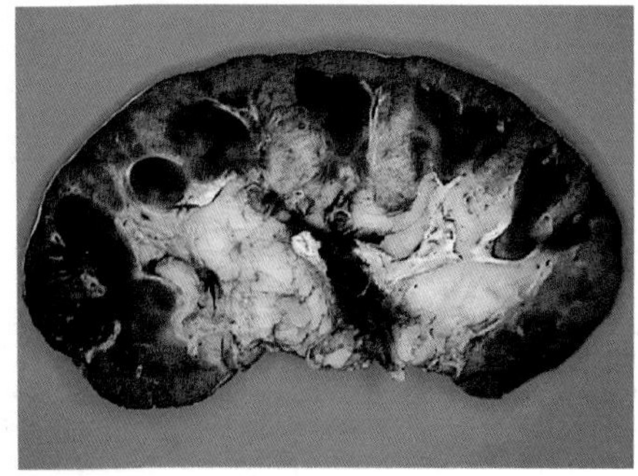

Fig. 9.4 This case of renal cortical necrosis due to bacteraemic shock shows diffuse mottling and pallor of the renal cortex peripherally.

Ischaemia

This is due to reduced blood flow to the kidney with reduced renal perfusion. It may follow a number of situations including blood loss due to trauma and reduced circulatory volume due to loss of plasma in severe burns. Hypotensive shock may also occur in bacteraemic shock (Fig. 9.4). The epithelial damage is due to reduced perfusion of the kidney.

Toxin exposure

Exposure to a large number of toxins may cause renal damage with renal tubular necrosis. Examples are listed below:

- Drugs, including antibiotics such as sulphonamides.
- Non-steroidal anti-inflammatory drugs.
- Organic chemicals: ethylene glycol, carbon tetrachloride.
- Other chemicals: paraquat, heavy metals.

Table 9.2 Causes of nephritis

Toxic (heavy metal)
Immunological
Metabolic (urate in gout)
Physical (obstruction)
Neoplastic (myeloma)
Analgesic nephropathy (aspirin and phenacetin)
Other drugs (sulphonamides, methicillin, other antibiotics
Radiation
Obstruction (may result in hydronephrosis)
Infection (pyelonephritis)
Calculi

Interstitial renal disease

This term describes conditions of a kidney which involve the connective tissue between the tubules. The most frequent interstitial renal disease is interstitial nephritis. Pathologically, there is a chronic inflammatory reaction in the connective tissue between tubules with associated fibrosis and tubular atrophy. One of the most common causes of interstitial nephritis is chronic renal obstruction. Drugs and toxins are also implicated in some causes of interstitial nephritis. Antibiotics are frequently implicated as a cause of interstitial nephritis. Streptococcal infection may result in interstitial disease. Examples of causes of interstitial renal disease (nephritis) are given in Table 9.2.

Other conditions that are associated with interstitial disease include amyloidosis and diabetes.

Infection

The most common source of infection of the kidneys is via the urine in urinary tract infection. Bacteria are the most frequent cause of this.

Acute pyelonephritis. This may be due to spill of bacteria into the kidneys from the urine or from the bloodstream. Infection of the urine is due to reflux from the bladder up the ureters into the renal pelvis. Common sources of haematogenous spread include infective endocarditis or septicaemia. There may be the development of multiple abscesses within the cortex and medulla of the kidney.

Chronic pyelonephritis. This is most frequently associated with so-called reflux-nephropathy. This is a condition which often begins in childhood with a congenital abnormality of the ureters or bladder which allows reflux of urine up the ureters into the kidney during micturition (vesico-ureteric reflux). Reflux of bacteria into the kidneys via the tubules causes chronic interstitial nephritis with marked fibrosis and chronic inflammation. There is also marked atrophy of areas of kidney probably due to ischaemia. Large scars develop over the renal surface with involvement of respective deformed calyces.

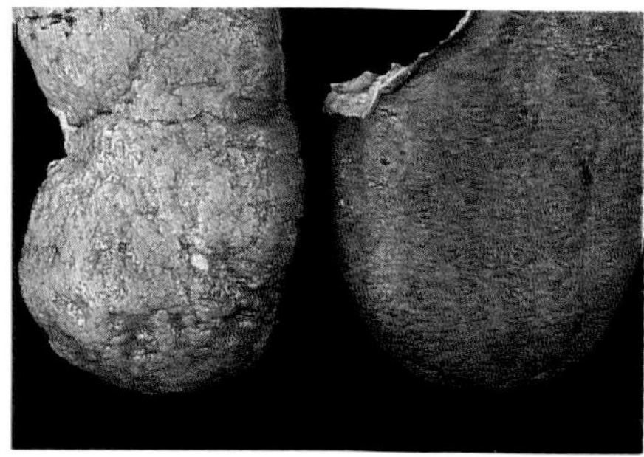

Fig. 9.5 The left kidney is taken from a case of essential hypertension and shows marked scarring and granularity. This is compared with a normal kidney on the right taken from another case.

A similar atrophy is seen in essential hypertension. There is arteriolosclerosis of interlobular arteries causing ischaemic atrophy of the cortices. The kidneys become granular and scarred (Fig. 9.5).

Diabetes

Diabetes is a very important disease with regard to the kidneys in that this condition is a very common cause of renal failure. There are a number of manifestations of diabetic nephropathy and two of these are listed below:

1. Accelerated arteriolosclerosis
2. Glomerular disease, including basement membrane thickening, mesangial proliferation and fibrosis, and nodular glomerulosclerosis (Kimmelstiel–Wilson

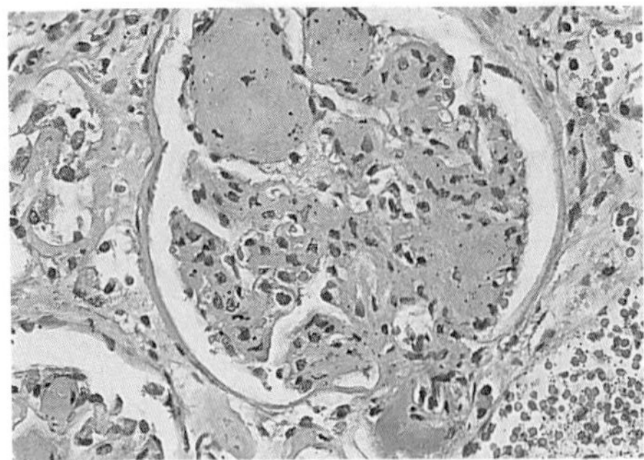

Fig. 9.6 Large pink deposits are seen replacing the glomerulus in this diabetic kidney.

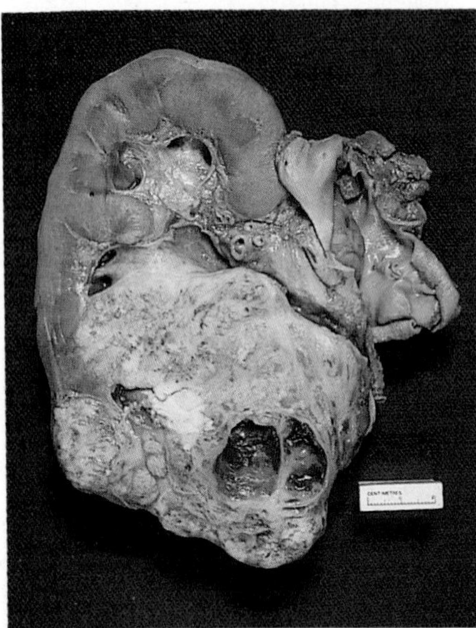

Fig. 9.7 A renal cell carcinoma arising in the lower pole of the kidney.

Syndrome, Fig. 9.6). There is frequently reduced blood supply with ischaemia of the renal papillae and subsequent renal papillary necrosis. The papillae literally fall off the renal medulla into the renal pelvis.

Kidney tumours

Renal cell carcinoma (Fig. 9.7)

This is the most common primary renal tumour in adults and occurs predominantly in men over the age of 50 years old. It represents about 3 per cent of all visceral tumours. It is a tumour that has a very wide range of presenting symptoms. In many cases these symptoms may be extremly vague. The most common presenting symptoms are blood in the urine (haematuria), pain in the loin, and a palpable mass. Patients may also show an increased haemoglobin (polycythaemia) because of increased erythropoietin production. A renal cell carcinoma may also cause hypertension or hypercalcaemia. Renal cell carcinoma is particularly associated with smoking.

A pathological specimen of a renal cell carcinoma typically shows a well-circumscribed but invasive solid tumour which is frequently a yellow colour because of the high-fat content of these tumours. Histologically, this high-fat content frequently gives a typical lace-like or network appearance, the cells appearing very clear. The tumour has a great tendency to invade the renal vein. The other name for renal cell carcinoma is clear cell carcinoma, because of the marked fat content which gives a clear appearance on histology.

Nephroblastoma (Wilms' tumour)

This is the most common tumour of the abdomen in young children below the age of 10 years. The highest incidence of Wilms' tumour is in children aged 1–4 years old. It is one of the 'small cell tumours' of childhood and is a very primitive embryonal tumour that attempts to imitate the fetal kidney. It has a high proliferation rate and therefore has a good response to treatment, particularly radiotherapy and chemotherapy. A Wilms' tumour is a solid tumour within the renal substance which shows invasion. Histologically, the appearance of the tumour resembles that of fetal kidney. The tumours appear to arise from residual primitive embryonal renal tissue which persists after birth (known as blastema).

Transitional cell carcinoma of the kidney

This is an epithelial tumour arising from the transitional cell lining of the renal pelvis. It represents about 10 per cent of all renal tumours. It is typically a tumour that grows outwards from the surface of the renal pelvis, a so-called exophytic pattern of growth. It frequently causes haematuria. Transitional cell carcinoma of the renal pelvis and of the bladder is particularly associated with smoking and certain carcinogens, such as aniline dyes, and certain drugs, in particular analgesics.

THE URINARY BLADDER

Bladder tumours

The most common tumours of the bladder arise from the transitional epithelium and are known as transitional cell carcinomas. There is a whole range of differentiation of transitional cell carcinomas from well-differentiated (grade 1) to poorly differentiated type (grade 3). They tend to be multifocal, suggesting that the same carcinogenic influence is present throughout the bladder. Of note, is that transitional cell carcinoma is of higher incidence in cases of carcinogen exposure to the bladder, in particular aniline dyes and organic chemicals involved in the plastic and rubber industry. Exposure to the cytotoxic drug cyclophosphamide also gives an increased risk of transitional cell carcinoma. It is also associated with chronic irritation due to schistosomiasis (these tend to be squamous cell carcinomas arising from metaplastic bladder epithelium). It frequently presents as haematuria and pain on passing urine (dysuria). In view of the nature of the epithelium growing into a cavity, the majority of bladder tumours initially show a papillary finger-like pattern of growth. They are still called *carcinomas* despite the absence of invasion at this early stage in view of their recurrent behaviour. The more poorly differentiated tumours tend to show a solid pattern of growth (Fig. 9.8). The precursor to many transitional cell carcinomas is carcinoma-*in situ*.

Transitional carcinomas of the bladder are staged by assessing the depth of invasion of the tumour into the bladder wall and distant spread. The UICC TNM system is summarized in Table 9.3. The survival rate from transitional cell carcinoma of the bladder is closely related to the tumour stage (Table 9.4).

Adenocarcinomas occasionally arise from the bladder, usually in association with congenital urachal remants derived from the fetal umbilical cord.

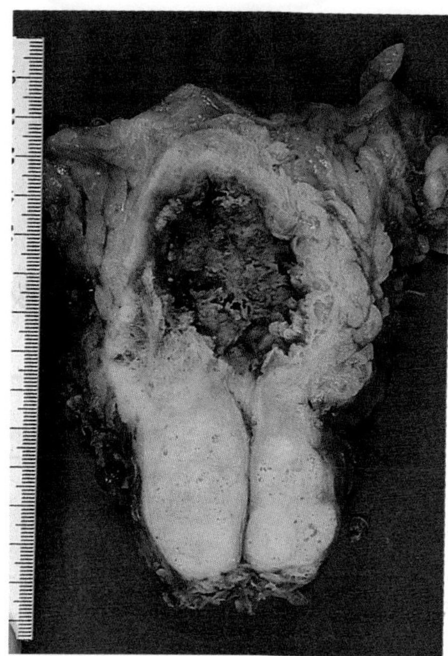

Fig. 9.8 A transitional cell carcinoma extensively involving the bladder. The prostate can be seen below.

Inflammation (cystitis)

Inflammation of the bladder is usually due to infection. It may also be due to physical agents such as urinary catheterization, radiation, or drugs. Stones may develop in association with infection. Hypercalcaemia may also induce stones.

Table 9.3 The staging of bladder cancer

Tcis	Carcinoma-*in situ*
Ta	Papillary non-invasive
T1	Invasion of lamina propria only
T2	Invasion of superficial muscle
T3a	Invasion of deep muscle
T3b	Invasion through the full thickness of bladder wall
T4	Tumour fixed or involving adjacent pelvic structures

PROSTATE

Prostatitis

This may be due to sexually transmitted organisms such as gonococcus or *Chlamydia*, or may be due to Gram-negative organisms introduced during surgical procedures.

Benign nodular hyperplasia

Androgens and oestrogens are involved in the cause of this condition. It is characterized by nodular enlargement of the prostate around the urethra (Fig. 9.9), and commonly results in bladder outflow obstruction. This may cause bladder wall hypertrophy (Fig. 9.10), an increased risk of urinary tract infection, and, in severe cases, hydronephrosis of both kidneys (Fig. 9.11). The normal prostate weighs about 20 g, but in nodular hyperplasia glands of more than 100 g may result. The incidence of the condition increases with age, from 70 per cent of 60-year-olds to 90 per cent of 90-year-olds.

Table 9.4 Five-year survival rates of transitional cell carcinoma of the bladder

Ta	95%
T1	80%
T2	50%
T3	40%
T4	20%

Adenocarcinoma

This is the second most common cancer in males. It is a disease of men over 50 years of age, and is a common cause of male cancer death. It arises in the peripheral zone of the prostate (Fig. 9.12), and is very frequent incidental finding at post-mortem. The

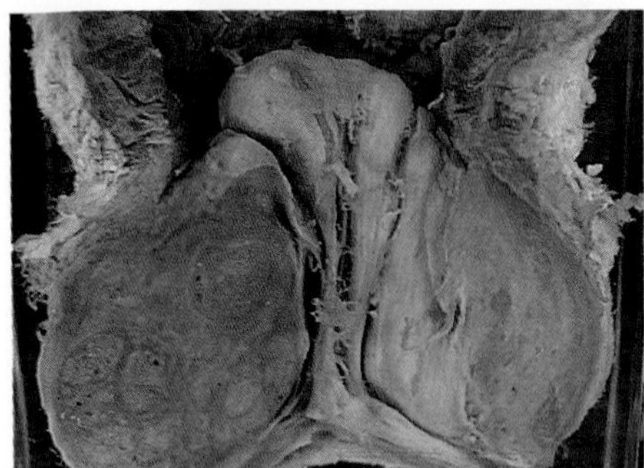
Fig. 9.9 Benign nodular hyperplasia of the prostate showing marked enlargement of the median lobe centrally.

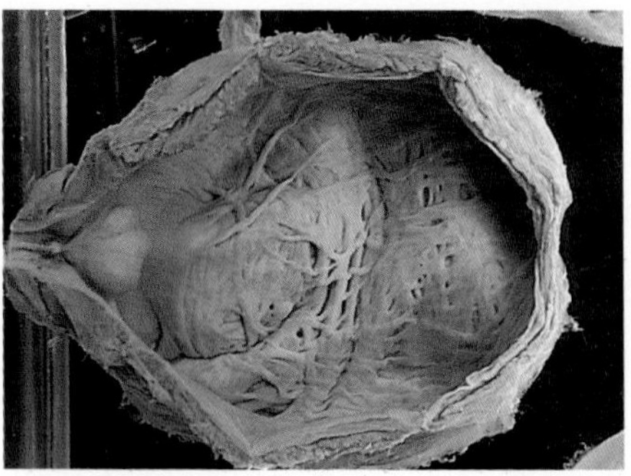
Fig. 9.10 A large dilated and hypertrophic bladder due to outflow obstruction due to prostate hyperplasia.

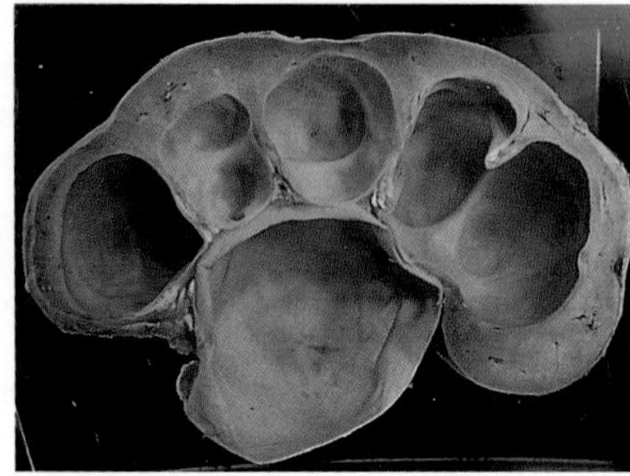
Fig. 9.11 A hydronephrotic kidney.

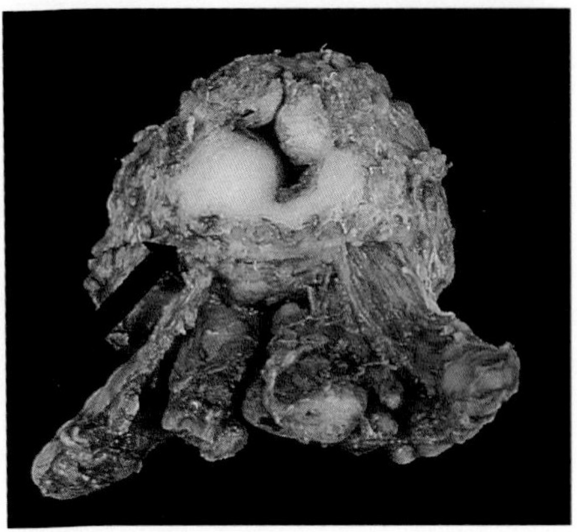
Fig. 9.12 Solid white prostate carcinoma to the left of the urethra.

development of the tumour is a testosterone-dependent. The marker, *prostate-specific antigen*, is raised in the serum in cases of prostatic cancer, and is a useful diagnostic marker for diagnosing and monitoring the disease. It initially spreads locally and then typically spreads via the bloodstream to involve bones. The metastases in bone are typically associated with an increase in bone formation, termed osteosclerosis.

Studies have shown that up to a third of men over 50 harbour foci of prostate carcinoma. This increases by up to 80 per cent in men over the age of 75. One problem with prostate cancer is early detection. Established prostate carcinoma is palpable at rectal examination. The majority of prostatectomy specimens show marked direct spread within the prostate gland, particularly to the capsule. There may be lymphatic involvement with spread to sacral, para-aortic, and iliac lymph nodes. Bloodstream spread occurs to bone, lungs, and liver. Staging of prostate cancer related to prognosis. This is summarized in Table 9.5.

Table 9.5 The staging of prostate cancer

Stage A	Incidental (latent) carcinoma
Stage B	Tumour confined to prostate
Stage C	Tumour extended outside of prostate but no distant metastases
Stage D	Distant metastases

TESTES

Important pathological conditions of the testis are detailed below.

Undescended testis

This is also known as cryptorchidism, and is a failure of the testis to descend from the inguinal canal during development. The affected testis becomes atrophic if it is not placed in its normal position. There is also an increased risk of testicular tumours in these testes.

Infections

Well-recognized testicular infections are shown in Table 9.6.

Tumours

The three most common tumours of the testes are: the *teratoma*, occuring in young men (Fig. 9.14); the *seminoma*, occurring in middle-aged men; and *lymphoma*, a tumour of the elderly. These are listed in Table 9.7.

Testicular tumours are usually staged to aid the planning of treatment and prognosis. The staging is summarized in Table 9.8.

Table 9.6 Testicular infections

Tuberculosis (Fig. 9.13)
Mumps virus
Syphilis
Gram-negative bacteria
Gonococcus
Salmonella

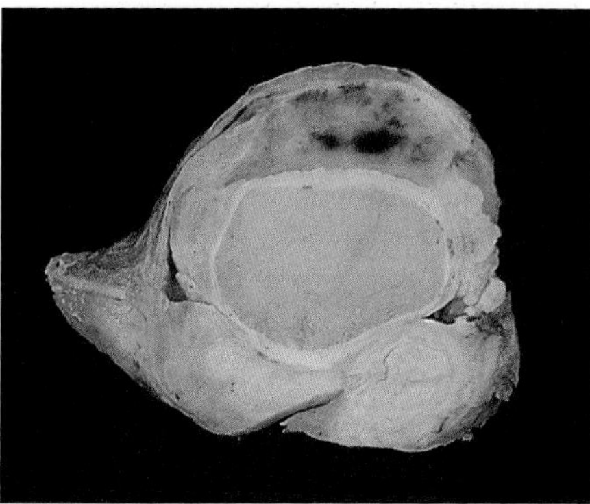

Fig. 9.13 Tuberculosis of the testis showing dense granulomatous inflammation and fibrosis surrounding the testicle.

Table 9.7 Testicular tumours

Germ cell tumours (Fig 9.14):
Seminoma
Teratoma (usually mixed with embryonal carcinoma)
Embryonal carcinoma
Yolk sac (endodermal sinus) tumour
Choriocarcinoma
Non-germ cell tumours
Lymphoma
Leydig cell tumour
Sertoli cell tumour

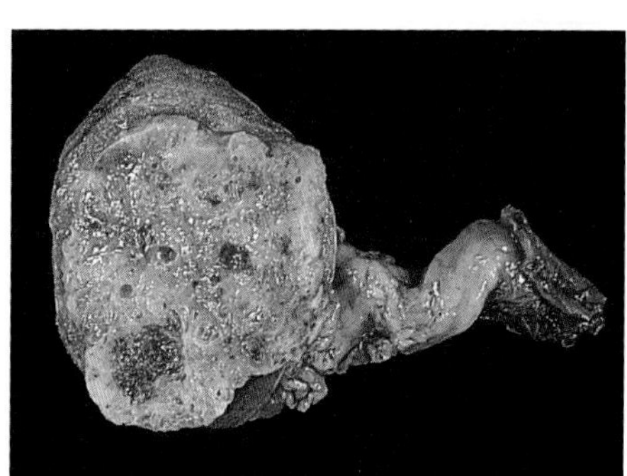

Fig. 9.14 A teratoma of the testis which almost completely replaces the organ. The teratoma shows numerous mucus-filled cysts as well as solid white areas.

Table 9.8 The staging of testicular tumours

Stage 1	Tumour confined to the testis
Stage 2	Tumour involving testis and para-aortic lymph nodes
Stage 2a	Radiological evidence of nodal metastasis
Stage 2b	Retroperitoneal disease
Stage 3	Mediastinal and/or supraclavicular lymph node involvement
Stage 4	Visceral metastases

SUMMARY

Kidney

Congenital abnormalities: these are relatively common. Examples include:

–agenesis

–cystic disease of both infants and adults

Glomerular disease: glomerulonephritis is the most common primary glomerular disease. There are many types, classified by morphological features. Most glomerular disease is of immunological origin.

Tubulo-interstitial disease

Renal tumours

–renal cell carcinoma
–transitional cell carcinoma
–nephroblastoma (Wilms' tumour)

Urinary bladder: the most common pathology of the bladder is:

–cystitis
–transitional cell carcinoma

Prostate: important pathology of the prostate includes:

–prostatitis
–benign nodular hyperplasia
–adenocarcinoma

Testis: important pathological conditions of the testis are:

–undescended testis
–infections
–tumours (particularly of germ cell origin)

10 The female genital tract

10 The female genital tract

VULVA

Vulval dystrophy

The term vulval dystrophy applies to quite a wide range of pathology involving the skin of that area. The term leukoplakia describes a white appearance of the skin and has no specific pathological meaning. It is really a manifestation of increased keratinization. Vulval dystrophy may either be hyperplasic or dysplastic.

Hyperplastic vulval dystrophy

This includes simple hyperplasia of the epidermis, termed squamous hyperplasia. The other form of vulval dystrophy in this group is lichen sclerosis. This is a condition of unknown cause which characteristically shows marked fibrosis of the dermis with a chronic inflammatory infiltrate superficially.

Malignant vulval tumours

The most common tumour of the vulva is squamous carcinoma which arises typically in elderly women. Melanoma has a higher incidence in the vulva than would be expected for that site. There is a form of intra-epithelial adenocarcinoma that occurs within the epidermis of the vulva called Paget's disease. This appears to arise from adnexal glands in that area.

UTERINE CERVIX

Squamous cell carcinoma

Squamous carcinoma of the cervix is the most common tumour at this site (Fig. 10.1). The tumour shows a pattern of incidence that suggests that a transmissible agent underlies its cause. Risk factors include multiple sexual partners, early age at first intercourse, and smoking.

A manifestation of human papilloma virus is the development of warts, either on the cervix or vulva. Human papilloma virus types 6, 11, 16, and 18 show a particular association with the lower female genital tract. HPV 6 and 11 are associated with benign genital warts. HPV 16 and 18 are, however, associated with neoplasia of the cervix.

The early preneoplastic changes in the cervix occur in the transformation zone between the ectocervical squamous epithelium and the endocervical mucinous columnar epithelium. A progression of dysplasia can be seen to develop from mild, moderate to severe (Figs 10.2, 10.3, and 10.4). The cytology screening programme aims to detect these pre-invasive neoplastic changes and to allow treatment before the development of overt squamous carcinoma.

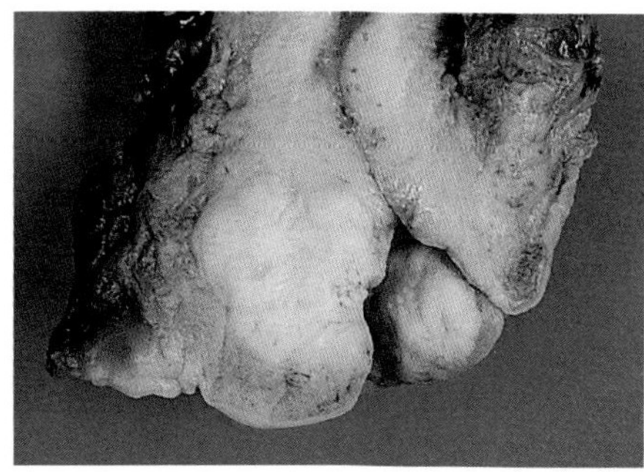

Fig. 10.1 Carcinoma of the cervix appearing as a white tumour involving one side of the cervical os. The tumour deeply invades into the cervical stroma.

Invasive squamous carcinoma occurs when there is invasion of dysplastic epithelial cells through the basement membrane into the subepithelial connective

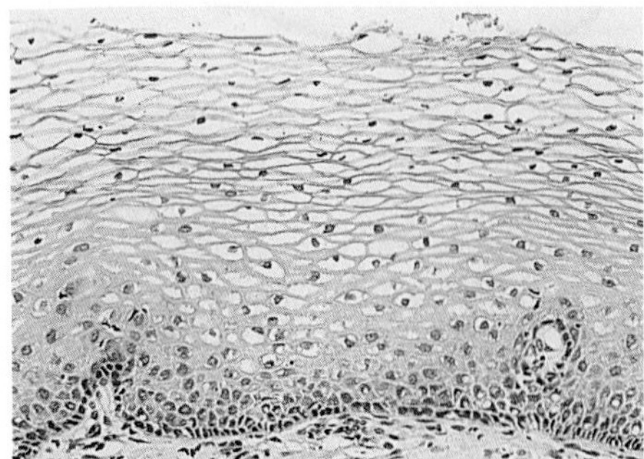

Fig. 10.2 Normal ectocervical epithelium which is squamous in type and very similar to oral epithelium. The basal layer is very thin at the bottom.

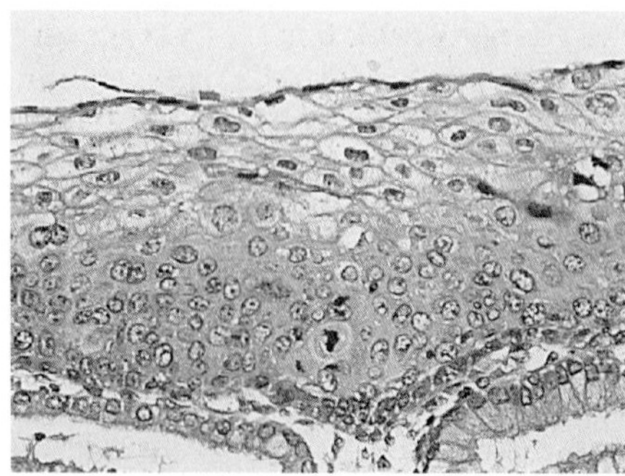

Fig. 10.3 Moderately dysplastic squamous epithelium of the cervix showing mitotic figures above the basal layer and increased numbers of basal cells which are atypical.

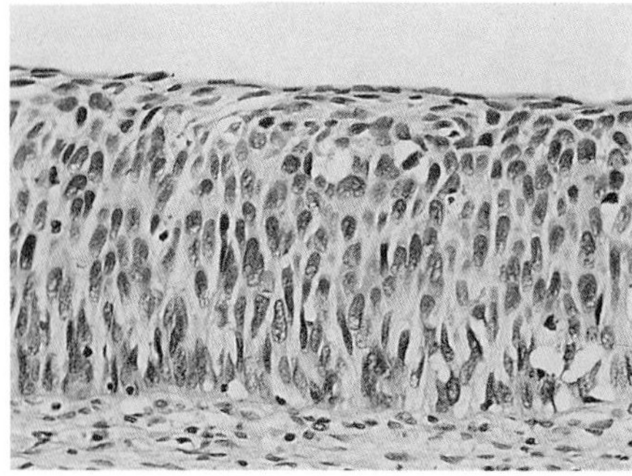

Fig. 10.4 Severe dysplasia of the cervical epithelium (carcinoma *in situ*) showing full thickness dysplasia. There is no invasion yet.

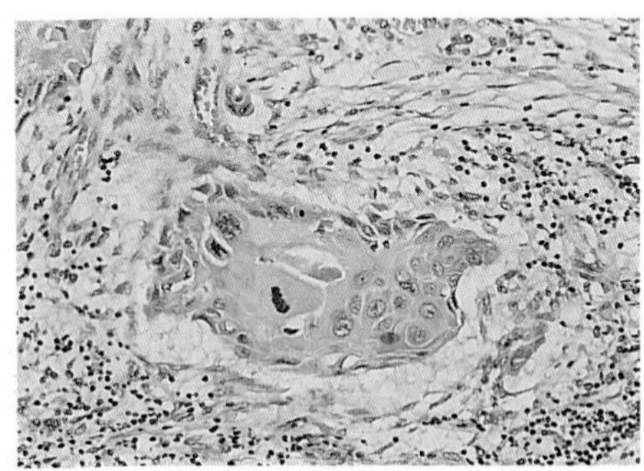

Fig. 10.5 Overtly invasive keratinizing squamous cell carcinoma invading into the stroma. There is a mitotic figure in the centre of the epithelial island.

tissue of the cervix (Fig. 10.5). The prognosis directly relates to the size and depth of invasion of the tumour and the absence or presence of lymph node metastases in regional sites.

Stage 1 cancer is confined to the cervix; stage 2 cancer extends beyond the cervix but not to the pelvic wall; stage 3 carcinoma involves the pelvic wall and lower third of the vagina; stage 4 cancer is when the tumour has extended outside the gynaecological tract.

Dysplasia and invasive carcinoma in the endocervical mucinous epithelium is becoming increasingly common. An equivalent premalignant phase within the endocervical tract can be seen, termed glandular neoplasia. This also shows a similar spectrum from mild to severe disease before overt invasive adenocarcinoma.

UTERUS

Endometrium

The endometrium is the lining of the endometrial cavity which is composed of two elements, glandular and stromal tissue. Both are sensitive to the hormonal environment, in particular, levels of oestrogen and progestogen. There are two main phases to the menstrual cycle, a proliferative phase and a secretory phase. In the proliferative phase, which is in a oestrogenic environment, there is proliferation of glandular epithelium. Ovulation then occurs and there is a switch to a progestogen environment where glands show marked secretory activity in preparation for possible implantation of an embryo. The endometrium is shed at menstruation. In view of the hormonal sensitivity of the endometrium many pathological processes in this tissue relate to the hormonal environment.

Endometrial hyperplasia

This is a process where there is a disproportionate increase in endometrial glands within the endometrial mucosa. It generally occurs with unopposed oestrogen secretion. It may be simple, complex, or show atypical features. If atypia is present there is a higher incidence of malignant change.

Endometrial adenocarcinoma

This is the most common malignancy of the endometrium and is strongly associated with unopposed oestrogen secretion. It is primarily a post-menopausal tumour. The depth of invasion of the myometrium of the uterus is the most important prognostic factor in the disease. Surgical excision is the main form of treatment. Stage 1 disease is when the tumour is confined to the uterus body; stage 2 is when the cervix is also involved; stage 3 is when the tumour has penetrated the uterus but is not outside the pelvis; and stage 4 is when there is involvement of the bladder, rectum, or sites outside the pelvis.

Adenomyosis

This is effectively endometriosis occurring within the muscle of the myometrium. It may be superficial, when endometrial glands and stroma are present rather deeper than is normally seen in the myometrium. Overt adenomyosis may form a tumour-like lesion which resembles a so-called fibroid. Strictly, endometriosis is defined as the presence of endometrial stroma, glands, and evidence of haemorrhage due to menstrual activity. There is often striking smooth muscle hypertrophy associated with adenomyosis.

Myometrium

The most common pathology affecting the myometrium is the so-called fibroid which represents a smooth muscle tumour (leiomyoma) arising from the smooth muscle of the uterus. Fibroids occur during late reproductive life and around the time of the menopause. They show an oestrogen-dependent growth in many cases, explaining their age distribution. They are seen as well-circumscribed pale masses within the myometrium, with a very characteristic whorled appearance (Fig. 10.6). If they get very large they may show central degeneration. They may vary from 0.2 cm up to 30 cm or more in diameter. They are almost always benign. Smooth muscle tumours with a high mitotic rate have a higher incidence of metastasis. Clinically, they are associated with menstrual irregularity, infertility, and may cause obstetric problems if very large.

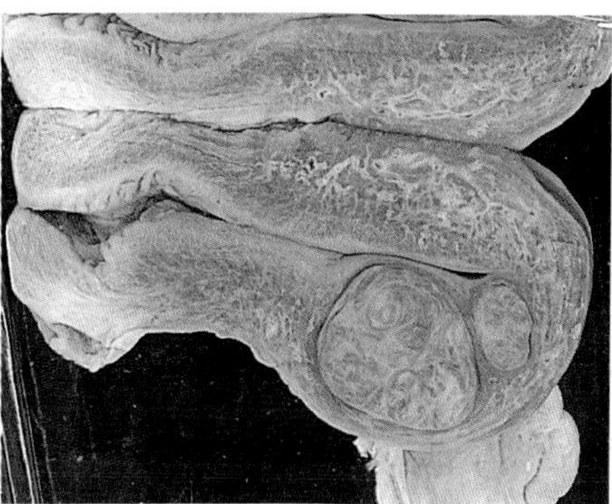

Fig. 10.6 Typical uterine fibroids in the wall of the uterus.

OVARIES

Endometriosis

This is the presence of endometrium outside of the normal situation within the endometrial cavity. The ovary is a frequent site of deposition of endometriosis. Other sites include the peritoneum adjacent to the uterus, including the pouch of Douglas posteriorly. It may also occur in the adjacent bladder and small and large bowel. Histologically, there is deposition of endometrial glands and stroma with associated haemorrhage. There is also frequently fibrosis and muscle hypertrophy associated with the endometriotic foci. Large blood-filled cysts may develop. Many of the problems of endometriosis relate to the striking scarring and recurrent haemorrhage that occurs in the condition.

Ovarian cysts

These are a very common discovery at laparotomy and are frequently removed. They may be physiological, in the sense that they develop from a normal developing follicle or corpus luteum during the menstrual cycle (Fig. 10.7). They also may be developed from pathological processes, such as endometriosis and, as will be discussed later, they may be derived from tumours. Benign epithelial lined cysts of the ovary are relatively common.

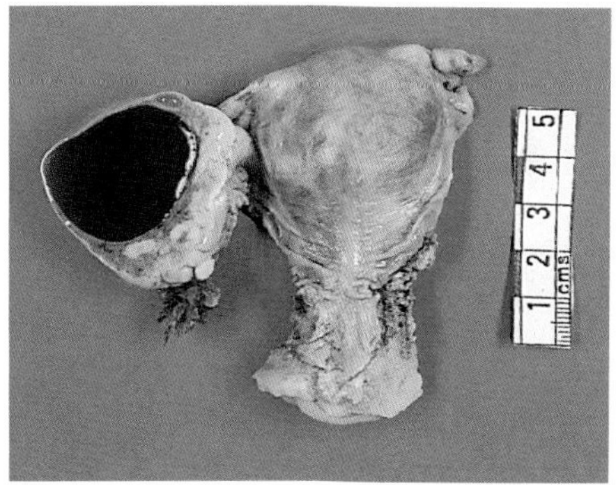

Fig. 10.7 The ovary contains a benign functional cyst contaning brown fluid.

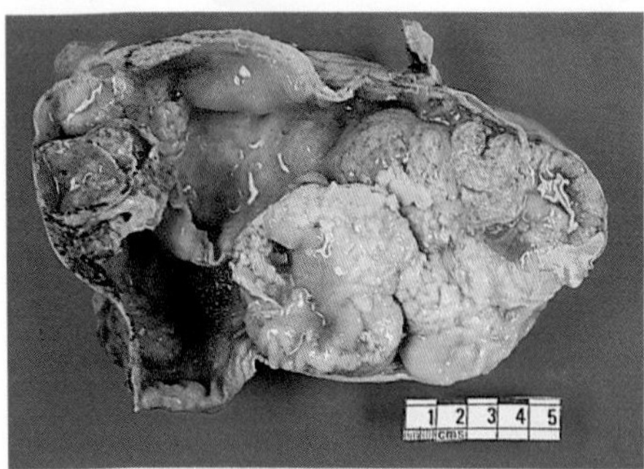

Fig. 10.8 An ovarian carcinoma showing extensive solid areas as well as cystic regions.

Tumours

Epithelial-derived tumours

An important concept in the understanding of epithelial tumours of the female genital tract is that Müllerian epithelium is capable of differentiating towards any of the types seen in the normal endocervix, endometrium, or uterine tube. Epithelial tumours of the ovary therefore can be of mucinous, endometrioid or serous type, respectively. Mucinous tumours of the ovary predominantly show a columnar mucus-secreting epithelium resembling that in the endocervix. Endometrial-like tumours (endometrioid) show a glandular structure resembling that of endometrium. Serous tumours show tubal-type epithelium which is a mixed ciliated and non-ciliated epithelium. Any of the three types of epithelial tumours can either be of benign type, overtly malignant, or show features of possible malignant potential, known as borderline change. Borderline tumours may show nuclear dysplasia but do not show the invasion seen in overt invasive carcinoma.

The benign ovarian cysts are totally cystic with no solid areas. Carcinoma, in contrast, shows solid invasive areas (Fig. 10.8).

Tumours derived from germ cells

The ovary, as with the testis, is unique in having a population of cells which are primarily a reservoir of genetic information. They are cells which, by their very nature, are capable of differentiation in many pathways, particularly in all three pathways of a developing embyro (ecto-, meso-, and endoderm). The term applied to this phenomenon is totipotent. In general, germ cell tumours of the ovary are similar to germ cell tumours of the testis. The most common types are listed below:

–dysgerminoma
–teratoma
–tumours resembling placental tissue (extra-embryonic)

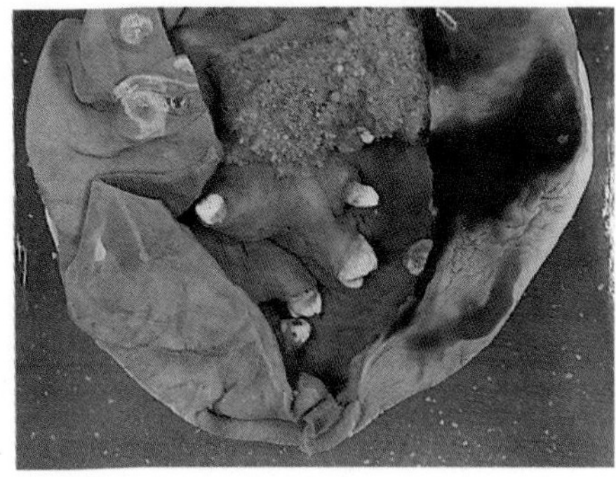

Fig. 10.9 A cystic teratoma of the ovary (dermoid cyst) containing teeth.

Dysgerminomas resemble testicular seminomas. A teratoma is a tumour in which there is a mixture of elements which are not normally found at the site of the tumour. Teratomas may also be entirely benign and in the ovary tend to express mainly skin-type elements and are known as dermoid cysts. They often contain hair, and occasionally teeth (Fig. 10.9). Less frequently, teratomas of the ovary may be malignant. Extra-embryonic-type tumours include the so-called yolk sac tumour and choriocarcinoma.

Stromal tumours

The ovary has a specialized stroma which is hormonally sensitive and tumours may be derived from this. The most frequent tumours of this type are fibroma-thecomas, tumours derived from the granulosa layer of developing follicles (granulosa cell tumours), and tumours derived from normal Leydig cells that are present in the ovary (Leydig cell tumours).

It is important to remember that the ovary is a common site of metastasis, in particular from the breast and stomach, so-called 'Krukenberg' tumours.

UTERINE TUBES

Salpingitis, which is inflammation of the uterine tube, is relatively common. It occurs as part of the spectrum of pelvic inflammatory disease. Cysts are relatively frequent which are derived from the tubal epithelium. Another important phenomenon occurring in the uterine tubes is ectopic pregnancy. This is when a pregnancy abnormally implants outside the endometrial cavity, within the tubal epithelium. This presents when the embryo has developed to a size at which the tube is distended and frequently may present as acute rupture with life-threatening intra-abdominal haemorrhage.

SUMMARY

Vulva

The vulva is covered with skin and is therefore prone to diseases seen elsewhere on the skin surface. Conditions which are limited to the vulva are:

–hyperplastic dystrophy
–lichen sclerosis
–intraepithelial neoplasia

Uterine cervix

Important lesions of the cervix are:

–cervical intraepitheleial neoplasia (CIN)
–squamous cell carcinoma

CIN is a pre-malignant dysplastic lesion which develops at the transitional zone of the cervix between the squamous and glandular epithelium. CIN is part of the progression to overt invasive squamous cell carcinoma and is graded mild, moderate, and severe (I, II, and III). The human papillomavirus (HPV) is closely related to the development of squamous cell carcinoma of the cervix.

Uterus

Endometrium: by its very nature the endometrium is sensitive to hormones. Many conditions of the endometrium relate to this hormonal sensitivity. Important conditions are:

- *Endometrial hyperplasia*: this generally occurs in an environment of unopposed oestrogen secretion. If there is dysplasia there is a risk of malignancy.
- *Endometrial adenocarcinoma*: this is the most common malignancy of the endometrium. It is a tumour that develops in post-menopausal women.
- *Myometrium*: the most common pathology affecting the myometrium is the fibroid, representing a smooth muscle tumour (leiomyoma).

Ovaries

Important non-neoplastic conditions of the ovary are:

Endometriosis: this is the presence of endometrium outside of its normal situation. It is defined as endometrial glands, stroma, and evidence of haemorrhage within an abnormal site.

Ovarian cysts: particularly of functional origin, are common and are frequently physiological. However, many tumours of the ovary are cystic.

Tumours: common ovarian tumours are summarized below:

- *Cystadenoma*: these benign cystic tumours may be either of mucinous (endocervical type) or serous (tubal type).
- *Cystadenoma-benign/borderline*: this is a benign epithelial derived ovarian cyst. The term borderline is applied when there is cytological and architectural atypia, but no invasion of the stroma.

- *Cystadenocarcinoma*: this is a malignant epithelial tumour of the ovary. It may be mucinous or serous.

Germ cell tumours: these are tumours in which the germ cells show neoplastic change and are capable of differentiation in multiple cell minds. Typical examples are the:

–teratoma (benign dermoid cyst)
–dysgerminoma
–yolk sac tumour
–choriocarcinoma

Stromal tumours:

–leydig cell tumour
–fibroma-thecoma

Uterine tubes

The most common pathology of the uterine tubes is salpingitis (acute or chronic) and ectopic pregnancy.

11 The breast

11 The breast

THE breast can be thought of as being an adapted sweat gland, in that it has a ductal and lobular structure. The development, function, and regression of the breast is under hormonal control, particularly by oestrogens and progestogens.

The secreting elements of the breast are contained within lobules. A lobule consists of a grape-like structure, lined with cuboidal secretory epithelium and surrounded by a specialized muscle layer called myoepithelium. Ducts and lobules therefore have a double cell layer. The myoepithelium is capable of contraction and aids milk production during pregnancy. Groups of lobules form lobular ducts which connect with interlobular ducts. A number of interlobular ducts join together to form lactiferous ducts. There are approximately 20 lactiferous units within the breast, each opening with a single duct on the nipple. A large amount of fatty tissue is present in between the lobules and ducts.

The normal breast undergoes cyclical changes during normal menstrual cycles. Oestrogens and progestogens induce proliferative activity in the epithelium of the breast. As will be seen later, many benign and malignant epithelial conditions are under some degree of hormonal control. During pregnancy, particularly under progestogen influence, the acini of the breast show secretory activity, and lobules undergo marked hyperplasia.

The major part of the lymphatic drainage of the breast (about 75 per cent) is to the axillary lymph nodes. The rest goes to internal mammary lymph nodes beneath the medial part of the chest wall. This is an important surgical point with regard to the treatment of breast cancer. The presence of metastases in axillary lymph nodes has a marked effect on prognosis.

BENIGN CONDITIONS

Inflammatory conditions

Mastitis

By its very nature breast milk is a very good culture medium for bacteria. During pregnancy and breast-feeding the breast is particularly prone to bacterial infection via the nipple which induces acute mastitis. Common organisms causing acute mastitis are *Staphylooccus aureus*. Other organisms frequently implicated are streptococci. A breast abscess may be the result of acute mastitis.

Duct ectasia

This is characterized by an enlargement of the large ducts of the breast, with retention of secretions. Frequently, the ducts are distended by a large amount of thick green mucinous fluid. There is frequently associated infection. It frequently presents as a nipple discharge in 50- to 60-year-old women, and therefore a diagnosis of malignancy is sometimes considered at presentation. It is a benign condition of unknown cause, but may have an underlying hormonal cause in that there is an association with increase prolactin secretion by the pituitary.

Trauma

A frequent result of trauma to the breast is a localized necrosis of the breast tissue. Fat necrosis may present as a well-defined firm mass and may imitate a tumour.

Fibrocystic disease

This term encompasses quite a wide range of appearances. It is sometimes known by other names such as fibroadenosis, cystic mastopathy, or cystic disease. The characteristic pathological features are epithelial hyperplasia, fibrosis, and glandular proliferation. It is a disease that affects women most frequently between the ages of 35 and 55, particularly in the peri-menopausal age group. It is very common and frequently presents as pain or lumpiness of the breast, with variation throughout the menstrual cycle. It is entirely benign. The underlying cause is probably due to loss of normal co-ordination of the breast epithelium and stroma, both of which are under hormonal influences.

The most striking feature on histology is fibrosis, with hyperplastic regions within ducts and lobules. The hyperplasia can be very striking and may fill and obstruct ducts. Large cysts may develop containing trapped secretion.

Hyperplastic lesions also develop in the lobules. The hyperplastic lesions involve both the epithelium and the myoepithelium. This involvement of the two components of the breast is the most helpful feature in determining whether or not the process is benign or malignant. Malignant proliferation involves the epithelial structures of the breast, and does not involve the myoepithelium. The fibrosis may constrict and trap lobules, imitating a carcinoma on histology.

The condition frequently comes to the attention of surgeons because of its tendency to form discrete nodules which imitate tumours. Surgical management of the disease is either drainage of cysts or removal of distinct nodules.

If there is marked epithelial hyperplasia, there is a slightly higher risk of the development of breast carcinoma.

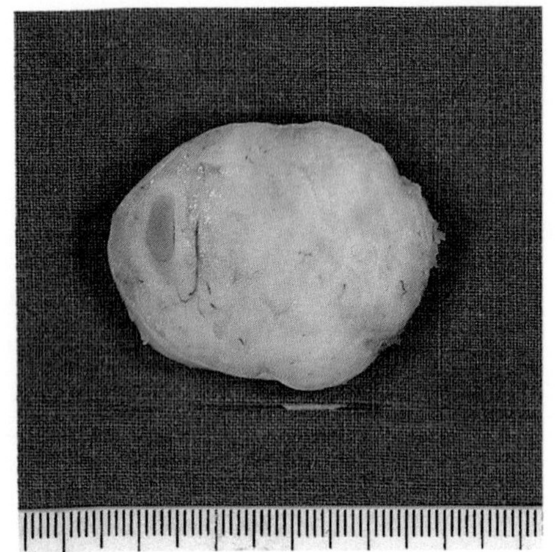

Fig. 11.1 A fibroadenoma of the breast. The well-circumscribed nature of the tumour and the lack of invasion indicate its benign nature.

Tumours

The most common benign breast tumour is the fibroadenoma. This occurs in women of reproductive age and presents as a discrete well-circumscribed mobile lump, often termed a 'breast mouse'. It is formed from both fibrous and glandular components, hence the name 'fibroadenoma' (Figs 11.1 and 11.2). Occasionally the connective tissue element of a fibroadenoma may be atypical in that it may be more cellular than normal and show mitotic activity. The term phylloides tumour is applied in this case. The term phylloides tumour really represents a low grade malignant connective tissue tumour (sarcoma).

Another characteristic benign tumour of the breast is an epithelial tumour that grows within a duct with a papillary pattern called a duct papilloma. They often occur in older women and may present as a nipple discharge in view of the high surface area produced by the papillary proliferation of epithelium.

Other less common benign tumours of the breast arise from connective tissue such as fat-forming lipomas, or blood vessels forming haemangiomas.

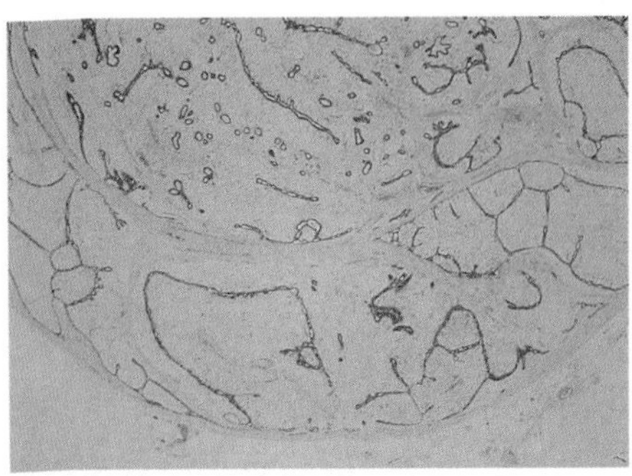

Fig. 11.2 Histology of a fibroadenoma shows thin epithelium within abundant connective tissue. No atypia is seen, and there is no invasive activity.

MALIGNANT CONDITIONS

Carcinoma

Breast carcinoma is the most common malignancy in women, being one-fifth of all cancers that develop in females. In the United Kingdom, approximately 1 out of every 14 women will develop a breast carcinoma, and has its highest incidence around the menopause. Breast cancer results in about 17 000 deaths a year in the United Kingdom. It is well-described as running in families.

The risk of breast cancer increases with the total cumulative time that the breast is exposed to unopposed oestrogen stimulation. In other words, any factor that increases the length of reproductive life increases the risk of breast cancer. Risk factors of importance are an early menarche and late menopause. Other risk factors are obesity, oestrogen drug treatment, and atypical proliferative lesions of the breast. Breast carcinoma is more frequent in women who have not had children compared to those who have.

Most cancers of the breast are of epithelial type—carcinomas. They may either be confined to the ductular system with no basement membrane invasion, when they are termed *in situ* or intraductal carcinomas. If the malignant change has penetrated the basement membrane to involve the stroma, then the term invasive carcinoma is used. The classification for breast cancer is summarized in Table 11.1.

The naked eye appearance of a breast carcinoma is of a very firm irregular mass which appears to infiltrate the surrounding breast tissue in a series of irregular projections (Figs 11.3 and 11.4). These resemble a crab, the origin of the term 'cancer'. There is often a striking proliferation of connective tissue within these tumours giving them a gritty cut surface. Microscopically, almost all malignant breast lesions are adenocarcinomas (Figs 11.5, 11.6, and 11.7). As with all carcinomas, breast carcinomas tend to spread through local lymph nodes (Fig. 11.8) before spreading to distant sites. Common sites of distant metastasis are

Table 11.1 Classification of breast cancer

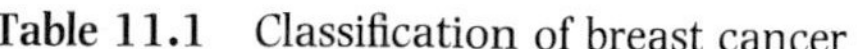

In situ lesions
Intraductal carcinoma
Intraductal papillary carcinoma
Lobular carcinoma (lobular neoplasia *in situ*)
Invasive lesions
Ductal carcinoma
Lobular carcinoma
Medullary carcinoma
Mucinous carcinoma
Colloid carcinoma
Paget's disease
Tubular carcinoma
Papillary carcinoma

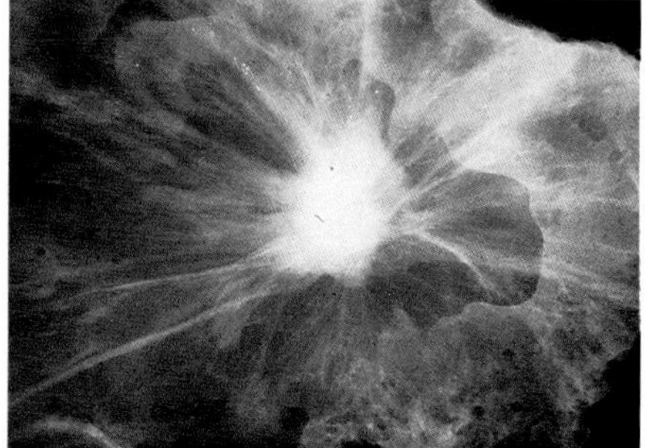

Fig. 11.3 A radiograph of a breast carcinoma showing radiating spurs of invasive tumour. Mammographic images of a carcinoma are very similar to this.

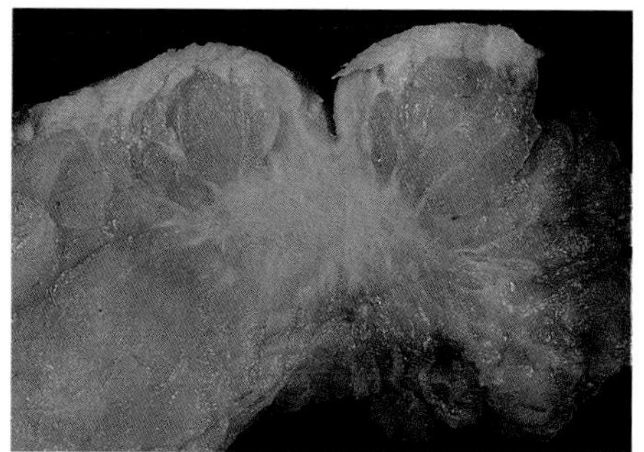

Fig. 11.4 A cut surface of a breast carcinoma showing a dense white invasive tumour. Tumour invades the skin at the top.

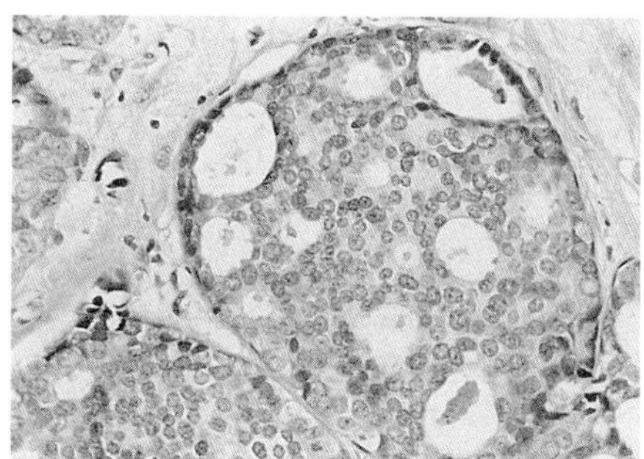

Fig. 11.5 This shows intraductal carcinoma (carcinoma *in situ*). The duct is filled with atypical cells with loss of the normal two-layered epithelium (see Fig. 11.6), but there is no invasion.

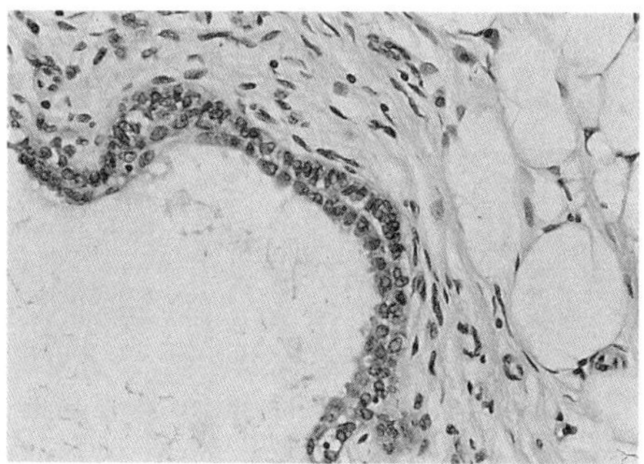

Fig. 11.6 Normal ductal epithelium. There are two layers; an outer myo-epithelium and an inner epithelium. Malignant tumours develop from the inner epithelium.

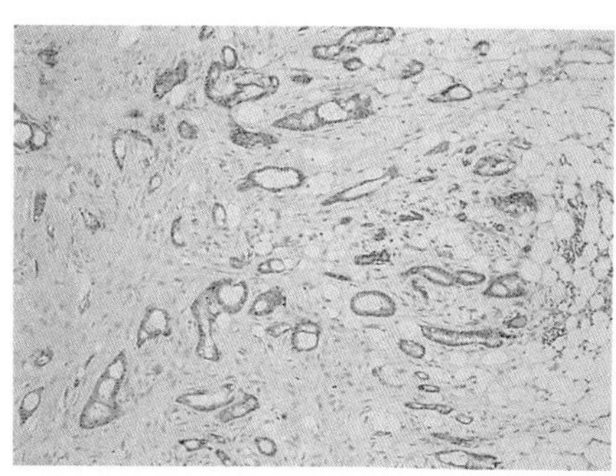

Fig. 11.7 Invasive, ductal adenocarcinoma.

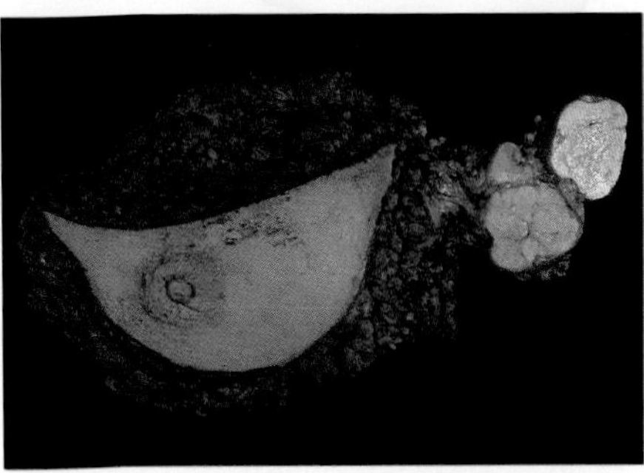

Fig. 11.8 A left mastectomy specimen with metastases in axillary lymph nodes from a breast carcinoma.

Table 11.2 Staging of breast carcinoma

Stage 1	The tumour is less than 5 cm diameter with no nodal spread and no distant metastases
Stage 2	This is a tumour less than 5 cm diameter with axillary lymph node involvement but with no distant metastases
Stage 3	Any size of tumour involving the skin or underlying muscles or involvement of axillary lymph nodes which are fixed to surrounding tissues. No distant metastases, however
Stage 4	Distant metastases present

Table 11.3 The TNM system for breast cancer

T1	Tumour 2 cm or less in diameter. No skin attachment or nipple distortion
T2	Tumour 2–5 cm, or tumour less than 2 cm involving the skin
T3	Tumour 5–10 cm or less than 5 cm, but with fixation of the tumour to adjacent structures
T4	Tumour greater than 10 cm in diameter, ulceration or deep chest wall involvement
N0	No nodes involved
N1	Axillary nodes involved but mobile
N2	Axillary lymph nodes involved but fixed to adjacent structures
N3	Lymphatic obstruction with oedema of arm or involvement of supraclavicular nodes
M0	No distant metastases
M1	Distant metastases present

Table 11.4 Five-year survival rate from breast carcinoma

Stage 1	80%
Stage 2	65%
Stage 3	40%
Stage 4	10%

the bone, liver, lung, and brain. The most important clinical feature that gives an indication of the future progression of the disease is the extent of lymph node involvement. This is still the most important prognostic feature of breast carcinoma. There are four stages used in the assessment of a breast carcinoma (Table 11.2). The UICC TNM system is summarized in Table 11.3. The five-year survival rates are given in Table 11.4.

The underlying biological problem with breast carcinoma is by that the time the tumour is clinically evident there are probably already microscopic distant metastases of tumour. Small tumours less than 2 cm in diameter, however, have a very good prognosis. Also tumours with no lymph node involvement have a good prognosis. As can be seen above, involvement of the lymph nodes dramatically reduces the survival rate. The type of tumour has a minimal effect on prognosis except for particular special types, such as the medullary tumour which has a very florid host immune response, and the mucin-dominated 'colloid' carcinoma. Tumours that have a high expression of oestrogen receptor on the cell surface of the tumour cells have a good response to hormonal manipulation. Generally, tumours that have a high expression of oestrogen receptors have a better prognosis than those with little expression of oestrogen receptors. The grading of the tumour, which reflects the rate that the tumour is proliferating, and to some degree the underlying nuclear abnormality, has prognostic significance. High-grade tumours, that is, rapidly growing tumours, have a poorer prognosis than low-grade tumours.

THE MALE BREAST

It is worth pointing out that 1 per cent of breast carcinomas occur in men, and in view of the proximity to the chest wall tend to have a poorer prognosis than in females. Hormonally dependent enlargement of the male breast may occur, and is called *gynaecomastia*.

SUMMARY

The breast is a glandular organ composed of lobules and ducts, both lined by epithelium which is surrounded by myoepithelium.

Benign lesions

–mastitis
–duct ectasia

Fibrocystic disease: this is a very common disorder of the breast and is characterized by a range of changes from fibrosis, inflammation, epithelial proliferation, and cyst formation.

Benign tumours: fibroadenoma.

Malignant tumours
Breast carcinoma is the most common malignancy in women. The risk of breast cancer is closely related to the total time the breast is exposed to unopposed oestrogens.

Breast carcinomas are either of ductal type or lobular type; the most common being ductal. Both types of tumour go through an *in situ* phase before invasive malignancy. These *in situ* phases are referred to as ductal carcinoma *in situ* (DCIS) or lobular carcinoma *in situ* (LCIS), respectively.

The most important prognostic factor for breast carcinoma is the presence or absence of metastases in local lymph nodes.

12 The endocrine system

12 The endocrine system

An endocrine gland is defined as a gland in which the product is secreted directly into the blood with no intervening duct. A ducted gland is known as an exocrine gland. The endocrine system can be defined into two parts: (1) the diffuse endocrine system; and (2) endocrine organs. All organs of the body, particularly the lung and gastrointestinal tract, contain an endocrine cell population which is involved in local monitoring of factors such as oxygen and control of function such as muscle activity in the case of the intestine. This local endocrine cell population is termed the diffuse endocrine system. Endocrine organs generally produce a hormone which has an effect on distant tissues. Hormones act on cells via receptors of a cell surface membrane which are specific for that particular hormone. Some hormone receptors may also be in the cytoplasm or nucleus, as in the case of steroid hormones. When a hormone receptor binds to each particular specific hormone (the ligand) this sets off a chain of intercellular messages which then affect the activity of enzymes or other metabolic products which then have an effect on cell growth function (see p. 000).

A cell may produce a hormone which then acts on its own receptors, and this is known as an autocrine effect. This is of particular relevance in some malignant tumours. A paracrine effect is when a hormone is produced by a cell and acts locally within adjacent cells within the same tissue.

There are many diagnostic problems in endocrine pathology in which the application of a few rules can assist the finding of a solution:

1. When assessing pathology, such as a nodule in an endocrine gland like the thyroid, *the uninvolved background gland is investigated* (or the other organ in a paired gland such as the adrenals). For example, an adenoma by definition occurs in normal or suppressed gland, whilst nodular hyperplasia involves the whole gland.

2. In the assessment of the benign or malignant nature of a tumour, the appearances of individual cells are usually not helpful. The behaviour of the tumour, particularly at the margins, is more important; features such as *vascular and capsular invasion* are far more significant. The size and weight of a tumour are all important as predictive factors in some organs such as the adrenal. In some cases, the only way to tell if a tumour is benign or malignant is to follow-up the patient after excision. The diagnosis is therefore retrospective; benign tumours will not give further trouble, malignant tumours will metastasize.

3. The result of many diseases of the endocrine system is the *under-production or over-production of hormones* and the appearance of clinical hypo- or hyperfunctional states. Endocrine cells have morphological features that show either the cells are hyperplastic and active, or atrophic and inactive.

4. Endocrine organs are under the control of feedback systems operating at various levels. Hypersecretion may result from 'autonomy' by a primary endocrine organ (for example, pituitary adenoma) or in an end-organ (for example, parathyroid adenoma). Autonomy in this sense means independence from normal control mechanisms. *Most functionally autonomous lesions are benign or malignant neoplasms*. Reduced function may be due to destruction of the pituitary (for example, trauma) or the end organ (for example, adrenal tuberculosis).

5. If one endocrine organ is involved, the other endocrine organs must be investigated. A multiple endocrine neoplasia (MEN) syndrome may be present.

Certain pathological processes unify the endocrine glands. All may show:

Diffuse hyperplasia, for example:

–*thyroid*: Graves' disease, iodine-deficient goitre, dyshormonogenesis
–*adrenal*: Cushing's disease due to basophil adenoma of the pituitary, Cushing's syndrome due to small cell carcinoma of the lung

Nodular hyperplasia (multiple nodules in the whole or both glands), for example:

–*thyroid*: nodular goitre (colloid goitre)
–*adrenal*: bilateral nodular hyperplasia
–*parathyroids*: nodular hyperplasia (all four glands)

Solitary nodule (adenoma), if this is functional the background gland may be suppressed. There should not be other nodules. (If there are other nodules then the possibility of nodular hyperplasia should be considered.), for example:

–*thyroid*: follicular adenoma
–*adrenal*: adrenal cortical adenoma
–*pituitary*: adenoma
–*parathyroid*: adenoma (one gland only)

Another clinical condition that emphasizes links between different endocrine glands is the syndrome of *multiple endocrine neoplasia* (MEN). There are two main types:

MEN I (Wermer syndrome)—hyperplasia and/or adenoma of pituitary, thyroid, parathyroid, adrenal *cortex*, pancreatic islet.

MEN II (Sipple syndrome)—multiple pheochromocytomas of adrenal *medulla* and medullary carcinoma of thyroid. The term MEN IIb or III is applied to MEN II with the addition of mucocutaneous neuromas.

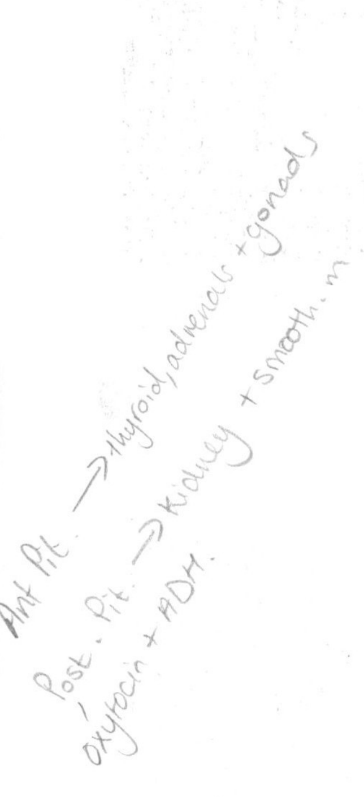

PITUITARY

The pituitary is effectively the king of the endocrine system in that it produces hormones which have an affect on a number of endocrine organs. It weighs approximately a gram and is situated beneath the brain, adjacent to the hypothalamus and lies in a bony cavity above the sphenoid sinus. Surgical access is possible through the roof of the sphenoid sinus from the nose. The pituitary is split into two parts: (1) the anterior and posterior pituitary known as the adenohypophysis; and (2) the neurohypophysis. The anterior pituitary produces hormones which have effect on the thyroid, adrenals, and the gonads. The posterior pituitary produces hormones which have effect on the kidney and smooth muscle, in particular oxytocin and vasopressin (antidiuretic hormone). The anterior pituitary has a portal blood supply from the hypothalamus. The hypothalamus produces various stimulatory or inhibitory factors which act on the anterior pituitary. The posterior pituitary is effectively a mass of modified neurones that are capable of secretion into the blood.

Increased function

The most common cause of increased function of the pituitary is a tumour which secretes a particular hormone in high concentration (Fig. 12.1). They are in most cases benign and may be derived from any one of the different populations of hormone-producing cell types found in the pituitary. Prolactin-screting (25–30 per cent), growth hormone (20–25 per cent), and adrenocorticotrophic hormone-secreting (10–15 per cent) adenomas make up to 90 per cent of functional tumours. Up to 30 per cent of tumours do not produce a measurable hormone.

If there is excessive adrenocorticotrophic hormone secretion, Cushing's syndrome will result, characterized by obesity, diabetes mellitus, hypertension, poor healing, osteoporosis, and hypercalcaemia, among other features. If growth hormone is produced in excess, acromegaly will develop, characterized by growth of the skull, mandible, and hands. There is also soft tissue growth in acromegaly, particularly of the face.

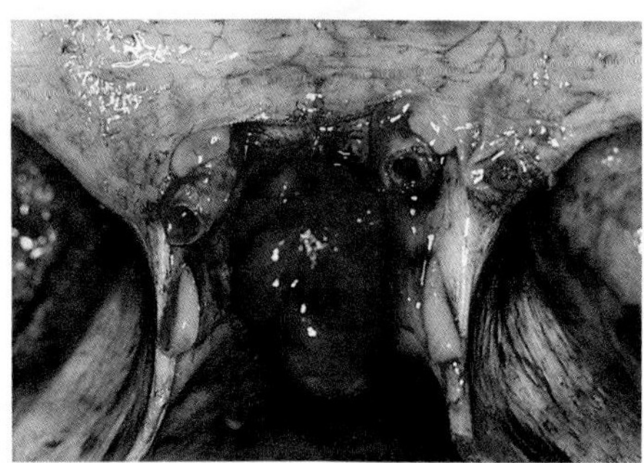

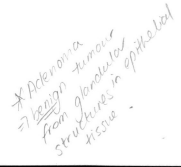

Fig. 12.1 A pituitary adenoma projecting out of the pituitary fossa.

Decreased function

Decreased function of the pituitary is most frequently due to destruction or damage of the pituitary by a tumour, compression by adjacent lesions, and trauma. Loss of antidiuretic hormone (vasopressin) results in diabetes incipidus, which is associated with reduced ability to concentrate urine.

THYROID

The thyroid gland weighs approximately 25 grams and is a bilobed organ which lies in front of the thyroid cartilage of the larynx. Four parathyroids lie behind the gland, a superior and inferior pair (Fig. 12.2). It develops in the area of the foramen caecum on the posterior part of the tongue (residual thyroid tissue is sometimes found here), and descends down the thyroglossal duct. Thyroglossal cysts occasionally develop in embryonic remnants of this duct. The thyroid is closely adherent to the trachea via its fascia. The major part of the thyroid gland comprises spherical follicles which are composed of a single cell layer of secretory epithelium which enclose spaces containing a protein called thyroglobulin. Thyroglobulin is effectively a storage material which is then metabolized by the thyroid epithelium to produce thyroid hormones which are then secreted into the closely adjacent capillaries of the thyroid. The thyroid gland is a highly vascular organ. There is also a smaller population of cells called C cells which lie within follicles, each follicle having about 6–8 such cells (Fig. 12.3). C cells produce calcitonin which reduces blood calcium.

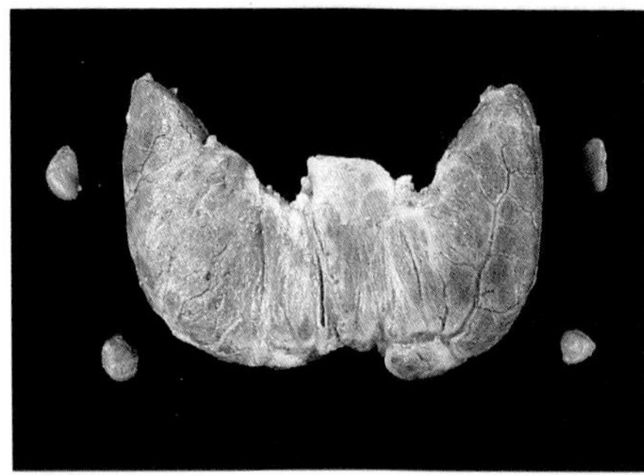

Fig. 12.2 Two pairs of parathyroids lie behind the thyroid. The two lobes of this normal thyroid can be seen.

Increased function

Ninety-five per cent of cases of hyperthyroidism are due to either Graves' disease, a toxic nodular goitre, or a benign follicular tumour known as an adenoma.

Hyperthyroidism presents with increased metabolic rate, with heat intolerance, weight loss, increased appetite, anxiety, and increased heart rate.

Graves' disease

This is an example of an autoimmune thyroiditis in which the patient has produced antibodies to the thyroid-stimulating hormone receptor which bind specifically to this receptor and cause inappropriate stimulation. The thyroid then behaves as if it is being chronically stimulated by thyroid-stimulating hormone from the pituitary and becomes hyperplastic and produces large amounts of thyroid hormone. There is a marked goitre and the patient becomes strikingly thyrotoxic. These patients also present with symptoms not always directly relating to the thyrotoxicosis, the most common one being protrusion of the eyes known as exophthalmos. Graves' disease

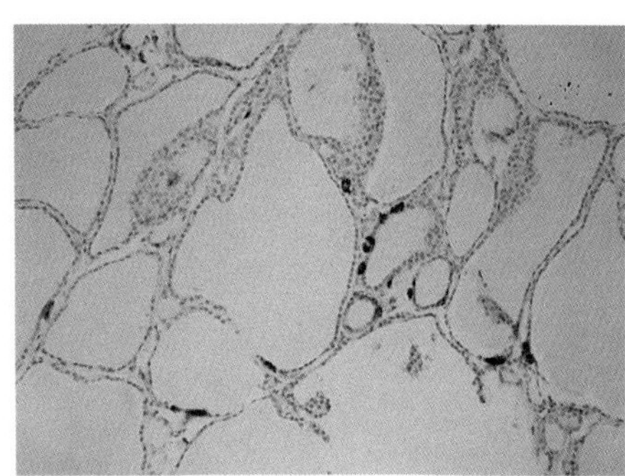

Fig. 12.3 C cells stained in a normal thyroid with an immunoperoxidase stain using an antibody to calcitonin. This emphasizes the thyroid as being two glands in one. The follicles can be seen in the background.

has a tendency to occur in females and is associated with human leucocyte antigen (HLA) type DR3.

Toxic nodular goitre

Toxic nodular goitre is when a goitre produces excessive thyroid hormones. Nodular goitre is discussed below. Hyperthyroidism is an uncommon presentation of a benign follicular adenoma. This tumour is also covered below.

Decreased function

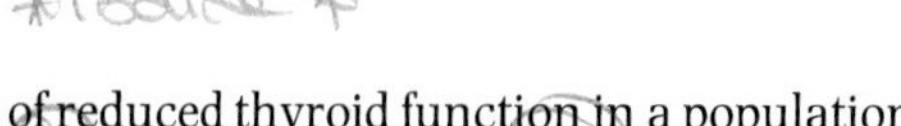

The most common causes of reduced thyroid function in a population where there is normal iodine in the diet are Hashimoto's disease and destruction of the thyroid due to surgical removal or radioactive treatment.

Hypothyroidism presents with increased weight, dry skin, tiredness, reduced sweating, and a puffy face. In children, the syndrome of *cretinism* may occur. Hypothyroidism is a cause of retarded eruption of deciduous or permanent teeth.

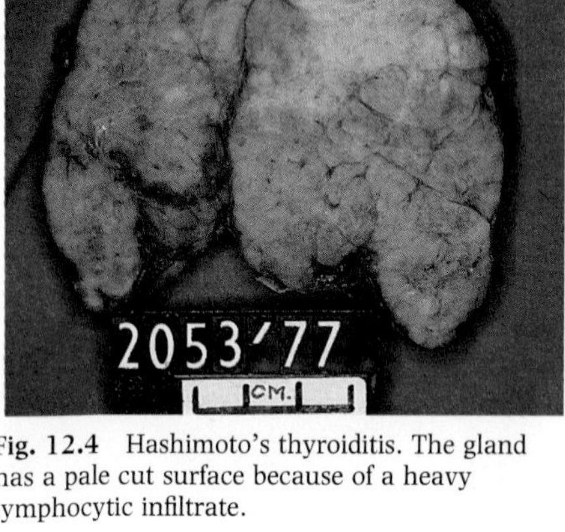

Fig. 12.4 Hashimoto's thyroiditis. The gland has a pale cut surface because of a heavy lymphocytic infiltrate.

Hashimoto's thyroiditis

This is an autoimmune condition in which there is T cell destruction of thyroid epithelium which is induced by loss of suppressor T cell activity. There is frequently a circulating antibody in these patients which is directed against thyroglobulin and certain intercellular organelles.

Pathologically, there is a mild to moderate goitre with pale discoloration of the gland (Fig. 12.4). Microscopically, there is a very striking lymphocytic infiltrate with destruction of thyroid epithelium. These patients may present initially with increased thyroid function; this rapidly changes to a situation where there is decreased thyroid function due to loss of thyroid-secreting epithelium. It is associated with HLA type DR5.

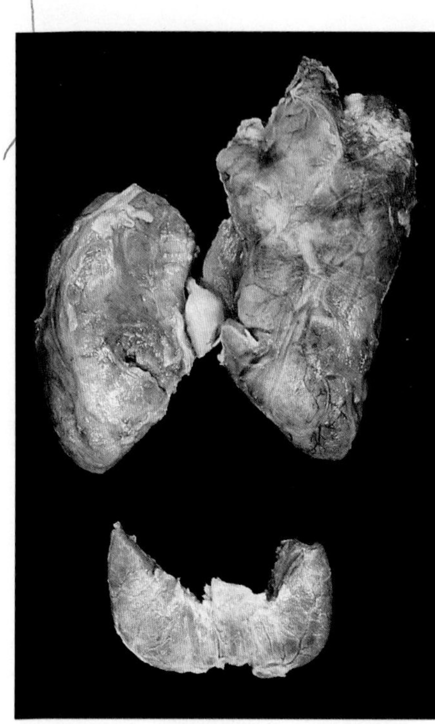

Fig. 12.5 A nodular goitre (above) compared to a normal thyroid (below). The whole of the gland is nodular and fibrotic.

Goitre

Diffuse goitre

This may occur in several situations; physiological goitre in the case of increased size of the thyroid at puberty or during pregnancy, and certain dietary factors (goitrogens) such as vegetables of the Brassica family are associated with increased thyroid size. Certain inherited inborn errors of metabolism (dyshormonogenesis) involving certain thyroid enzymes may present as a goitre with associated reduced thyroid functions. Iodine deficiency is classically associated with increased size of the thyroid.

Nodular goitre

This is a relatively common condition in which there is enlargement of the thyroid with a striking nodularity (Fig. 12.5). In most cases, there is no change in thyroid function, although it is a well-recognized cause of thyrotoxicosis. It is entirely benign and has no increased incidence of malignancy. It is of unknown cause although it may be related to some factor in the diet. Pathologically, there can be very large goitres, up to a kilogram or more. There is nodularity of the cut surface of the gland with areas of fibrosis, calcification, and haemorrhage. Microscopically, there is marked loss of co-ordination of function in the gland with areas of increased function and decreased function occurring simultaneously. Thyroidectomy is usually performed for cosmetic reasons.

Tumours

In view of the close proximity of the thyroid to the oral cavity, tumours of the thyroid may be evident to a dental practitioner.

Benign

The best-recognized benign thyroid tumour is the so-called follicular adenoma. This is defined as a follicular tumour which is of different appearance to the normal background gland. It has a well-defined fibrous capsule with no evidence of vascular or capsular invasive activity by the tumour (Fig. 12.6).

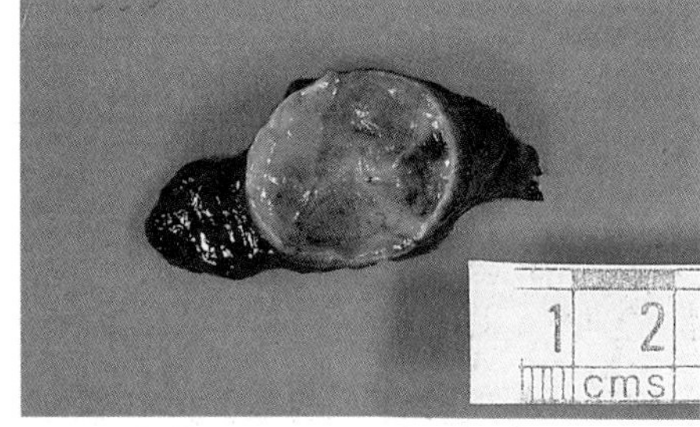

Fig. 12.6 A follicular adenoma which shows no capsular or vascular invasion. The background gland is normal.

Malignant

Malignant tumours contribute to less than 5 per cent of the causes of all cancer and, generally, the tumours are slow-growing and associated with a good prognosis. The majority of thyroid tumours arise from the follicular epithelium, but in the case of medullary carcinoma the tumour arises from the calcitonin-producing C cells.

Papillary carcinoma

This is the most common type of thyroid carcinoma, accounting for up to 70 per cent of cases. It is derived from the follicular epithelium, but as its name suggests, the tumour grows in frond- and finger-like projections known as papillae (Fig. 12.7). It is as if the thyroid follicles are growing inside-out. It occurs generally in young people and has a striking tendency to spread via the lymphatics to local lymph nodes (Fig. 12.8). The primary tumour is often small with extensive nodal metastasis, although the presence of metastases does not affect the prognosis. The outlook for this tumour is excellent. A typical presentation is a young person who presents with a lump in the neck which is found to be a lymph node containing metastatic papillary carcinoma. The thyroid is then removed and the small primary focus found.

Follicular carcinoma

This is less common and occurs in the older population, usually late to middle age and accounts for up to 20–25 per cent of thyroid cancer. It presents as an

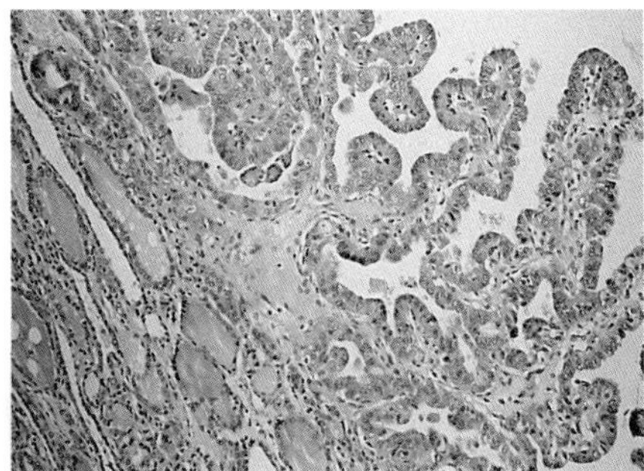

Fig. 12.7 Papillary carcinoma is named because of the finger-like papillary way in which the neoplastic epithelium grows. Uninvolved follicles can be seen in the bottom left.

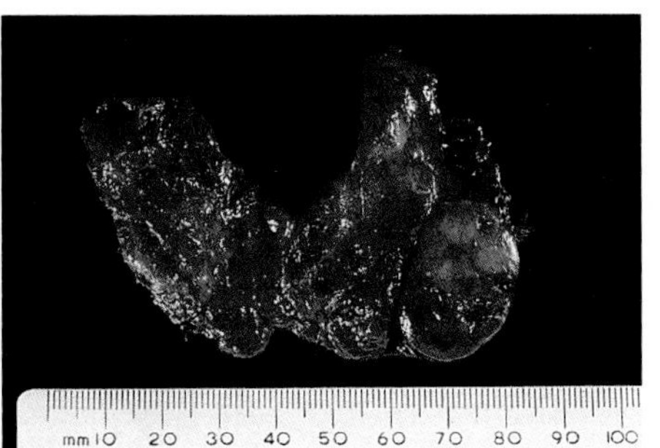

Fig. 12.8 A lymph node (below right) is enlarged by metastatic papillary thyroid carcinoma. The primary tumour was found to be in the upper pole of the left lobe and has spread via lymphatics.

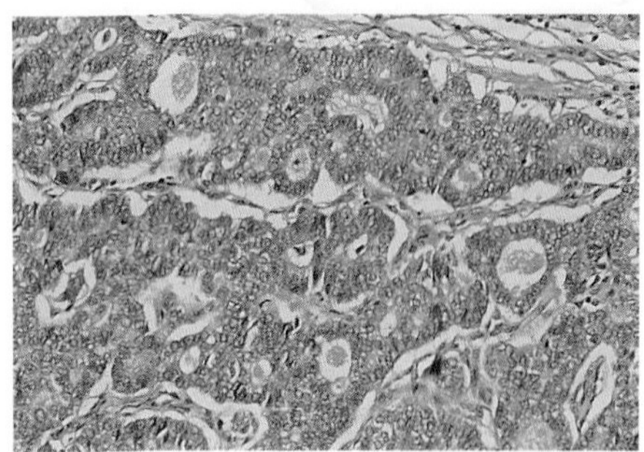

Fig. 12.9 Follicular carcinoma shows by definition capsular and/or vascular invasion.

aggressively growing invasive follicular tumour which has a tendency to invade the blood vessels and spread to distant sites (Fig. 12.9), particularly the lung and bone (Fig. 12.10). It has a poorer prognosis than papillary carcinoma, although the outlook is generally still good, in view of the sensitivity of thyroid epithelium to destruction by radioactive iodine.

Anaplastic carcinoma

This accounts for up to 10 per cent of thyroid cancer and typically occurs in an elderly person who has a history of a goitre which suddenly increases. Pathologically, there is an extensively infiltrating carcinoma which microscopically appears to show no specific differentiation. In most cases, some evidence of thyroid differentiation can be found using special techniques. It has a very poor prognosis.

Medullary carcinoma

This, in contrast to the thyroid tumours already discussed, is derived from the C cells. It presents as a generally rapidly growing malignant tumour. It has a bimodal age distribution at presentation in that there is a population who present at a young age with a very high tendency to have a family history of the disease. Patients who present in later middle life tend not to have a family history. It is now known that there is gene defect which strongly predisposes patients to the disease and these patients have an associated family history. They develop a pre-malignant condition at an early age, known as C cell hyperplasia. Medullary carcinoma comprises part of one of the multiple endocrine neoplasia syndromes (MEN). MEN II is a syndrome in which there is an association between medullary carcinoma and a tumour of the adrenal medulla called a phaeochromocytoma.

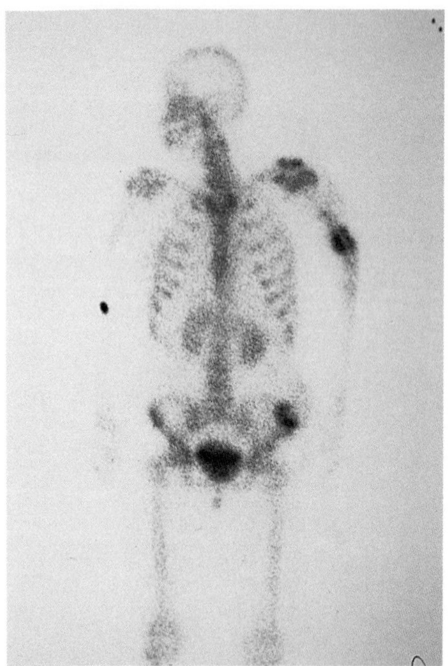

Fig. 12.10 Follicular thyroid carcinoma has spread to the left shoulder and upper arm in this bone scan (dark areas), via the blood.

Lymphoma

This tends to be of B cell type and has similarities to so-called mucosal-associated lymphomas seen in the gastrointestinal tract or lungs. It has an increased incidence in the thyroid with a previous history of thyroiditis such as Hashimoto's disease. The clinical staging of thyroid cancer is shown in Table 12.1.

PARATHYROIDS

The parathyroids are four small glands, each normally weighing no more than 12 milligrams. They lie in pairs, the superior pair lying behind the superior thyroid notch, and the inferior pair lying just behind the lower poles (Fig. 12.2). They have an important role in calcium metabolism, in that their secretion, called parathyroid hormone, has a strong action in raising blood calcium. A raised blood calcium is a common finding in parathyroid disease.

Table 12.1 Staging of thyroid cancer

Stage	Pathology
1	Tumour entirely within thyroid
2	Tumour not fixed but node metastases
3	Local fixation/cervical nodes fixed
4	Distant metastases

Increased function

This is frequently due to a benign tumour known as an adenoma, or parathyroid hyperplasia. An adenoma is defined as one large parathyroid gland showing a well-defined tumour within it with compression of background suppressed gland (Fig. 12.11). The other three glands also show suppression.

Parathyroid hyperplasia is seen when a number of parathyroid glands show increased size with nodularity. The situation of increase parathyroid function due to pathology within the glands is known as primary hyperparathyroidism. Parathyroid carcinoma is a very rare tumour in which the parathyroid tissue can be seen invading adjacent tissues. Secondary parathyroid hyperplasia occurs in situations of increased demand, such as in renal failure or malabsorption of calcium.

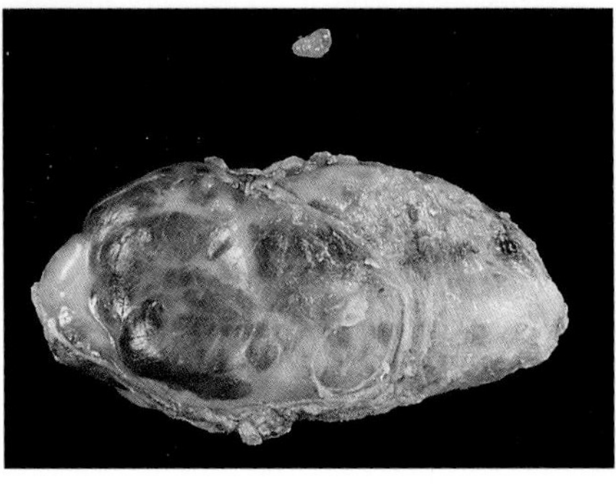

Fig. 12.11 A parathyroid adenoma weighing 12 g. A normal parathyroid is shown for comparison (top: normal weight 12 mg).

Decreased function

The most common reason for decreased function of the parathyroids is removal or disturbance in the case of a thyroidectomy.

ADRENALS

The adrenal glands are paired organs lying above the kidneys, each weighing approximately 5–7 grams. They are divided into the cortex and medulla (Figs 12.12 and 12.13). The cortex is also split into two parts; one part secretes aldosterone which is involved in sodium metabolism (the zona glomerulosa) and the other part is involved in the secretion of glucocorticosteroids (the zona fasciculata and reticularis). The medulla is involved in the secretion of adrenaline and noradrenaline.

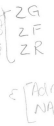

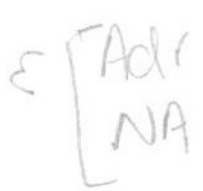

Adrenal cortex

Increased function

The most common reasons for increased function of adrenal cortex are: adrenal nodular hyperplasia (Fig. 12.14); adrenal adenoma (Fig. 12.15); and adrenal cortical carcinoma (Fig. 12.16). The hormones secreted may be any of the steroid hormones produced by the adrenal cortex. Diffuse adrenal hyperplasia is closely associated with a pituitary adenoma which is producing excessive adrenalcorticotrophic hormone. This is known as Cushing's disease.

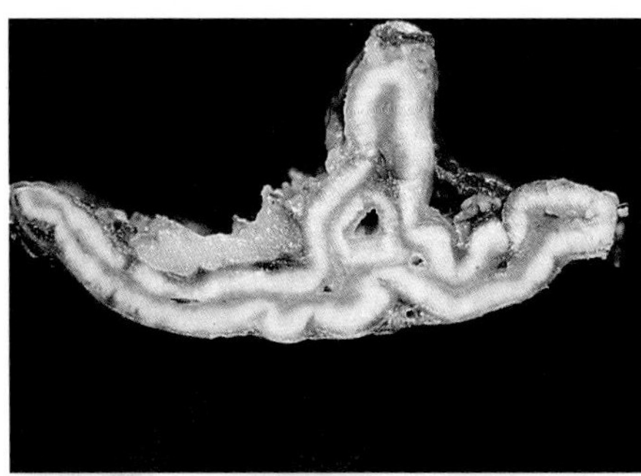

Fig. 12.12 An adrenal gland showing a yellow fat-filled cortex. A single central vein can be seen.

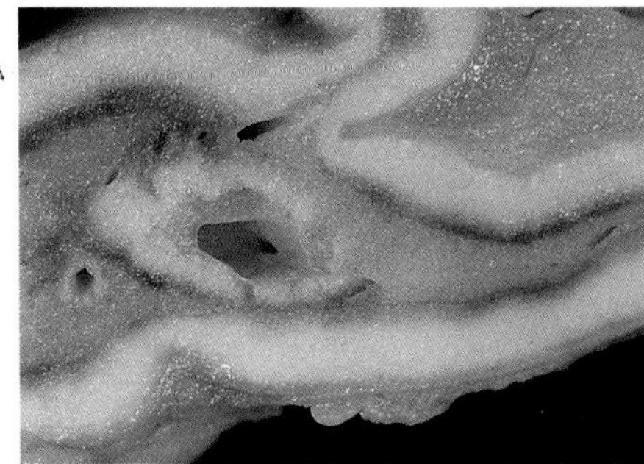

Fig. 12.13 On a closer view the thin inner part of the cortex is brown and the thick outer part is yellow. The medulla is grey in colour. Cortex also surrounds the central vein.

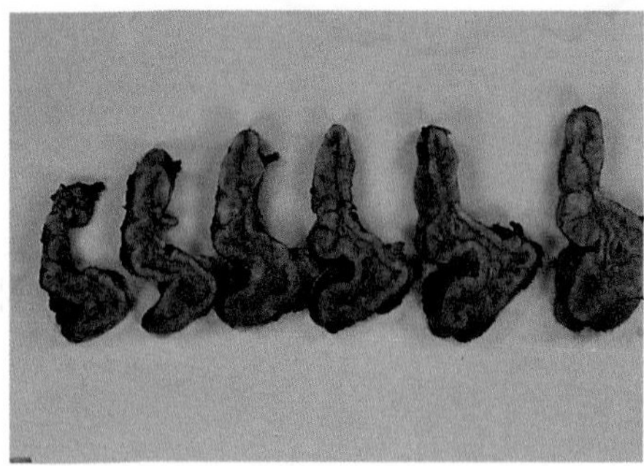

Fig. 12.14 An adrenal has been cut into multiple slices and shows nodularity throughout.

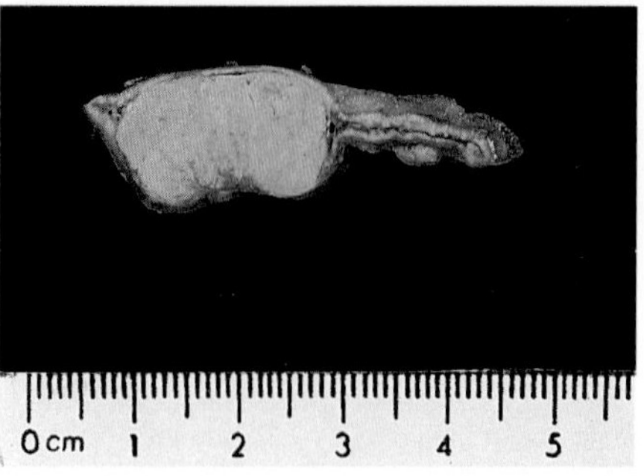

Fig. 12.15 This is an adrenal cortical adenoma. The background cortex is thin due to suppression.

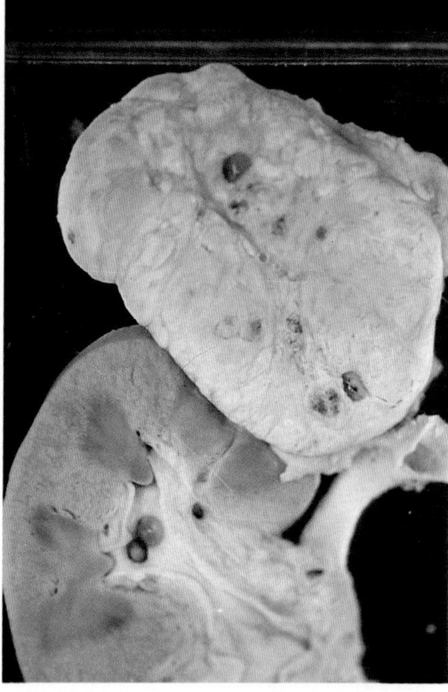

Fig. 12.16 An adrenal cortical carcinoma, with a kidney below. Malignancy is predicted because of its large size and weight.

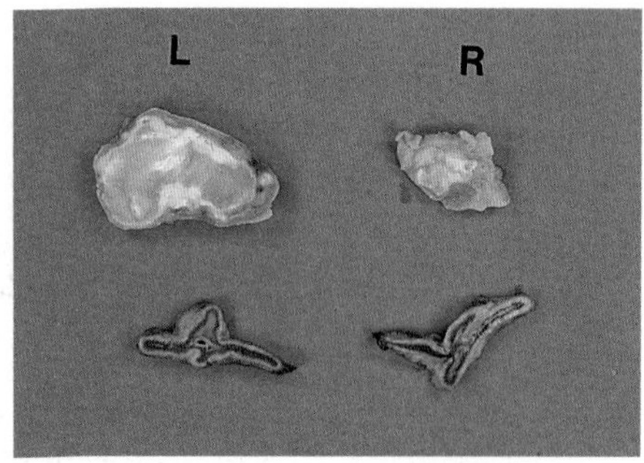

Fig. 12.17 The upper two adrenal glands have been destroyed by tuberculosis; two normal glands are included below for comparison.

Decreased function

Decreased function of the adrenal cortex is most frequently due to autoimmune destruction by lymphocytes, known as Addison's disease. Other causes include infections such as tuberculosis (Fig. 12.17), and destruction by metastatic tumour. Adrenal haemorrhage can occur in septic shock. Adrenals are suppressed with long-term steroid treatment.

Adrenal medulla

The most important lesion of the adrenal medulla that is recognized is the primary tumour which secretes excessive adrenaline and noradrenaline, known as the phaeochromocytoma (Figs 12.18 and 12.19).

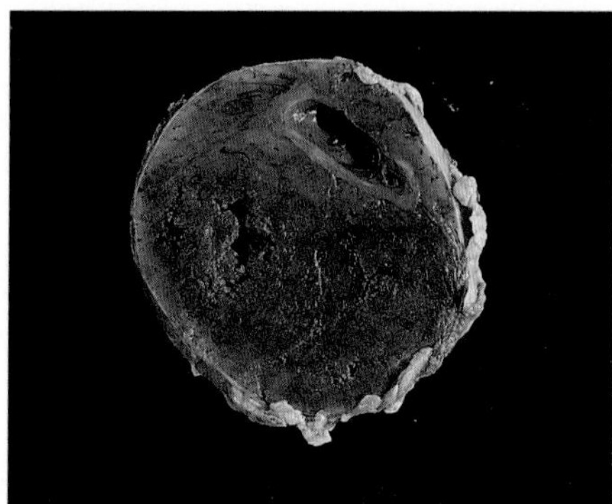

Fig. 12.18 A phaeochromocytoma (literally meaning a 'brown-coloured tumour'). It goes brown in oxidizing fixatives.

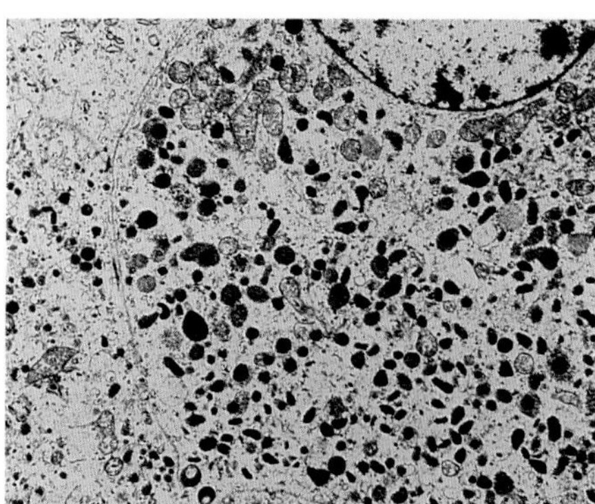

Fig. 12.19 Electron microscopy at high power shows endocrine granules associated with adrenaline and noradrenaline storage.

ENDOCRINE PANCREAS

The pancreas is effectively two glands in one, with an exocrine component which secretes pancreatic enzymes to the pancreatic duct into the duodenum. The endocrine pancreas is composed of multiple small collections of endocrine cells known as the islets of Langerhans. The normal pancreas weighs approximately 75 grams, the majority of which comprises the exocrine pancreas. A normal pancreas has only about 1–2 ml of islets of Langerhans within it representing about 1–2 g. The islets of Langerhans are composed of a number of cell types as listed in Table 12.2.

Table 12.2 Cell types in pancreatic islets

Alpha cells secreting glucogen
Beta cells secreting insulin
Delta cells secreting somatostatin
Pancreatic polypeptide

The most important disease of the endocrine pancreas is diabetes in which there is reduced function of the beta cells. The most important cause of increased function of the pancreatic islets is benign tumours (Figs 12.20 and 12.21).

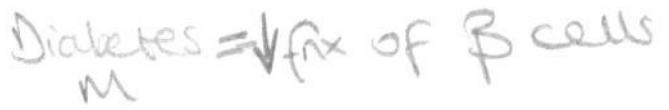

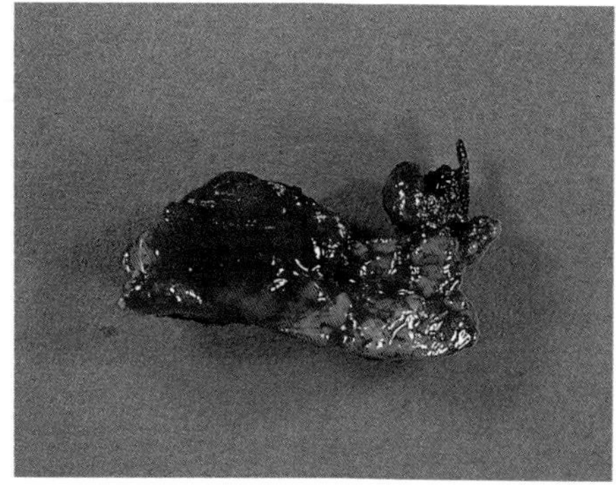

Fig. 12.20 This islet cell tumour ('insulinoma' because it produced excessive insulin) was only 1 cm diameter, yet it was life-threatening due to induced hypoglycaemia.

DIABETES

This is defined as a condition which is a state of chronic hyperglycaemia. The underlying physiological cause is a deficiency of insulin which leads to defects in carbohydrate metabolism.

There are two major types of diabetes seen in the population. These are type 1, insulin-dependent diabetes and type 2, non-insulin-dependent diabetes. Non-insulin-dependent diabetes is associated with obesity. Diabetes mellitus is one of the most common chronic diseases in the population, and it has been estimated that diabetes is present in up to 5 per cent of the population. The types of diabetes is summarized below.

Type 1 (insulin-dependent)

This is also known as juvenile onset diabetes as it typically presents in childhood or young adult life. The underlying defect is an inadequate secretion of insulin by the beta cells of the endocrine pancreas. Many of these patients have circulating antibodies to islet cells. There is also an association with other autoimmune disease. The autoimmune reaction may be induced by a viral infection. Coxsackie virus B has been implicated in the causation of this type of diabetes. Pathologically, there is a marked reduction in the number of insulin-producing beta cells in the pancreas and an associated lymphocytic insulitis is frequently seen. This suggests that there is an autoimmune destruction of beta cells. However, some beta cells remain unaffected. Genetic factors are also involved in that there is association with certain HLA types, particularly HLA type DR4.

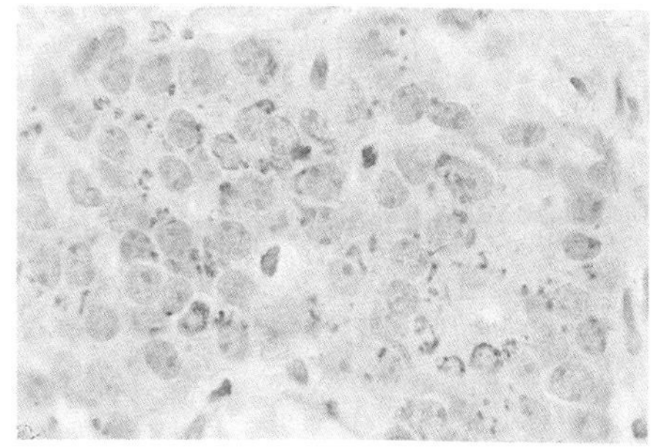

Fig. 12.21 The islet cell tumour in Fig. 12.20 contanined insulin on immunohistochemistry.

Type 2 diabetes (non-insulin-dependent)

This occurs in a much older age group than type 1 diabetes and is more common, usually presenting in late middle age. It is particularly prevalent in the obese. The actual production of insulin by the pancreas may be normal, or increased and the underlying abnormality appears to be an increased requirement for insulin in most cases. Proinsulin, a precursor of insulin, shows increased secretion from the islets. This increased requirement may be due to decreased numbers of insulin receptors on cells. There is a close link with genetic factors in that there is frequently a family history and identical twins show nearly a 100 per cent concordant risk of developing the disease.

Many of these patients show deposits of amyloid in the pancreatic islets which seems to correlate with the severity of the disease. Fibrosis of islets with islet cell regeneration is occasionally seen.

Diagnosis of diabetes

If a fasting glucose blood test is taken and the blood glucose is greater than 7.8 mM/l then a diagnosis of diabetes can be made (normal random glucose is between 4.2 to 6.4 mM/l). A glucose tolerance test may be performed, and is abnormal if the blood glucose goes above 11.1 mM/l.

Complications of diabetes

In summary, the underlying problem that is seen in all tissues and organ systems of the body in diabetes is basement membrane thickening. Although the basement membranes are thicker, there is increased permeability. The most common complication is therefore small blood vessel disease with ischaemia. The complications are summarized below.

Blood vessels

Diabetics have an increased risk of atherosclerosis. This may result in myocardial infarction, cerebrovascular accidents, severe ischaemia of peripheral limbs, and gangrene. The basement membrane involvement of small vessels leads to damage, particularly in the retina and nerves. The kidney is also a site of diabetic disease. Diabetics are particularly prone to infection, and autonomic nerve damage.

SUMMARY

Pituitary

Anterior pituitary: the most common pituitary pathology is the adenoma. Most adenomas secrete a single hormone.

Prolactinoma	30%
Growth hormone	17%
Mixed growth hormone/prolactin	10%
Adrenocorticotrophic hormone	15%
Non-functional	25%

Tumours producing gonadotrophins or thyroid-stimulating hormone occasionally occur.

Other lesions of the anterior pituitary include Sheehan's syndrome, which is pituitary infarction following shock, usually associated with obstetric causes.

Posterior pituitary: the most significant abnormality of the posterior pituitary is deficiency of antidiuretic hormone which produces diabetes insipidus.

Thyroid

Common causes of over-activity of the thyroid are:

–Graves' disease
–multinodular goitre
–toxic adenoma

Common causes of reduced thyroid function are:

–Hashimoto's disease
–surgical or medical treatment
–iodine deficiency

Autoimmune disease: the two most common autoimmune diseases of the thyroid are *Graves' disease* (an antibody is produced which binds and stimulates the TSH receptor), and *Hashimoto's disease* (there is autoimmune lymphocyte-mediated destruction of the thyroid).

Diffuse goitre: a diffuse enlargement of the thyroid occurs at adolescence, in pregnancy, associated with some dietary factors, and classically iodine deficiency.

Nodular goitre: a common condition of unknown cause with striking diffuse nodularity of the thyroid. May cause increased thyroid function.

Tumours—benign: the most common benign thyroid tumour is the *follicular adenoma*.

Tumours—malignant: most malignant tumours of the thyroid are of epithelial origin.

Papillary carcinoma	70%
Follicular carcinoma	20%
Medullary (from the calcitonin-producing C cell)	5%
Anaplastic carcinoma	5%

Parathyroids
Parathyroid gland pathology usually presents with a raised serum calcium. The most important lesions of the parathyroids are:

–adenoma
–hyperplasia
–carcinoma

These are causes of *primary hyperparathyroidism*.

Secondary hyperparathyroidism: is over-activity of the parathyroids associated with another disease, most commonly renal failure. It may also occur in vitamin D deficiency and malabsorption.

Adrenals

Adrenal cortex: causes of over-activity of the adrenal cortex are:

–pituitary adenoma causing diffuse hyperplasia (Cushing's disease)
–adrenal adenoma
–adrenal carcinoma
–diffuse nodular hyperplasia

Common causes of reduced adrenal function are:

–autoimmune destruction (Addison's disease)
–infection
–bacteraemic shock
–metastatic carcinoma
–surgery

Adrenal medulla: the most important pathology of the adrenal medulla is the development of a phaeochromocytoma, a tumour of which produces excessive adrenaline and noradrenaline.

Diabetes mellitus
This is a very common disease which can involve the kidney. Manifestations of diabetic nephropathy are:

–accelerated arteriolosclerosis
–glomerular disease

The pathology of diabetes can be summarized as basement membrane thickening with increased permeability. The basement membrane changes involve predominantly small vessels (microvascular angiopathy).

13 Haematology

13 Haematology

THE cells in the blood all derive from the bone marrow. They develop and mature from a continually dividing population of stem cells. In a normal bone marrow there are a number of distinct cell lines which arise from the stem cells and produce distinct populations of mature cells (Fig. 13.1). These are erythroid cells, myeloid cells producing neutrophils, mononuclear–phagocytic cells, megakaryocytes producing platelets, mast cells, and lymphocytes of B and T type. When produced by the stem cell population they mature within the bone marrow. Bone marrow tissue in the adult is mainly found in the sternum, vertebrae, pelvis, and long bones. Immature T cells (pre-T cells) mature in the thymus, and B lymphocytes (pre-B cells) mature probably in the liver. Many cells produced by the bone marrow have a relatively short life span and are then engulfed by phagocytes or die. There is therefore a continual production of bone marrow cells which is balanced by the continuing loss. It has been shown that the stem cells in the bone marrow are capable of forming various types of blood cell—they have a multiple potential for development. The stem cell population of the bone marrow is a very small percentage (less than 0.001 per cent) of the total number of cells found in the bone marrow. There is a tremendous reserve of stem cells, an individual stem cell undergoing very infrequent division. Most of the proliferative activity will be taking part in the maturing compartment of the bone marrow. It is possible to show that colony-forming cells can be derived from the bone marrow. Colony-forming cells can either form a mixture of different cell types, for example, red cells, white cells, and macrophages, or they may be dedicated to the production of one cell type. Growth factors are very important in the control of the production and maturation of these colony-forming cells. Important growth factors are erythropoietin which is involved in stimulating red cell production, many interleukins which are involved in the maturation of lymphocytes and mast cells, for example, and specific growth factors which act on

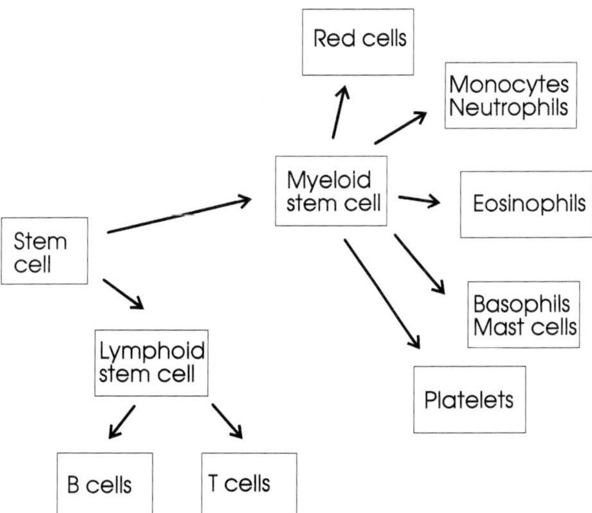

Fig. 13.1 Bone marrow cell lines.

Table 13.1 Symptoms and signs of anaemia

Increased heart rate (tachycardia)
Breathlessness (dyspnoea)
Heart murmurs
Tiredness, faintness
Pallor of skin, oral mucosa, nail beds
Smooth atrophic tongue
Swallowing difficulty (dysphagia), oesophageal webs—Paterson–Kelly syndrome

Table 13.2 Causes of anaemia

Chronic blood loss
Increased red blood cell destruction
Decreased red blood cell production

Table 13.3 Normal haematological results

Haemoglobin	
Male	16 g/100 ml
Female	14 g/100 ml
Red cell numbers	
Male	$5.4 \times 10^6/\mu l$
Female	$4.8 \times 10^6/\mu l$
White cell numbers (per μl)	
Total	**4.5–10 000**
Neutrophils	1500–6000
Eosinophils	1–700
Basophils	1–150
Lymphocytes	1500–4000
Monocytes	200–1000
Platelets	140 000–400 000

Table 13.4 Types of anaemia

Iron deficiency
Megaloblastic
Haemolytic
Haemoglobinopathies (disorders of the haemoglobin molecule structure)—thalassaemia, sickle-cell anaemia
Chronic disease causing reduced bone marrow function
Bone marrow failurc

specific maturing colony-forming cells. These specific factors are known as colony-stimulating factors.

ANAEMIA

Anaemia is a term which is used to indicate a reduced haemoglobin concentration in the circulation; symptoms and signs are shown in Table 13.1. The main groups of causes of anaemia are listed in Table 13.2. The normal haemoglobin in a normal adult male is about 14–16 g per 100 ml, the normal female range is slightly lower at 12–14 g per 100 ml (Table 13.3). Anaemia can be due to a reduced production of red cells in the bone marrow or an increased loss of blood cells from the circulation. The major types of anaemia are listed in Table 13.4.

Anaemia due to iron deficiency

The body is very efficient at conserving iron and recyling it. Only about 1 milligram of iron is required in the diet each day. Iron deficiency anaemia occurs when there is not enough iron to maintain haemoglobin production. As well as having a reduced haemoglobin concentration, the red cells become smaller in size. This is termed microcytic anaemia. The major causes of iron deficiency anaemia are listed below:

–excessive loss of haemoglobin due to blood loss
–reduced dietary intake
–increased iron requirement
–malabsorption

The most frequent cause of iron deficiency anaemia is some form of chronic blood loss. This includes heavy menstrual loss in females, which is a common cause of iron deficiency anaemia. Also other areas well recognized as sites of chronic blood loss are peptic ulcers, either in the stomach or duodenum. Inflammatory bowel disease and carcinoma is a common cause of blood loss. Diet is an uncommon cause of anaemia but vegetarian diets are inherently short of iron, and also iron is poorly absorbed within such a diet. Increased demand for iron occurs in some physiological situations, particularly in childhood and pregnancy. Malabsorption may follow inflammatory bowel disease or intestinal resection. Coeliac disease is also a cause of iron deficiency anaemia.

Megaloblastic aenamia

This is associated with a deficiency primarily of two vitamins, vitamin B_{12} or folic acid. Both of these compounds are involved in DNA synthesis. The effects of the deficiency of vitamin B_{12} and folic acid are therefore seen predominantly in rapid dividing cells. In megaloblastic anaemia, the red cells show an increased size. They also vary in size. Both of these factors are derived in the diet. In particular vitamin B_{12} (cobalamin) is derived from protein by proteases and then the vitamin binds to a specific protein called intrinsic factor which is produced by the gastric parietal cell. It is then able to be absorbed by the small bowel.

Vitamin B_{12} is derived from meat, being absent in a strict vegetarian diet. If there is severe loss of parietal cells there is failure to absorb vitamin B_{12}. Pernicious anaemia is a megaloblastic anaemia which is due to deficiency of vitamin B_{12} as a result of malabsorption of this vitamin. This is due to an autoimmune gastric atrophy. This often runs in families. It may also be associated with other autoimmune diseases. In the majority of patients there are antibodies to gastric parietal cells, causing parietal cell destruction. Antibodies also occur to intrinsic factor produced by the stomach.

Haemolytic anaemia

This is where there is anaemia due to increased destruction of red cells which overcomes the ability of the bone marrow to produce cells. With an increased destruction of red cells there is an increase in the breakdown products of haemoglobin in the circulation, particularly bilirubin. A frequent cause of haemolytic anaemia is the presence of antibodies produced against red cells. The antibodies bind to the red cells and either activate complement to cause red cell destruction or cause the red cells to be phagocytosed by macrophages in the spleen. Haemolytic anaemia may also be due to inborn abnormalities of red cells. It is more commonly acquired and may be autoimmune or induced by drugs. Artificial heart valves, infections, burns, an enlarged spleen, and vitamin E deficiency are causes of acquired haemoloytic anaemia. Congenital abnormalities of haemoglobin or red cell enzymes may also cause haemolysis. It is important to point out that red cells given to an incompatible recipient at a blood transfusion will haemolyse, the free haemoglobin causing renal failure.

Haemoglobinopathies

These are abnormalities of the structure of the haemoglobin molecule.

Thalassaemia

Normal adult haemoglobin A has a molecular structure comprising two alpha chains and two beta chains which are bound together. Thalassaemia syndromes are a situation where there is reduced or absent production of either alpha chains (alpha thalassaemia) or beta chains (beta thalassaemia). Red cells are reduced in size and number and show low levels of haemoglobin (hypochromic microcytic anaemia), with a relative excess of the unaffected haemoglobin. Haemoglobin alpha chains are coded for by two pairs of genes on chromsome 16, and beta chains by two pairs of genes on chromosome 11. The severity of the disease depends on the number of abnormal genes, as each gene contributes a quarter of the total amount of haemoglobin chain.

Alpha thalassaemia

This occurs among Asian and African populations. The excess, free beta chains bind together in adults to form tetramers (haemoglobin 'H'). In infants, however, the fetal type haemoglobin predominates (gamma), forming tetramers (haemoglobin 'Barts'). If all the genes are abnormal, the fetus does not survive to term (hydrops fetalis). If three genes are abnormal, haemoglobin H disease occurs with anaemia and an enlarged spleen. Alpha-thalassaemia trait (two involved genes) and a carrier state (one involved gene) also occur; these show no clinical symptoms.

Beta thalassaemia

This occurs in Mediterranean populations, and some areas of South East Asia and Africa. The excess alpha chains form complexes of abnormal haemoglobin which cause cell damage and increased loss in the bone marrow during red cell development. Fetal-type haemoglobin is increased in the red cells. Depending on the number of involved genes, the disease may be severe, requiring constant blood transfusions (thalassaemia major), or clinical symptoms may be mild (thalassaemia minor).

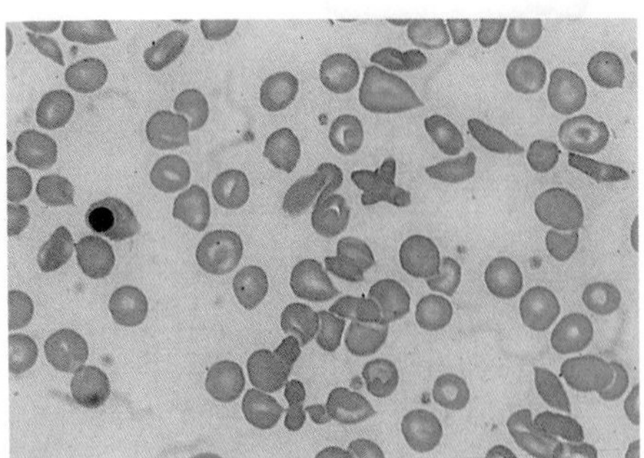

Fig. 13.2 Sickle cells in a blood smear.

Sickle-cell disease

This is characterized by the presence of an abnormal haemoglobin with an abnormal amino acid substitution due to an inherited gene defect. The most common type is haemoglobin S, with the substitution of valine for glutamic acid at position 6 on the beta chain. In areas of low intravascular oxygen, the haemoglobin polymerizes and causes distortion of the red cells into a characteristic sickle shape (Fig. 13.2). This sickling causes a haemolytic anaemia, and ischaemia in many sites due to occlusion of small blood vessels. Organs involved include the bones, eye, spleen, lungs, and brain. If both beta genes are involved, severe disease results. If only one gene is abnormal, sickle-cell trait is present; this has only mild symptoms.

Occurrence of the sickle-cell gene is common among populations of African descent.

Table 13.5 Systemic conditions associated with anaemia

Chronic infection or inflammatory disease (normochromic or hypochromic/normocytic or microcytic)
Chronic renal disease (normochromic/normocytic)
Alcoholism (macrocytic)

Anaemia of chronic disease (Table 13.5)

Anaemia is frequently seen in association with chronic disease such as chronic sepsis, tumours, and rheumatoid arthritis. The anaemia may also be caused by renal failure because of reduced erythropoietin production by the kidney.

Marrow failure

Cytotoxic drugs and other therapeutic drugs are recognized causes of severe marrow failure involving all cell lines of the bone marrow. Radiation and viruses may also induce marrow failure.

POLYCYTHAEMIA

Polycythaemia is an increase in haemoglobin and red cell mass due to an increased production of red cells. It may be physiological in the case of a polycythaemia secondary to chronic low oxygen tension such as in living at a high altitude. It may also occur secondary to some tumours which produce erythropoietin such as renal cell carcinoma. Secondary polycythaemia also occurs in chronic lung disease and in heavy smokers. Polycythaemia also occurs in association with some neoplasms of the bone marrow. This is termed polycythaemia rubra vera.

NEUTROPAENIA

This is a situation where there is a reduced number of neutrophils in the circulation. Neutrophils are predominantly phagocytic in nature and a reduced neutrophil count in the blood predisposes the person to a high risk of infection, particularly of bacterial and fungal type. There is an increased incidence of periodontitis with neutropaenia. The term lymphopaenia refers to a specific reduction in lymphocytes. Neutropaenia may be reduced to reduced produced of neutrophils in the bone marrow by, for instance, viral infection, drugs, such as cytotoxic agents, some autoimmune diseases, and replacement of the bone marrow by malignant tumour or a malignant proliferation of bone marrow cells as in leukaemia. In the case of bone marrow destruction, anaemia is frequently seen.

NEUTROPHILIA

This is when there is increased numbers of neutrophils in the circulation and this is most commonly associated with bacterial infection. Neutrophilia is also frequently associated with any form of trauma, accidental or surgical. Marked neutrophilia is usually seen in association with malignant diseases of the bone marrow involving cells of the neutrophil line, so-called myeloid cells. Lymphocytosis refers to an increase in lymphocytes specifically, and it is typically seen in viral infection. A marked increase in lymphocytes may be seen in some forms of leukaemia involving the lymphoid cell lines. An increase in eosinophils is associated with parasitic infection and allergy.

HAEMATOLOGICAL NEOPLASMS

Leukaemia

This is uncontrolled proliferation of bone marrow cells, which is associated with an imbalance between cell production and cell maturation, and is frequently associated with an excess of one or more of the cell lines in the circulation. The malignant change may be seen early on in the differentiation of the bone marrow cell, and this is termed an acute leukaemia. Acute leukaemias show a high proportion of rapidly proliferating primitive 'blast' cells in the bone marrow, often forming at least 30 per cent of the total population of the bone marrow cells. If the malignant change results in an increase in mature cells it is termed chronic leukaemia. The underlying problem in chronic leukaemia is a loss of negative feedback to the stem cells. Leukaemias occur in different cell lines. The most frequent involve the lymphoid and myeloid cell lines. The bone marrow becomes dominated by the particular malignant cell line, suppressing the production of other bone marrow cells (Fig. 13.3).

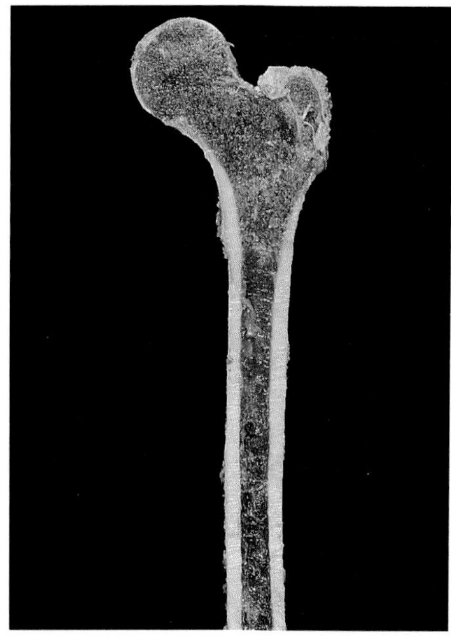

Fig. 13.3 Bone marrow extends down the full length of the femur in this case of leukaemia. Normally the shaft of the femur contains only yellow fat.

Acute lymphoblastic anaemia

This is diagnosed by the presence of lymphoblasts in the peripheral circulation and in the bone marrow. These are primitive lymphocytes with large nuclei but no granules in the cytoplasm. There appears to be an uncontrolled proliferation of these primitive cells in the bone marrow, with an apparent block in differentiation. The bone marrow, and then the peripheral blood is swamped by this proliferation of primitive cells. There is replacement of the normal cells of the bone marrow with resulting marrow failure. This manifests itself as anaemia, bleeding disorders due to low platelets, and infection due to low neutrophil counts. It is from this vast increase in white cells in the peripheral circulation that the name leukaemia is derived.

This disease is most common in childhood between the ages of 1 and 6 years, and may be of either T cell or B cell type.

Chronic lymphocytic leukaemia

This is a less aggressive form of leukaemia occurring in later life, being uncommon in children. It either is discovered on blood film, where there is vastly increased count in mature lymphocytes or discovered on clinical presentation with enlarged lymph nodes or spleen. In almost all cases there is an uncontrolled proliferation of lymphocytes of B cell type, which replace normal bone marrow elements, causing bone marrow failure. There is frequently anaemia, low platelets or a low neutrophil count. The cells of chronic lymphocytic leukaemia are much more mature than those seen in childhood, acute lymphoblastic leukaemia. Chronic leukaemia has a tendency to transform to a more aggressive acute leukaemia with time.

Acute myeloid leukaemia

In this there is an autonomous or uncontrolled proliferation of cells of the myeloid series, cells on some part of the pathway of differentiation towards the granulocytes producing polymorphs. Acute myeloid leukaemia is relatively rare in children and becomes more frequent in the older age group. As with other leukaemias there is an increase in primitive and abnormal myeloid cells in the peripheral blood and bone marrow which replace normal cell elements. Blast cells are found in the peripheral blood. The myeloid cells can be classified according to their differentiation, some sharing monocytic, platelet, or red cell type differentiation.

Chronic myeloid leukaemia

In this there is an increased proliferation of production of mature myeloid cells, the usual finding being an increase in relatively mature cells of the granulocyte series in the peripheral blood. It is a disease of a very slow progression compared to the other leukaemias. Chronic myeloid leukaemia illustrates its monoclonality in that there is consistent chromosomal abnormality in all the neoplastic cells. The consistent chromosomal abnormality seen in chronic myeloid leukaemia is a translocation of part of chromosome 22 to chromosome 9. This is known as the Philadelphia chromosome.

Other myeloid disorders

There are other problems in stem cell differentiation manifesting themselves as myeloid abnormalities, the most frequent are polycythaemia rubra vera, myelofibrosis, and thrombocythaemia.

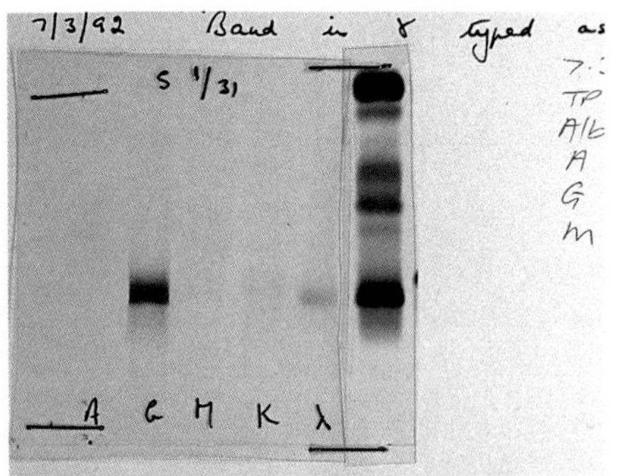

Fig. 13.4 A dominant monoclonal band can be seen in the lower part of the strip on the right. The band stains for IgG and lambda light chain (strips to the left).

Myeloma

There are some proliferations of lymphoid cells where the malignant cells show marked differentiation towards plasma cells. Plasma cells by their very nature produce immunoglobulins, and a frequent manifestation of this is a production of just one type of immunoglobulin at the expense of the others. This is seen in the plasma protein as a monoclonal band in a protein strip (Fig. 13.4). It is a malignant B cell proliferation where plasma cells are prominent. It is a disease of the elderly.

DISORDERS OF HAEMOSTASIS

Blood coagulation

Blood, of course has to remain fluid in the circulation, but has to become solid when blood vessel damage occurs to prevent life-threatening haemorrhage. Dentists frequently cause vascular damage, for instance when extracting a tooth. On damage to small capillaries and arteries, the first mechanism to control blood loss is a transient period of vessel constriction of spasm. This can also be seen in damage to larger vessels such as muscular arteries. Plugging of small defects by platelet aggregates then occurs within minutes, known as *primary* haemostasis. Exposure of subendothelial connective tissue and tissue factors, such as Hageman factor and platelet-activating factor, cause rapid platelet aggregation. Platelets accumulate over the site of endothelial damage. This mass of platelets then acts as a focus for the production of fibrin which is a polymer that plugs the vessel. When the platelets fuse and are welded together with fibrin, a *secondary* haemostatic plug is formed.

Platelets adhere to subendothelial tissue using mechanisms that require von Willebrand factor. If this factor is deficient, platelets show a reduced ability to aggregate. The platelets then contract using changes in the cytoskeleton involving myosin and actin filaments. They release substances such as fibrinogen, fibronectin, and platelet-derived growth factor from *alpha* granules. Platelets also express platelet factor 3 on their surface which acts as a focus for the formation of factor X in the intrinsic blood-clotting cascade. The *dense* bodies release histamine, adrenaline, serotonin, and adenosine diphosphate (ADP). Serotonin is a potent vasoconstrictor, and ADP is involved in platelet aggregation. Platelets also release calcium which is involved in the intrinsic blood clotting system.

Endothelium produces substances that inhibit clotting such as prostaglandin I_2, tissue plasminogen activator, thrombomodulin (which activates protein C and S), and heparin-like substances. Endothelium also produces substances that induce clotting such as tissue factor, factor V, inhibitors of fibrinolysis, von Willibrand factor, and platelet-activating factor. The thrombotic and antithrombotic processes are normally held in balance.

Fibrin is produced from fibrinogen, which is a precursor molecule. There is a cascade of proteins acting in an amplification manner. The majority of these factors are produced in the liver. Defects in blood clotting may be due to a deficiency of one or more of the blood clotting factors, or an abnormality of platelets may be present. Some congenital disorders, for example protein C deficiency, in contrast give an *increased* risk of abnormal thrombosis. The blood clotting cascade is summarized in Fig. 13.5 and Table 13.6.

The fibrinolytic system acts as a method of removing blood clot and acts also as a protective balance against inappropriate clotting. Other mechanisms, such as clearance of activated factors from the circulation, and the dilution of clotting factors act to protect against excessive fibrin production. There are also circulating inhibitors of blood clotting including antithrombin III, C′1-activator (a complement pathway inhibitor), and protein C.

The most important enzyme in the fibrinolytic system is *plasmin*, produced by the action of factors on *plasminogen* (see p. 000). Factors that inhibit clotting and factors that promote clotting (procoagulants) are shown in Table 13.7. The causes of bleeding disorders are summarized in Table 13.8.

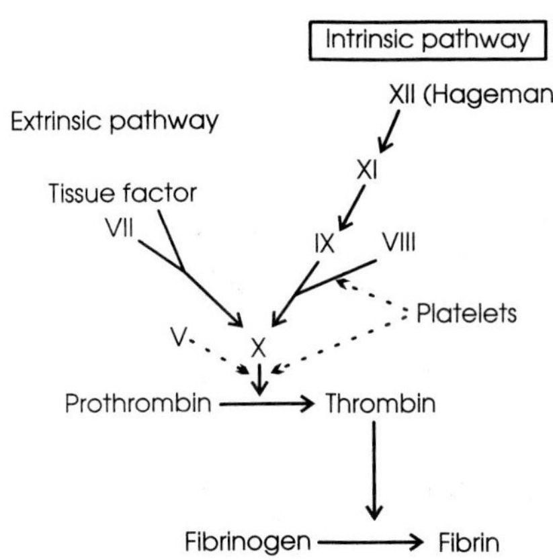

Fig. 13.5 The blood clotting cascade.

Coagulation factor deficiencies

The majority of these are inherited bleeding disorders. They frequently present as excessive bleeding or bruising after injury. One feature that may suggest a bleeding tendency is abnormal bleeding from a tooth socket after an extraction. The most common type of congenital bleeding disorder is haemophilia A, which is a deficiency of factor VIII. This is a gene defect which is linked to the X chromosome, and therefore affects males but is carried by females. The reduced manifestation of haemophilia in females is due to the presence of two X chromosomes in the cells, one of which only has the abnormal gene present. There is almost always a remaining normal gene producing some factor VIII. Along with a lot of blood clotting factors, factor VIII is mainly produced in the liver. The most common clinical presentation of this disease is repeated episodes of bleeding into joints and muscles, and extensive haemorrhage after superficial injury which persists. The disease is of most importance when surgery is considered, where patients need additional factor VIII replacement before and during surgery. Bruising into the skin (purpura) does not occur, in contrast to that seen in platelet abnormalities. The bleeding time (the time

Table 13.6 Clotting (coagulation) factors

I	Fibrinogen
II	Prothrombin
III	Tissue factor
IV	Calcium
V	Labile factor
VI	Proconvertin
VII	Antihaemophilic factor
VIII	Christmas factor
IX	Stewart–Prower factor
X	Thromboplastin
XI	Hageman factor
XII	Fibrin-stabilizing factor

Table 13.7 Blood clotting

Anticoagulant	Procoagulant
Herparin-like molecules	Coagulation system
Plasminogen activators	Fibronectin
Thrombomodulin	Plasminogen activator inhibitors
Prostacyclin	Tissue factor
	Platelet-activating factor

Table 13.8 Causes of bleeding disorders

Coagulation factor deficiency
Haemophilia A; reduced factor VIII
Haemophilia B; reduced factor IX
Von Willebrand's disease
Liver disease with reduced production of coagulation factors
Vitamin K deficiency
Disseminated intravascular coagulation (DIC) with reduced fibrinogen levels
Platelet abnormalities
Reduced platelet numbers (thrombocytopaenia)
Abnormal platelet adhesion (Von Willebrand's disease)
Abnormal platelet granules
Abnormal blood vessels
Vascular damage due to infection or inflammation
Connective tissue abnormalities (vitamin C deficiency, excessive steroids)
Multiple haemangiomas (hereditary haemorrhagic telangiectasia)

taken for a small skin incision to stop bleeding) is normal, reflecting a normal platelet function. However, the clotting time of blood is very prolonged.

A congenital deficiency of factor IX occurs in haemophilia B (Christmas disease). The clinical symptoms are the same as those for haemophilia A.

Von Willibrand's disease is another important congenital blood clotting disorder. In contrast to the haemophilias, it related to a gene on an autosome (non-sex chromosome); it has an autosomal dominant pattern of inheritance. It is a deficiency of the von Willibrand factor, which is a factor involved in the adhesion of platelets to exposed connective tissue under damaged endothelium. Von Willibrand's factor is also binds factor VIII in the circulation. As well as having an increased clotting time, because of the interference with factor VIII function, there is disturbance of platelet function, with an increased bleeding time.

Platelet abnormalities

If the platelet count is low (10–20 000/μl), there may be spontaneous bleeding from small blood vessels in the skin to form purpura, or from mucosal surfaces. The count may be low because of reduced production by the bone marrow (due to replacement of the marrow by leukaemia or tumour, aplastic anaemia, drugs, toxins, or infection), or increased destruction of platelets in the circulation or spleen (due to autoimmune disease, drugs, or disseminated intravascular coagulation).

Drugs, such as aspirin and non-steroidal anti-inflammatory drugs, renal and liver failure are associated with platelet abnormalities. There are also congenital defects of platelet function, abnormal glycoprotein expression, or adenosine diphosphate (ADP) that interfere with platelet aggregation.

Vascular abnormalities

The deposition of immune complexes within small blood vessels in type III hypersensitivity can cause bleeding into the soft tissue or skin, manifesting as purpura. An example is Henoch–Schönlein purpura, an illness in children often related to a viral infection.

Abnormal blood vessels may bleed; an example of such a condition is hereditary haemorrhagic telangiectasia where there is the development of large numbers of abnormally dilated capillaries in the skin, oral mucosa, the gastrointestinal tract, and viscera.

Acquired blood coagulation disorders

Reduced production of clotting factors

Vitamin K is important in the production of blood clotting factors II, VII, IX, and X by the liver. Therefore a deficiency of vitamin K due to a poor diet or reduced absorption may present a blood coagulation disorder.

In view of the fact that the liver is the main source of many of the blood clotting factors, one of the many manifestations of chronic liver failure is clotting disorders. Failure of coagulation is also seen in chronic renal failure and also in conditions where there is a reduction of platelet count. This reduction in platelets may occur in association with either severe viral infections or bacterial infections.

Disseminated intravascular coagulation (DIC)

There may be a widespread, inappropriate activation of the coagulation system in a number of systemic conditions, including Gram-negative bacterial infection, shock (particularly obstetric), injury, cancer, burns, and other major insults to the body. There are deposits of fibrin in small blood vessels, affecting mainly the kidneys, brain, and myocardium. This deposition of fibrin causes ischaemia to these organs. A result of all this clotting factor activation is that the clotting factors are depleted, giving rise to an abnormality in blood clotting. Patients with DIC develop purpura and other problems with haemostasis.

In DIC there is a reduced platelet count, red cell fragmentation, low blood fibrinogen levels, and increased clotting time.

Thrombotic thrombocytopaenic purpura and haemolytic uraemic syndrome are similar to DIC in that there is consumption of circulating platelets. In contrast to DIC there is not such a dramatic activation of clotting factors.

LYMPH NODES

The structure of the mormal lymph node has been covered in the chapter on immunology. This section will concentrate on the surgical pathology of lymph nodes. Lymph nodes are strategically placed in areas that drain sites at varying distances from the nodes. The lymph nodes in a particular region therefore screen for antigens taken to the node from these areas. There is frequent circulation between the lymph nodes and their respective drainage areas. This is particularly prominent in the gastrointestinal tract, where there appears to be specialized populations of lymphocytes that re-circulated from the mucosal surface to regional lymph nodes.

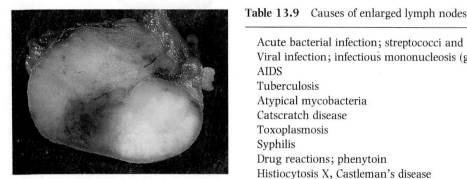

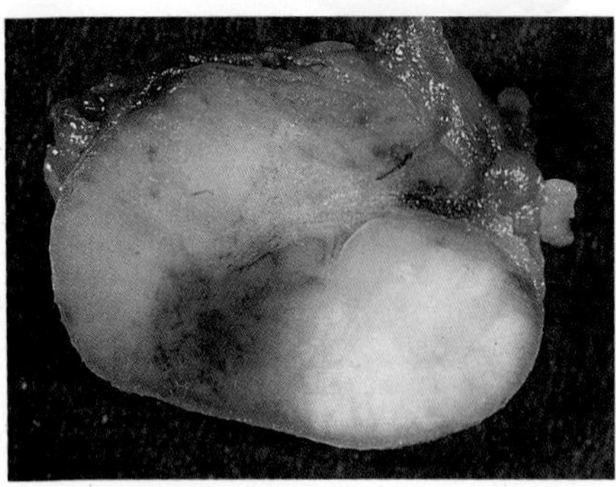

Fig. 13.6 A white nodule of metastatic carcinoma is seen in this lymph node (bottom right).

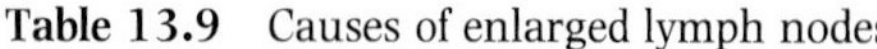

Table 13.9 Causes of enlarged lymph nodes

Acute bacterial infection; streptococci and staphylococci
Viral infection; infectious mononucleosis (glandular fever)
AIDS
Tuberculosis
Atypical mycobacteria
Catscratch disease
Toxoplasmosis
Syphilis
Drug reactions; phenytoin
Histiocytosis X, Castleman's disease
Malignant primary disease; lymphoma, Hodgkin's disease
Metastatic cancer (Fig. 13.6)
Granulomatous disease; sarcoidosis
Autoimmune disease; rheumatoid arthritis

Causes of enlarged lymph nodes

A frequent presentation of lymph node pathology is enlargement. The cause of an enlarged lymph node has a wide differential diagnosis, which is summarized in Table 13.9.

Lymphoma

Malignant proliferations in lymph nodes form into two main groups, both biologically and clinically. These are Hodgkin's lymphoma or non-Hodgkin's lymphoma.

Hodgkin's disease

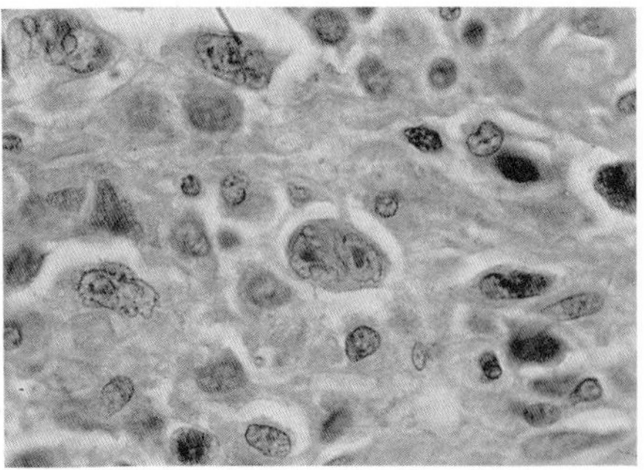

Fig. 13.7 Hodgkin's lymphoma; there is a proliferation of atypical cells, including a Reed–Sternberg cell (centre).

This is a distinct entity which is characterized by a malignant proliferation of large atypical lymphocytes within a reactive inflammatory background within a lymph node. It is still not clear which cell these malignant lymphoid cells are derived from, but the classification of a lymphoma as Hodgkin's disease has great clinical significance in that there is a distinct treatment regime for this disease. There are generally four basic types of Hodgkin's disease which correspond to the nature of the inflammatory reaction to the malignant cells. These are lymphocyte-predominant (10 per cent of cases), nodular-sclerosing (40 per cent, more common in females), mixed-cellularity (40 per cent), and lymphocyte-depleted (10 per cent). They are all characterized by this proliferation of atypical lymphoid cells with a very distinct histological appearance. The large atypical lymphocytes have very prominent nuclei and often have a binucleate form known as the Reed–Sternberg cell (Fig. 13.7). There is evidence that Reed–Sternberg cells are derived from B cells but the origin is not yet proven.

Non-Hodgkin's lymphomas

These are generally clinically classified into low-grade and high-grade types. Low-grade lymphomas tend to be slow growing, with low proliferative activity. They generally do not need treatment unless there are clinical symptoms. However, in view of their low proliferative activity they are relatively resistant to chemotherapy and radiotherapy. High-grade lymphomas are rapidly growing and progressive but in view of the higher proliferative activity of these tumours they are relatively sensitive to chemotherapy and radiation. The clinical stage of a lymphoma which

Table 13.10 The staging of lymphoma

Stage	Clinical findings
I	A single node region involved
II	Two or more node regions, same side of diaphragm
III	Involvement both sides of diaphragm. Spleen involved = stage S
IV	Disseminated lymphoma
A	No symptoms
B	Fever, night sweats, more than 10% weight loss

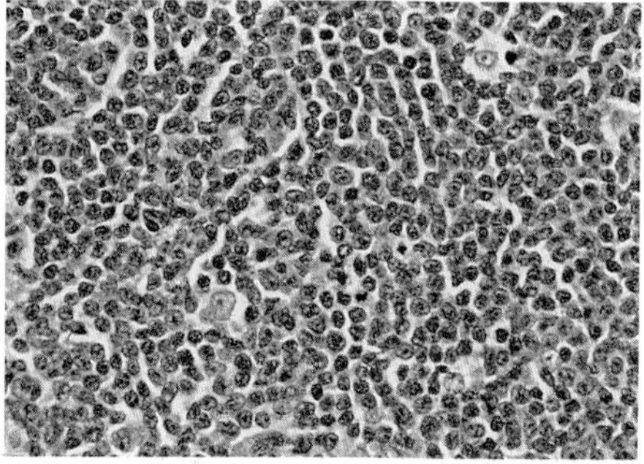

Fig. 13.8 The lymph node is replaced by a monotonous proliferation of malignant lymphocytes.

reflects the extent of disease is very important in determining the prognosis of a lymphoma. Lymphomas are classified by pathologists by the apparent cell of origin of the malignant lymphocyte. Low-grade lymphomas show well-differentiated cells which closely resemble their normal counterpart. Mitotic rate of these lymphomas is low and the cells generally small. High-grade lymphomas show large undifferentiated lymphocytes, often of blastic type in that they are rather primitive. High-grade lymphomas generally have a high mitotic grade. The most common type of non-Hodgkin's lymphoma is derived from B cells. T cell lymphomas are less common. Other rarer types appear to be derived from macrophages or monocytes.

On histology, lymphomas are recognized by destruction of the normal lymphocyte structure, with effacement by a proliferation of malignant lymphocytes (Fig. 13.8). There is frequently capsular invasion of the lymph node with extension into surrounding tissues.

Lymphomas can arise in sites other than lymph nodes, often referred to as extranodal lymphomas. Common extranodal sites are the gastrointestinal tract, the lung, salivary glands, and thyroid. Lymphomas may develop in the oropharynx, nasopharynx, and Waldeyer's ring (tonsils and adenoids). The skin is also a well-recognized site of lymphoma, mainly of T cell type. The prognosis of lymphomas depends on the type, the grade, and the stage of the disease. The system used in staging is shown in Table 13.10.

SPLEEN

Causes of an enlarged spleen (Fig. 13.9)

When the spleen shows increased function, it commonly enlarges from its normal 150 grams. Some common causes of an enlarged spleen are listed in Table 13.11.

Diseases of the spleen can be divided into those conditions which affect the red pulp, and those conditions which affect the white pulp. The red pulp contains the sinusoids and macrophages, and is affected, for example, by infective processes. The white pulp consists of T cell-dependent periarteriolar lymphoid tissue and B cell-dependent lymphoid follicles with germinal centres. Lymphoma and reactive immunological conditions affect the white pulp.

Loss of the spleen, most commonly due to removal following traumatic rupture (Fig. 13.10), increases the risk of septicaemia, particularly from encapsulated organisms such as pneumococci. Infection by *Haemophilus influenza* or meningococcus may also occur. Infection is most common in the first two years after loss of the spleen. The risk is particularly high among children, but persists into adult life. It is recommended that a person without a spleen should be on antibiotic cover and be vaccinated against pneumococcal strains.

The spleen is prone to infarction (necrosis due to ischaemia, Fig. 13.11).

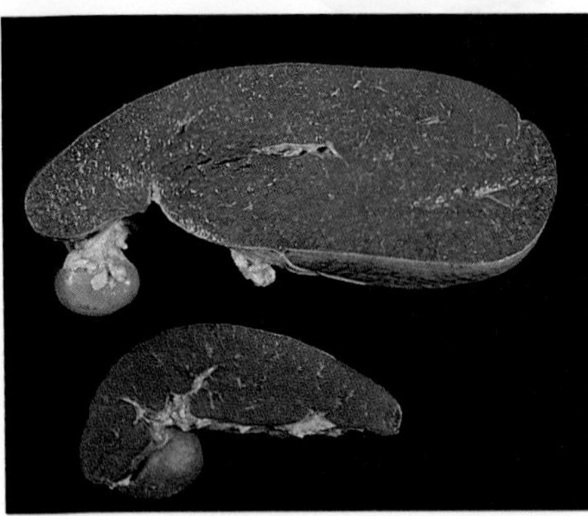

Fig. 13.9 How large some spleens can become compared with normal (below).

Table 13.11 Causes of an enlarged spleen (Fig. 13.9)

Reaction to infection: malaria, Epstein–Barr virus, hepatitis, AIDS, visceral leishmaniasis, infective endocarditis, tuberculosis
Infiltration by tumour: lymphoma, metastases
Increased function: haemolytic anaemia, production of blood cells (haemopoiesis) associated with bone marrow failure (e.g. myelofibrosis)
Vascular congestion: portal hypertension
Depositions: amyloid, Gaucher's disease
Autoimmune disease: rheumatoid arthritis

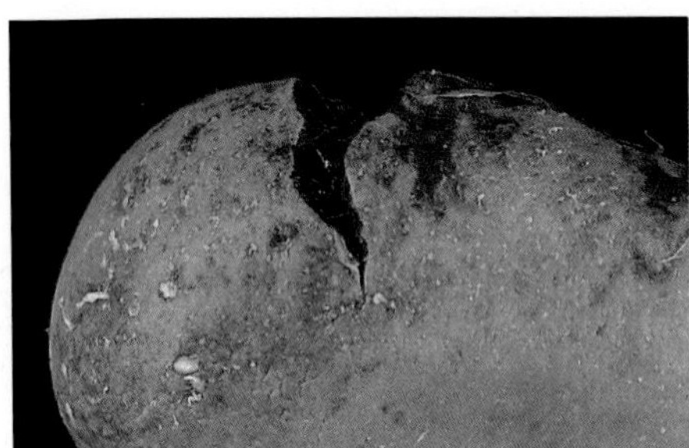

Fig. 13.10 A tear in the splenic capsule due to trauma.

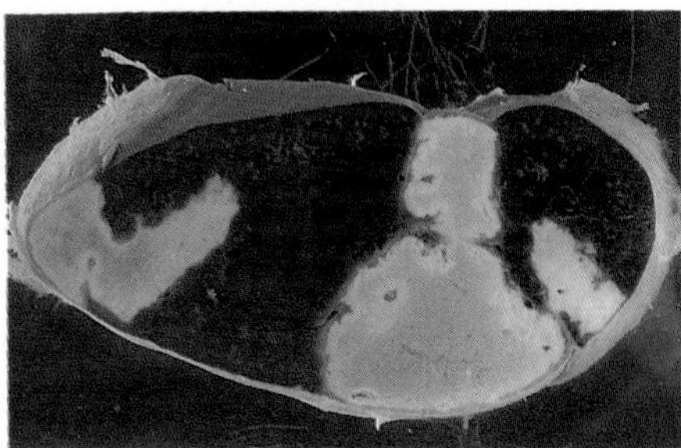

Fig. 13.11 White, wedge-shaped splenic infarcts due to emboli of vegetations from infective endocarditis.

SUMMARY

Anaemia

Major causes of anaemia are:

–iron deficiency
–folate and vitamin B_{12} deficiency (megaloblastic anaemia)
–haemolytic haemoglobinopathies
–chronic disease with reduced marrow function

Polycythaemia

This is an increase in haemoglobin and red cell mass. It is usually physiological and secondary to chronic low oxygen tension.

Haematological neoplasms

Leukaemia: this is an uncontrolled proliferation of bone marrow cells with abnormal maturation. The most frequent forms of leukaemia involve the lymphocytic and myeloid cell lines. Common forms of leukaemia are listed below:

–acute lymphoblastic leukaemia
–chronic lymphocytic leukaemia
–acute myeloid leukaemia
–chronic myeloid leukaemia

The term *acute* refers to the immature nature of the cells found in the circulation. The term *chronic* refers to the mature differentiated cells that are found in the circulation.

Causes of bleeding tendency

Abnormalities of haemostasis may be due to:

–vascular abnormality
–platelet abnormality
–coagulation factor abnormality

Pathology of lymph nodes

A frequent presentation of lymph node pathology is enlargement. There is a large number of causes of lymphadenopathy, which can be classified as:

–bacterial infection
–viral infection
–reaction to drugs
–primary neoplasia (lymphoma)
–metastatic cancer

Lymphoma: these can be divided into Hodgkin's lymphoma and non-Hodgkin's lymphomas. Non-Hodgkin's lymphomas are classified into low-grade and high-grade types. They are classified according to the differentiation of the neoplastic lymphocytes.

The spleen

Splenic enlargement is a common manifestation of splenic pathology. Diseases of the spleen can be divided into red pulp and white pulp pathology. There is a large number of causes of splenic enlargement, including reaction to infection, association with haematological disease, infiltration by tumour, and vascular disorders.

14 The nervous system

14 The nervous system

CENTRAL NERVOUS SYSTEM

Hypoxia

The brain has a very high metabolic rate and subsequently a very high oxygen consumption. Although the brain represents only 2 per cent of the body weight, it receives 15 per cent of the cardiac output. Hypoxia is a state of oxygen deficiency which is usually due to inadequate oxygen in the blood. The brain is very sensitive to hypoxia, and in normal situations it cannot survive more than four minutes without oxygen. The causes of hypoxia can be classified as below:

1. *Ischaemia*. The brain is particularly sensitive to ischaemia, which is a situation when there is reduced or absent blood flow to part of the brain. Ischaemia may be due to cardiogenic shock from haemorrhage or a myocardial infarct. Severe atherosclerosis of the cerebral arteries causing occlusion may also result in ischaemia. The brain can survive longer periods of ischaemia if the metabolic requirement of the brain is reduced by, for instance, cooling. This may occur in the case of immersion into cold water, where people have survived an hour or more in view of the cooling of the brain reducing the requirement for oxygen, as long as blood flow continues.

Episodes of ischaemia may cause infarction, which may be regional if an occlusion involves only one artery. If a person with widespread severe atheroma of the cerebral arteries has an episode of low blood pressure, there may be infarction only in areas where the cerebral circulation is normally relatively low—the so-called 'watershed' areas. The reduced blood pressure is enough to compromise these areas which are found where two regional circulations meet, for example between the middle and posterior cerebral circulations. This strip of cortex may be the only area affected. Infarction is dealt with in more detail later in this chapter.

2. *Systemic hypoxia*. Reduced blood oxygen may be a cause of cerebral hypoxia. Clinical conditions where this occurs include particularly respiratory failure due to lung disease or severe aneamia.

3. *Toxins*. Carbon monoxide replaces oxygen and binds strongly to haemoglobin, thereby inactivating it. This has the same metabolic efect as severe anaemia and cerebral damage may occur due to hypoxia.

4. *Metabolic causes*. The brain is also very sensitive to hypoglycaemia, in view of the fact that the main metabolic fuel of the brain is glucose. Hypoglycaemia may be induced by, for instance, insulin overdose.

Coma is a manifestation of a number of disorders listed in Table 14.1.

Table 14.1 Causes of coma

Cerebral
Trauma
Cerebral haemorrhage
Cerebral infarction
Subdural haematoma
Raised intracerebral pressure
Tumour
Abscess
Infection, including meningitis
Epilepsy
Cerebral malaria
Any midbrain disease
Systemic
Hypoxia
Ischaemia
Hypotension
Hypoglycaemia
Toxins: alcohol, drugs, e.g. barbiturates
Liver failure
Renal failure; uraemia
Endocrine gland failure; thyroid, adrenals

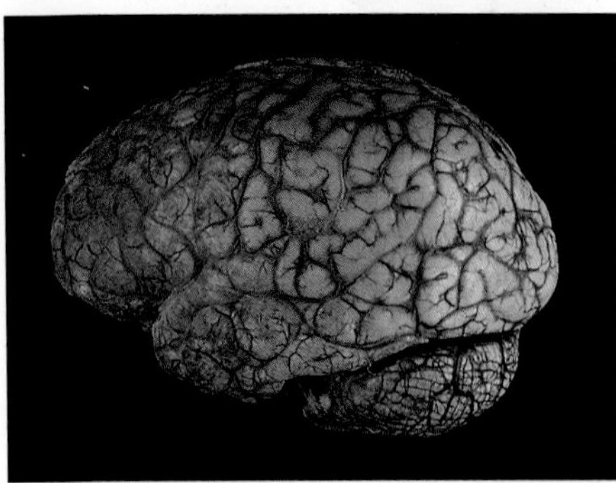

Fig. 14.1 Acute meningitis. Pus is seen over the frontal cortex (left).

Infections

Meningitis

This is inflammation of the meninges by bacteria, viruses, or fungi, which may reach the meninges via the bloodstream, or directly through trauma to the skull which allows entry of organisms from particularly the paranasal sinuses or the middle ear. Another source of infection is dental infection spreading to the maxillary sinus and then into the cranial cavity. An important point is that the roots of the upper premolars frequently project into the maxillary sinus. Clinically, meningitis may present as headache, fever, and associated neck stiffness. Meningitis can be divided into acute and chronic types, and the causative organisms vary depending on the age of the individual concerned.

Acute meningitis

Pathologically, features of acute inflammation are seen over the meninges and surface of the brain, including vascular congestion, swelling, and an inflammatory exudate composed of pus which comprises large numbers of neutrophils. There is also a striking exudate of fibrin (Fig. 14.1). The causative organisms can be identified within this purulent exudate and may be identified in samples of cerebrospinal fluid taken during lumbar puncture. As mentioned above the causative organisms depend on the age of the individual (Table 14.2).

Table 14.2 Causes of meningitis

Neonates
Group B streptococci
E. coli
Children under 10 years
Haemophilus influenzae
E. coli
Meningococcus
Pneumococcus
Adults
Meningococcus
Pneumococcus
Less frequent causes of meningitis include *Listeria*, staphylococci, and other coliforms.

Chronic meningitis

This occurs when there is a less virulent organism causing meningitis, with a much more prolonged clinical course and pathological organism. Frequently, the striking feature of chronic meningitis is fibrosis with obstruction of flow of cerebrospinal fluid through the foramina from the fourth ventricle. This results in a so-called communicating hydrocephalus where the third, fourth, and lateral ventricles become dilated due to pressure of cerebrospinal fluid produced by the choroid plexus. There may also be striking vascular changes in chronic meningitis with marked proliferation of the intima which may cause partial or complete occlusion of the lumen. This will then result in ischaemia or infarction of the area supplied by that artery.

Organisms causing chronic meningitis include tuberculosis, fungal infections, including *Candida* and *Aspergillus*, and yeast infections particularly cryptococcus and histoplasma. A historically important but now less frequent cause of chronic meningitis is tertiary syphilis which is manifested as a chronic obliterative inflammation of blood vessels called endarteritis obliterans. This in particular involves dorsal spinal roots clinically seen as so-called tabes dorsalis.

Acute meningitis may progress to a subdural empyema, or may be associated with or progress to a brain abscess. A subdural empyema occurs when pus accumulates within the subdural space and spreads over the surface of the brain. This may also induce vascular thrombosis within large veins over the surface of the brain including venous sinuses. Brain abscesses occur predominantly within the white matter and are associated particularly with spread from the paranasal and middle ear cavities with a subsequent temporal or cerebellar abscess. An abscess cavity develops, with features as seen within any abscess cavity within the body. The brain becomes liquefied and is surrounded by a reactive stromal response in the brain by the connective tissue cells of the brain, the glial tissue. Brain abscesses are frequently associated with cerebral oedema. Another source of infected material is the bloodstream, and a serious complication of infective endocarditis is septic embolism. Viral meningitis is relatively common and less clinically serious than bacterial meningitis. Pathologically, there tends to be a lymphocytic inflammatory response rather than a neutrophil inflammatory response and bacteria cannot be cultured from the cerebrospinal fluid. A more serious complication of virus infection of the nervous system is encephalitis.

Encephalitis

This occurs when there is direct infection of brain tissue by the virus which results in direct cell death and destruction of neurones. There is then an associated lymphocytic inflammatory response. Viruses which are commonly implicated in encephalitis are shown in Table 14.3.

Table 14.3 Causes of encephalitis

Herpes simplex types I and II (this typically is associated with a temporal encephalitis)
Herpes zoster
Cytomegalovirus (in this large intranuclear inclusions are frequently identified)
Epstein–Barr virus
Enterovirus (polio virus, coxsackie virus, ECHO)
Measles virus
Mumps virus
Rabies
Rubella
HIV
Other infrequent organisms causing cerebral infection include toxoplasmosis, toxocara, and malaria

Cerebral haemorrhage

Cerebral haemorrhage can be classified by the anatomical compartment into which the bleeding occurs.

Extradural haemorrhage

This is typically associated with cerebral trauma. Most cases show an associated skull fracture, particularly of the temporal bone and there is tearing of the underlying closely adherent middle meningeal artery. Bleeding may also occur from the fracture site. The pressure of bleeding strips the dura from the inside of the skull and forms a space-occupying mass which slowly enlarges, compressing the underlying brain. Clinically there may be a long delay between the time of trauma and subsequent clinical symptoms from the space-occupying lesion of the haematoma.

Subdural haemorrhage (Fig. 14.2)

Subdural haematomas develop when there is tearing of the thin communicating veins between the cerebral veins and the large venous sinuses. Subdural haematoma is associated with trauma with closed head injury. Subdural haematomas may be acutely associated with cerebral trauma, or may be very insidious and gradually develop over days or weeks following the time of injury. The haematoma forms a slowly enlarging mass with secondary damage to the underlying compressed brain. In a chronic subdural haematoma the surrounding tissue may become very fibrotic and walled-off. The clinical presentation of a subdural haematoma particularly of chronic type may be very insidious.

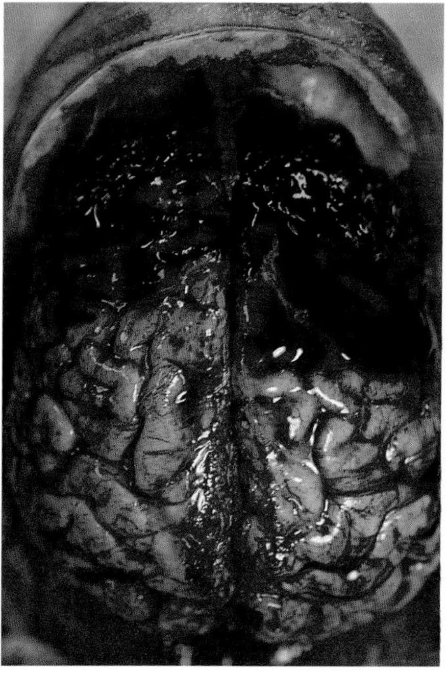

Fig. 14.2 A subdural haematoma following trauma.

Subarachnoid haemorrhage (Fig. 14.3)

Bleeding into the subarachnoid space is usually due to rupture of a berry aneurysm arising from a cerebral artery (Fig. 14.4). Berry aneurysms in 80 per cent of cases occur in the anterior circulation of the circle of Willis and are frequently seen at the branching points of cerebral arteries. Arteries that are commonly involved include the middle and anterior cerebral arteries. Berry aneurysms are seen in up to 2 per cent of the population and may be multiple. Because of the arterial nature of the bleeding, and the large potential space of the subarachnoid layer, the bleeding is often extensive and associated with severe underlying brain injury including cerebral oedema and midbrain compression. There may also be infarction in the area of brain supplied by the artery with the aneurysm. Ruptured cerebral berry aneurysms have a high mortality rate, almost a quarter of patients dying rapidly at presentation.

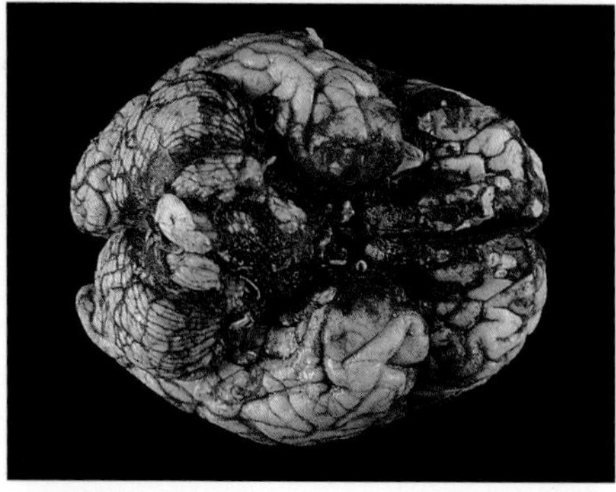

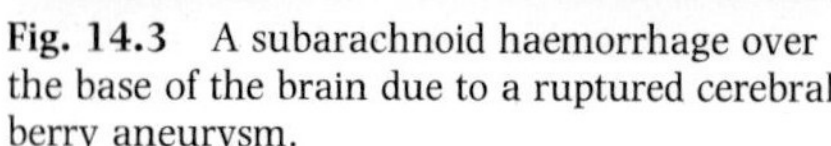

Fig. 14.3 A subarachnoid haemorrhage over the base of the brain due to a ruptured cerebral berry aneurysm.

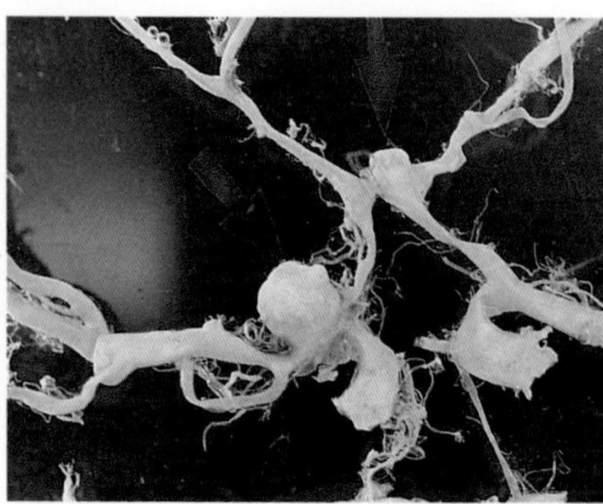

Fig. 14.4 Cerebral berry aneurysms (arrowed).

Less common causes of subarachnoid haemorrhage include arteriovenous malformations, which are abnormal and dilated communications between the arteries and veins, probably congenital in origin. Angiomas may also be responsible for subarachnoid haemorrhage.

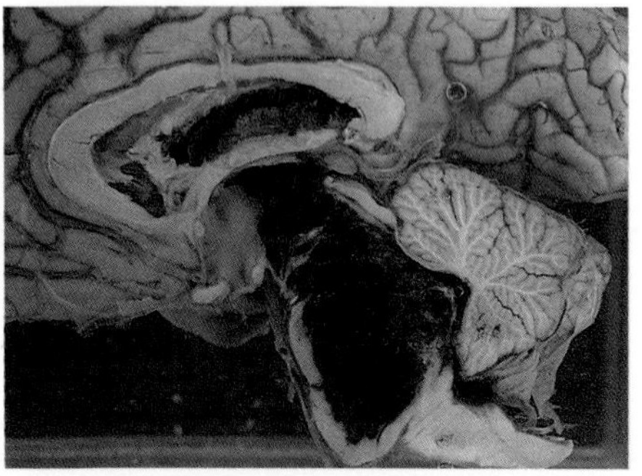

Fig. 14.5 An intracerebral haemorrhage involving the midbrain and pons.

Intracerebral haemorrhage (Fig. 14.5)

This is strongly associated with essential hypertension in the population and is commonly seen within the brain substance in the area of the basal ganglia. The haemorrhages appear to arise from small perforating branches arising from the middle cerebral artery called lenticulostriate arteries. Haemorrhage may also occur within the posterior part of the brain, including the brain stem and midbrain. Microaneurysms (often called Charcot–Bouchard microaneurysms) are associated with intracerebral haemorrhage, these being small outpouchings of arteries less than a millimetre in diameter which are associated with essential hypertension. They are seen more commonly in the older population, and are also seen occasionally in patients without a history of hypertension. Other causes of intracerebral haemorrhage include clotting disorders and trauma. Large intracerebral haemorrhages are frequently fatal. On slicing the brain a large circumscribed clot will be seen in the area of haemorrhage with severe compression of the surrounding brain. This compression frequently causes secondary neurological deficits and in fact may be responsible for midbrain compression and death.

Cerebral infarct

Cerebral infarction occurs when there is death of brain tissue due to compromised blood supply. It is the most common reason for a 'stroke', which is a sudden onset of a neurological deficit which lasts longer than 24 hours and is of vascular origin. Another name for this is a 'cerebrovascular accident'. Another cause for a stroke is an intracerebral haemorrhage. The term 'transient ischaemic attack' is used to describe neurological symptoms of vascular origin which last 24 hours or less.

The entire cerebral circulation is derived from the two vertebral and two carotid arteries and occlusion of any one of these vessels may result in infarction. In view of the marked collateral circulation of the circle of Willis, and the variable anatomy of this circulation, the distribution of infarction and the extent of infarction is very variable for any given occlusion of a cerebral artery. It is difficult to predict the extent of an infarct for a given occlusion of a cerebral artery. Occlusion of a cerebral artery may be due to local thrombosis, commonly overlying cerebral arteriosclerosis.

Occlusion may also be due to embolus from a distant source. Common sites of such emboli are thrombi arising from the heart, in association with myocardial infarctions or infective endocarditis. Atrial thrombus may also be present in the case of atrial fibrillation.

As with myocardial infarction, pathological changes take time to develop from the time of arterial occlusion. Naked-eye changes take approximately 24–36 hours to occur, the first change being haemorrhage and subsequent softening of the brain tissue due to capillary leakage from damaged endothelium (Fig. 14.6). Within 3–5 days, there is swelling of the infarct which may compress the surounding brain tissue. By 10–12 days, there is striking softening of the brain tissue and eventually the area of infarct may form a cyst with so-called liquefactive necrosis. A cyst may persist for many years afterwards, and often the surrounding brain tissue is slightly pigmented due to the deposition of iron pigment. Microscopically, necrosis of neurones is seen within 6–10 hours. As with other infarcts in other places in the body there is then a neutrophil infiltrate within 3–5 days, then macrophages migrate to clear necrotic debris, and eventually there is a connective tissue response. The connective tissue response within the brain occurs with a proliferation of astrocytes and the subsequent scarring is termed gliosis.

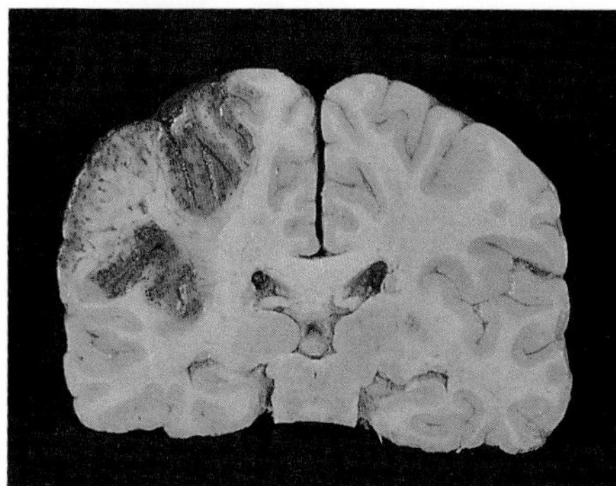

Fig. 14.6 Recent cerebral infarcts (left).

Cerebral tumours

The most common brain tumour is, in fact, metastatic disease from a primary site such as breast or lung carcinoma. An inherent clinical problem with brain tumours is the rigid nature of the skull and surrounding tissues of the brain which cannot yield to a space-occupying lesion. This means that even a benign tumour which is not invasive, may have serious clinical manifestations due to brain compression. Malignant tumours of the brain tend not to metastasize to sites distant from the skull. This is in contrast with malignant tumours in other places of the body. Most tumours of the brain develop from the connective tissue cells, the so-called glial cells. Neurones are highly specialized and stable cells incapable of further division or repair, and mature neurones do not form tumours themselves. A summary of the classification of cerebral tumours is shown in Table 14.4.

Table 14.4 Classification of brain tumours

Gliomas
- Astrocytomas
- Oligodendrocytomas
- Ependymomas
- Choroid plexus tumours
- Blastomas, including neuroblastomas and medulloblastomas
- Nerve sheath tumours including schwannomas (neurilemmomas)
- Neurofibromas
- Meningiomas
- Microgliomas

Neural
- Neuroblastomas
- Medulloblastomas

Vascular tumours

Germ cell tumours

Astrocytomas

These are tumours which arise from astrocytes, the 'nurse' cells of the neurones. They have a range of behaviour from very benign to very malignant, depending on cell type. Approximately 20 per cent of primary brain tumours are astrocytomas. The low-grade, slowly growing, and clinically benign astrocytoma commonly occur in children and tend to develop within the posterior part of the brain. At the other end of the spectrum, however, is the malignant astrocytomas which forms almost half of all glial tumours. This occurs in the fifth to sixth decade and commonly develops within the central part of the cerebrum within the white matter. They tend to occur anteriorly. They are typically very vascular and show areas of necrosis (Fig. 14.7). An older term for these malignant tumours is glioblastoma multiforme.

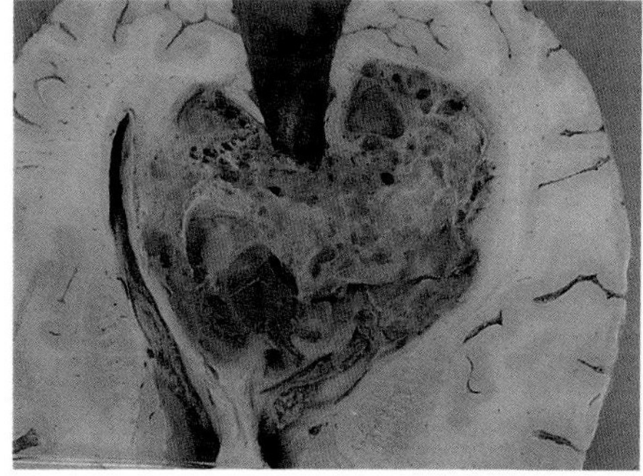

Fig. 14.7 A malignant astrocytoma.

Oligodendrogliomas

These are rare and are only seen in about 5 per cent of all gliomas and occur in the fourth to sixth decades. They tend to occur in the central part of the cerebrum and occur within the white matter. Oligodendrocytes in a normal situation produce myelin. They often calcify and may show on X-ray.

Ependymomas

These are the most common tumours that occur within the spinal canal and develop from the ependyma which is the epithelial-like lining of the spinal canal. They tend to be very slow-growing tumours.

Choroid plexus tumours

As with the normal choroid plexus within the lateral ventricles, these tumours tend to be very papillary and may produce large amounts of cerebrospinal fluid resulting in raised intracranial pressure.

Neuroblastomas

These are common childhood brain tumours and arise from primitive rests of embryonal neuroblasts which show malignant transformation. They also occur within the adrenals and sympathetic nervous system peripherally. The primitive neuroblasts may produce catecholamines.

Medulloblastoma

This is a primitive tumour developing within the cerebellum in children. As with neuroblastomas they appear to arise from primitive embryonal tissue which persists after birth.

Nerve sheath tumours including schwannomas (neurilemmomas). These are tumours that arise from the myelin-producing cells that surround cranial and peripheral nerves. Schwannomas are a pure proliferation of these Schwann cells and form a tumour which often is peripherally located and adherent to the particular nerve of origin. They are predominantly benign tumours and slow-growing and surgically may be removed with preservation of the nerve of origin.

Neurofibromas

These are also a tumour of cranial and peripheral nerves but in contrast to schwannomas involve many elements of the nerve tissue. These include Schwann cells, and connective tissue cells such as fibroblasts and perineural cells. It is difficult to preserve the nerve on surgical excision.

Both Schwannomas and neurofibromas may be multiple in association with von Recklinghausen's disease (neurofibromatosis).

Meningiomas

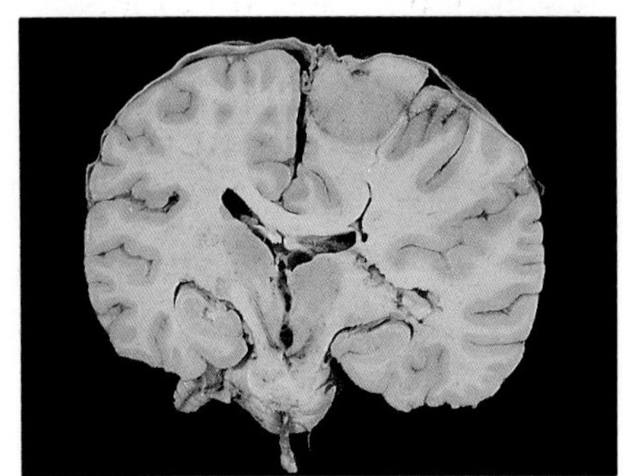

Fig. 14.8 A meningioma is seen in the top right of the picture. The right side of the brain is swollen.

These are relatively common tumours forming about 10 per cent of intracranial tumours. They have a very similar appearance to, and appear to arise from, the arachnoid granulations within the venous sinuses. They are therefore frequently associated with these venous sinuses and are attached to the dura. They are almost always benign and compress the adjacent brain tissue (Fig. 14.8). They can be surgically excised and shelled-out and do not show invasion of brain tissue.

Microgliomas

This is an old term which refers to lymphomas developing as primary tumours within the brain. These are rare, but are of increasing incidence in view of their association with immunosuppression, in particular, acquired immunodeficiency syndrome (AIDS) and patients who have immunosuppressive therapy for organ transplantation or treatment of malignancy.

Vascular tumours

These are important in view of their close association with spontaneous cerebral haemorrhage. Tumours include angiomas and arteriovenous malformations.

Metastatic tumours

Most metastatic tumours of the brain, which comprise at least 20 per cent of all brain tumours, are carcinomas. Common sites of origin are the lung, breast, kidney, gastroinestinal tract, and thyroid. Metastatic deposits in the brain are typically found at the junction between the cortical grey matter and the underlying white matter.

Demyelination

Myelin is the insulating material that surround nerve fibres in peripheral nerves, spinal cord, and the brain. The most important disease which involves loss of myelin is multiple sclerosis, although other demyelinating diseases are listed in Table 14.5.

Table 14.5 Demyelinating diseases

Multiple sclerosis
Post-infectious or post-vaccination demyelination
Progressive multifocal leucoencephalopathy
Toxic agents

Multiple sclerosis

This is a disease particularly seen in the northern hemisphere in temperate climates and has an incidence of about 10 per 100 000 of the population. There appears to be a strong environmental factor involved in that if a person moves from a high-incidence area to a low-incidence area the risk of getting the disease becomes that of the low-incidence area. It occurs at the highest instance in the first two decades. It has a slight female predominance. The clinical presentation of multiple sclerosis is very variable but typical presenting features are visual disturbances with retrobulbar neuritis or optic atrophy. Limb weakness may also be a presenting feature. The disease is typically cylical in its behaviour with periods of acute exacerbation followed by remission. It is typically a chronic disease which has a tendency to progression in most cases. The pathology of multiple sclerosis is characterized by focal areas of demyelination which can be seen in computed tomography scans or magnetic resonance scans clinically, and as areas of loss of white matter pathologically. The plaques are typically multiple and may be scattered throughout the cerebral hemispheres, brain stem, cerebellum, and spinal cord. Plaques are typically seen in areas surrounding the ventricles of the brain within the white matter (Fig. 14.9). During active plaque formation there is infiltration by mononuclear cells including lymphocytes and plasma cells. In inactive plaques there is less inflammation, the striking feature being the absence of myelin. There is evidence of myelin breakdown products with macrophages contaning foamy lipid material. Clinically, the distribution and number of plaques has a very poor relationship with the clinical features of the disease. The pathological features suggest that the disease is mediated by the immune system and is possibly of autoimmune nature.

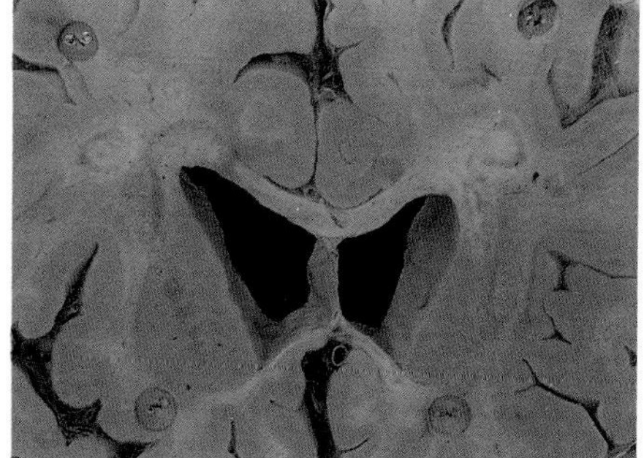

Fig. 14.9 Areas of white demyelination are seen above the ventricles.

Metabolic disorders

Toxic agents, including alcohol and drugs and several metals, are associated with damage to the nervous system. Also, several dietary deficiencies are associated with

Table 14.6 Metabolic causes of cerebral dysfunction

Toxins
- Alcohol
- Methanol
- Aluminium
- Arsenic
- Lead
- Mercury
- Insecticides

Dietary deficiency: in particular of vitamins A, B group, and C

Drugs (therapeutic): methotrexate, vincristine, gold, amphetamines, opiates

Solvent abuse
- Liver disease
- Renal failure
- Cardiovascular disease
- Diabetes mellitus

Connective tissue disease including polyarteritis nodosa, giant cell arteritis, systemic lupus erythematosus

Table 14.7 Causes of dementia

- Alzheimer's disease
- Lewy body disease
- Huntington's disease (chorea)
- Pick's disease
- Jacob–Creutzfeldt disease
- Multi-infarct dementia

neurotoxicity. Furthermore, there are many diseases which cause secondary neurological symptoms and damage. These are listed in Table 14.6.

Epilepsy

Epilepsy is frequently of unknown cause, but it is important to remember that a presenting feature of a cerebral tumour may be an epileptic fit.

Dementia

Dementia is a generalized and progressive reduction in higher brain function which causes loss of the intellect, disorientation, loss of memory, alteration in character, and speech disturbance. Important diseases which are characterized by dementia are shown in Table 14.7.

Alzheimer's disease

This is a very common cause of dementia which in many cases is pre-senile, in other words occurring before the age of 60 years. It causes about a half of all dementia in the population, occurring in up to 15 per cent of people over the age of 80 years. It is of unknown cause; it sometimes runs in families. It frequently occurs in Down's syndrome, and a similar condition has been described in aluminium toxicity in dialysis patients. Pathologically, there is atrophy of the brain with reduced weight, narrowing of cortical gyri, and widening of the sulci. The cerebral ventricles are enlarged. There is loss of cortical neurones. Typically, there are plaques of amyloid-like material associated with abnormal neuronal processes and so-called neurofibrillary tangles within the cortex of the temporal lobe and hippocampus. These tangles consist of accumulation of neurofilaments within neurones. Amyloid is also seen in superficial cortical and meningeal vessels. The number and distribution of these plaques and neurofibrillary tangles closely correlates with clinical extent of the disease.

The amyloid is derived from a protein which is normally produced by neurones and is encoded for by a specific gene on chromosome 21 (the amyloid precursor protein gene). This protein is called protein P. In familial Alzheimer's disease (about 15 per cent of cases) there are mutations in this gene.

Lewy body disease

This is similar to Alzheimer's but has a more rapid progression. There may be rigidity similar to that seen in Parkinson's disease. Numerous inclusions in neurones called Lewy bodies are seen. Lewy bodies are also seen in small numbers in Parkinson's disease, but Parkinson's disease is not typically associated with dementia.

Huntington's disease (chorea)

This is an inherited disease which presents at 40–50 years of age with dementia and involuntary movements (chorea). It has been shown that the disease is associated with an abnormality of a gene on chromosome 4. This gene which codes for a protein called Huntingtin normally has only 10–30 'CAG' base pair sequence repeats. In Huntington's disease there may be 100 or more accumulated repeats of this sequence, which interferes with gene expression.

Jacob–Creutzfeldt disease

The importance of this form of dementia is that it has been shown to be due to a transmissible agent which is strongly resistant to sterilization by normal methods. It has been shown to be transmissible by surgical instruments, corneal grafts, and growth hormone replacement which has been derived from human tissue. There is an important potential risk of transmission from dental instruments. The infectious agent appears to be a protein without any associated DNA, called a 'prion'. It is characterized clinically as a rapidly progressive dementia. There is frequently associated muscle spasm called myoclonus and characteristic electroencephalogram findings. In experimental situations, the incubation period for the disease is approximately 12–18 months. The disease is very similar to the spongiform encephalopathy or bovine spongiform encephalopathy (BSE) described in cattle. This appears to be due to its transmissible agent from sheep, possibly scrapic, which has previously been incorporated into the cattle feed.

The disease occasionally shows a family history, when a mutation occus in a gene called the human prion gene (*PrP* gene).

There is loss of neurones on pathological examination, with scarring (gliosis), and deposition of amyloid. There is also sponge-like microscopic vacuolation of the brain, described as a spongiform encephalopathy.

Multi-infarct dementia

Dementia may be associated with numerous small cerebral infarcts which accumulate over time. The dementia may be associated with overt localized neurological signs due to the occurrence of larger infarcts. The infarcts may sometimes be limited to the white (myelinated) matter. Other causes of dementia include poisoning by heavy metals, and metabolic causes.

Other 'degenerative' diseases

Parkinson's disease

This is a relatively frequent disease seen in the population. It occurs predominantly in late middle age and old age. The hallmark of Parkinson's disease is a resting tremor with marked rigidity in the limbs and difficulty in muscle extension. There is also striking slowness of movement. The disease is persistent and progressive but is not normally associated with dementia. Typical pathological features are loss of pigmentation of the substantia nigra within the midbrain. These pigmented cells are involved in the dopaminergic system. The disease responds to L-dopa reflecting the loss of dopamine in the substantia nigra.

Trauma

Closed head injury

Much of the cerebral damage in the case of closed head trauma is due to acceleration/deceleration forces alone. Movement of the brain within the skull causes cortical lacerations and bruising and is also responsible for the so-called *contre-coup* injury. This is particularly seen with a blow to the back of the head where injury is caused to the brain underneath the frontal lobes due to the normally rough orbital plate of the adjacent skull. In closed injury, there also may be extensive axonal damage which is not apparent to the naked eye. There is frequently extensive tearing of neurofibres. Cerebral oedema is frequently a serious complication of head injury, usually occurring 1–2 days after the injury. This swelling of the cerebrum can cause herniation of the singulate gyrus underneath the sagittal falx, or of the cerebellar tonsils or the midbrain through the foramen magnum. As described previously, cerebral haemorrhage is a frequent complication of cerebral injury, in particular extradural and subdural haematomas.

Cranial nerves

Two conditions that are particularly relevant to dentists are trigeminal neuralgia and Bell's (facial) palsy.

Trigeminal neuralgia

This is a disorder of the fifth cranial nerve root where there appears to be an over-sensitivity of the sensory neurones. The condition is seen in the elderly and is characterized by sudden short episodes of severe pain in the distribution of the fifth nerve. It may be precipitated by contact with 'trigger zones' on the face or in the mouth. It appears to be a form of 'epilepsy' involving a sensory nerve; it frequently responds to anti-epileptic drugs.

Bell's (facial) palsy

As with trigeminal neuralgia, this is of unknown cause. It is usually a self-limiting condition lasting a few weeks in which there is paralysis of the facial nerve. This is due to an inflammatory process involving the narrow path the nerve takes through the facial canal or stylomastoid foramen. It may be of viral aetiology; steroids are an effective treatment in the early stages.

PERIPHERAL NERVOUS SYSTEM

Neuropathy

The characteristic feature of neuropathy is death of nerve cells. Recognized clinical entities where this occurs are listed in Table 14.8.

Table 14.8 Causes of neuropathy

Motor neurone disease
Spinal muscular atrophy
Syringomyelia
Infection: poliomyelitis, herpes zoster, leprosy
Guillain–Barre syndrome
Tumours
Neuropathy associated with tumours in the body
Autonomic neuropathy, in particular diabetes
Toxins: alcohol, heavy metals
Vitamin deficiency
Bell's (facial nerve) palsy
Trauma

Tumours

The most common peripheral nerve tumours are the schwannoma (neurilemmoma) and the neurofibroma. They often calcify and may show on X-ray.

MUSCLE

Muscle pathology tends to be included under the heading of neuropathology, and is briefly mentioned here.

Muscular dystrophy

This is a group of intrinsic diseases of muscle, which are hereditary (Table 14.9).

Table 14.9 Muscle dystrophies

Duchenne muscular dystrophy
Limb girdle dystrophy
Facioscapulohumeral dystrophy
Myotonic dystrophy

Inflammation

Myositis may be infective in origin, or it may be associated with autoimmune disease or tumours. For example, myositis may be associated with systemic lupus erythematosus or lung cancer. Dermatomyositis, where there is also a dermatitis, is particularly associated with malignancy elsewhere in the body.

Prolonged steroid therapy may induce a myopathy, predominantly of proximal muscles.

SUMMARY

Central nervous system

Hypoxia: causes of hypoxia are:

–ischaemia
–systemic hypoxia
–toxins
–metabolic disorders

Infections

Meningitis: this is the most common infection of the central nervous system, usually due to bacteria, although viruses are also a recognized cause. There is acute and chronic forms of meningitis.

Encephalitis: this is direct inflammation of the brain tissue due to infection, usually by a virus.

Cerebral haemorrhage: this is classified by the anatomical compartment into which the bleeding occurs. Types of haemorrhaging are extradural, subdural, subarachnoid, intracerebral.

Cerebral infarct: this is death of brain tissue due to compromised blood supply. It is the most common reason for so-called 'stroke'.

Cerebral tumours: the most common cerebral tumour is a metastatic lesion from a primary site such as breast or lung. Primary brain tumours are mainly of connective tissue (glial) origin.

The important degenerative conditions of the central nervous system include:

–demyelination (multiple sclerosis)
–metabolic disorders
–epilepsy
–dementia
–Parkinson's disease

Trauma: the brain is a common site for accidental injury. Injury may either be secondary to skull fracture, or due to acceleration/deceleration injury in closed head trauma.

Cranial nerves: two relevant conditions that involve cranial nerves are:

1. Trigeminal neuralgia
2. Bell's (facial) palsy

Peripheral nervous system

Pathology that involves the peripheral nervous system includes neuropathy and tumours.

15 The skin

15 The skin

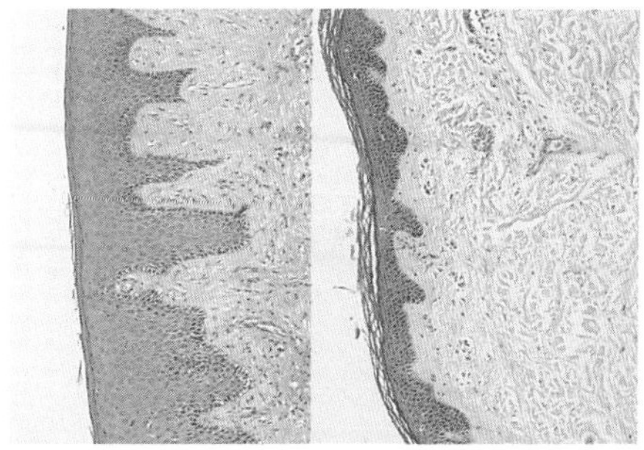

Fig. 15.1 The oral squamous epithelium (left) is thicker than the epidermis of the skin (right, same magnification).

ALTHOUGH the lining of the mouth and the surface of the tongue are covered by a mucosa which is a lot thicker than the epidermis (Fig. 15.1), the underlying structure of the oral and tongue epithelium is identical to the skin. The tongue and oral cavity are lined by squamous epithelium and are prone to many diseases which are also manifested on the skin. As with the skin, the squamous epithelium of the mouth also has a population of melanocytes. Many basic pathological processes occur in the oral mucosa as well as in the skin. These include hyperplasia, which manifests as a thickening of the epidermis of the skin or the oral mucosa which has similar appearances. Spongiosis also occurs in the mouth and skin, which is effectively oedema which separates the squamous cells. A complete breakdown of the squamous cells of the mouth and oral mucosa may occur, a process known as acantholysis. In this, epithelial cells can be seen lying within large spaces or bulla. There may also be abnormal proliferation of the epidermis or oral mucosa with abnormal keratinization. This is known as dysplasia and dyskeratosis. There may be similar forms of disruption of the basal layer of the epidermis or oral mucosa, which is often associated with specific disorders.

SKIN DISORDERS THAT MANIFEST IN THE MOUTH

Summarized below are skin diseases which are commonly manifested in the mouth.

Lichen planus

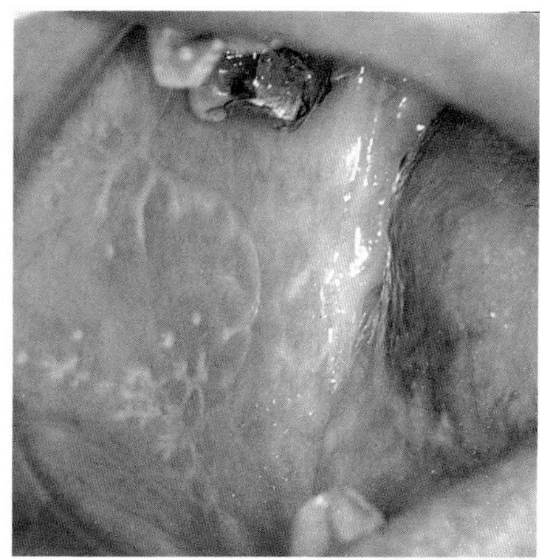

Fig. 15.2 Lichen planus.

This is a condition of unknown cause. It occurs in about 1 per cent of the population in the 30 to 50 year age group. In about a half of patients with skin involvement, lesions of the oral mucosa are seen. Clinically, it presents in the skin as a very itchy rash with small red papules which may persist for a long time, up to several years. In the mouth, it presents with red lesions, either with thinning and atrophy of the mucosa, or a lace-like pattern of white linear lesions (Fig. 15.2). White plaques giving the appearance of leukoplakia may be present.

It is characterized pathologically, both in the skin and the mouth, by a very typical band-like lymphocytic infiltrate which is superficial and appears to 'hug' the basal layer (Fig. 15.3). The epidermal cells express HLA class II, normally only seen on cells of the immune system. The lymphocytes are mainly of helper type; in long-standing disease suppressor/cytotoxic lymphocytes predominate. There is often marked disruption of the basal cell layer with frequent pink spherical bodies known as colloid bodies. The overlying epithelium or oral epithelium shows thickening with flattening of the underneath of the epithelial surface. There is a variant where blisters form, known as the bullous variety. There is also a variety where the epithelium or epidermis becomes very thick, known as the hypertrophic variant. There is an increased incidence of disordered maturation of the epithelium, known as dysplasia. There is an increased incidence of oral carcinoma with this condition.

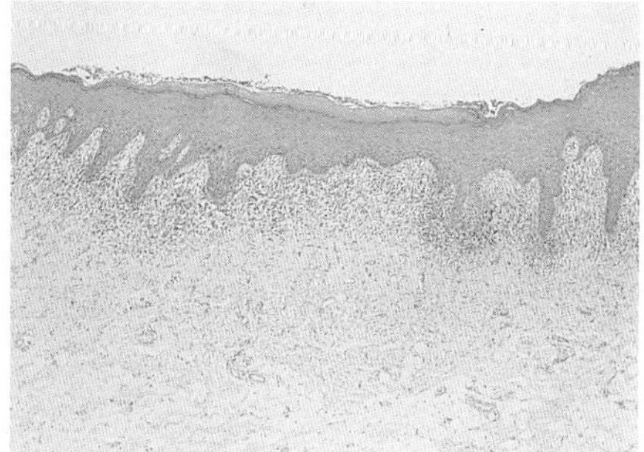

Fig. 15.3 Lichen planus.

Lichen planus is associated with some drugs, such as methyl dopa, and drugs used to treat malaria. It has been described in association with a variety of immunological

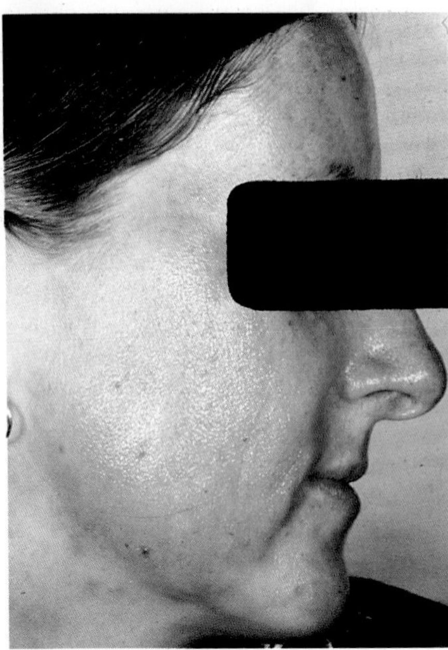

Fig. 15.4 SLE of the skin.

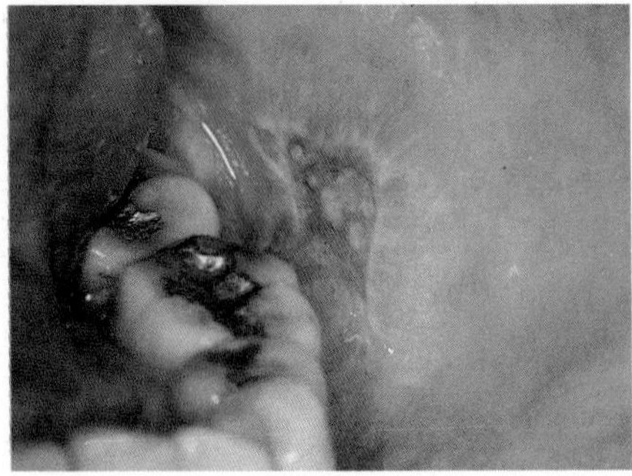

Fig. 15.5 SLE of the mouth.

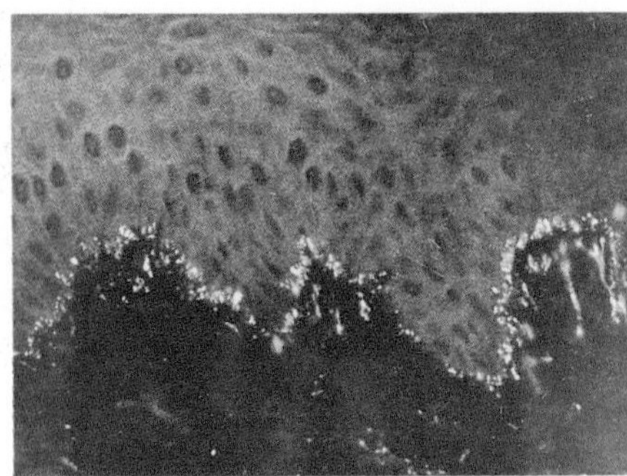

Fig. 15.6 There are granular deposits of antibody on the basement membrane in SLE.

conditions, such as diabetes mellitus, graft-versus-host disease in bone marrow transplants, and hypersensitivity to an antigen.

Systemic lupus erythematosus (SLE)

This is an example of an autoimmune disease. It is a multisystem disease which frequently affects the skin and oral mucosa. It also has a limited cutaneous form known as discoid lupus erythematosus. As with other autoimmune diseases, it is more common in females. Patients show auto-reactive antibodies to nuclear antigens; the cause of the disease is unknown. There is deposition of immune complexes in many organs, including the kidney, lungs, brain, and skin. A characteristic symmetrical rash develops on the face and other light-exposed areas (Fig. 15.4). The oral mucosa shows red pathes or superficial ulcers (Fig. 15.5). There is frequently an associated inflammation of blood vessels known as vasculitis.

Histologically, there is in the skin hyperkeratosis, atrophy of the epidermis, and basal cell layer disruption. Follicular plugging may be present. A heavy and deep lymphocytic infiltrate is present in the dermis. Immunochemistry shows granular deposits of immunoglobulins, usually IgG (Fig. 15.6). There may also be deposits of complement components.

Pemphigus

This is a disease characterized by blistering which can affect both the skin and the oral mucosa (Figs 15.7 and 15.8). In both the skin and the oral mucosa the bulla develop by breaking down intercellular bridges between the squamous epithelial cells. This is due to deposits of auto-reactive antibodies to components that hold the epithelial cells together. It is a disease which affects middle-aged people, mainly females, and may present in the mouth before skin lesions developed. The fragile blisters that develop are easily ruptured, leaving painful ulcers.

Histologically, there is splitting of epithelial cells as part of the development of bullae. In pemphigus vulgaris the splitting is low in the epidermis; in pemphigus foliaceus the splitting occurs just beneath the corneal layer. Frequently, after the development of a blister there is a layer of epithelial cells left on the basement membrane. On immunohistochemistry there is deposition of IgG antibody to intercellular material (Fig. 15.9). There may also be deposits of complement.

The prognosis of the disease without treatment by steroids is poor. There is another, very rare disease which shows splitting between epidermal cells called Hailey–Hailey disease. It runs in families and may also show oral involvement. Immunohistochemistry is negative, in contrast to pemphigus. Bullous (blistering) diseases and their immunology are shown in Table 15.1.

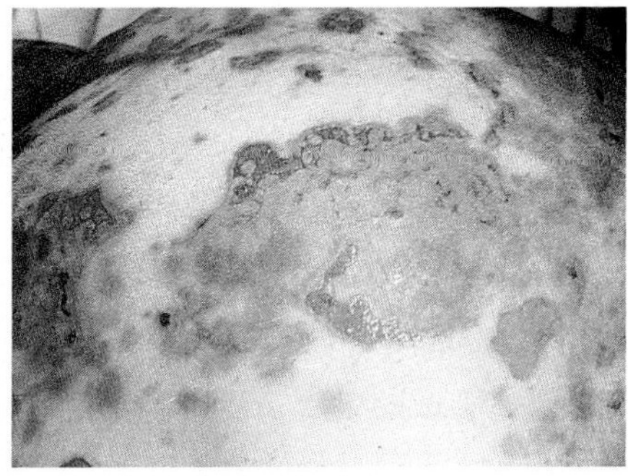
Fig. 15.7 Pemphigus of the skin.

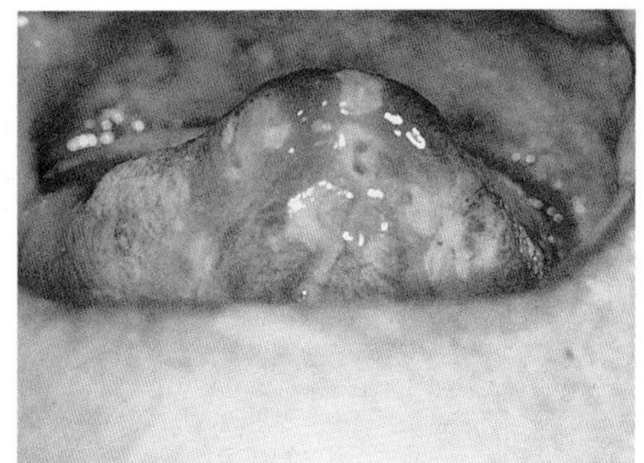
Fig. 15.8 Pemphigus of the mouth.

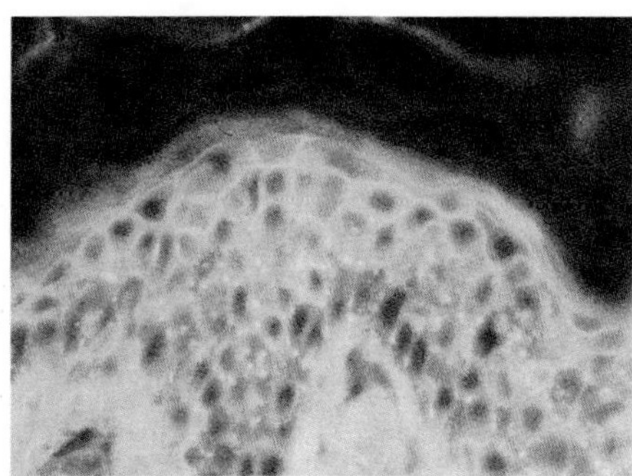
Fig. 15.9 Antibodies to intercellular material are seen in pemphigus.

Table 15.1 Immunology of blistering skin and oral disease

Disease	Site of blister	Immunology
Pemphigoid	Subepidermal (eosinophils)	Linear basement membrane; IgG
Pemphigus	Intraepidermal	Intercellular in epidermis; IgG
SLE	Epidermal and mucosal	Granular basement membrane; IgG, C3
Dermatitis herpetiformis	Subepidermal (neutrophils)	Granular basement membrane; IgA

Pemphigoid

This is another frequently recognized bullous disorder that affects the mouth and also the skin. It is a disease of middle-aged and elderly people, particularly females. There is a development of bulla which results from splitting of the basement membrane from the underlying connective tissue (Figs 15.10 and 15.11). The bulla are therefore subepidermal or subepithelial in type. Histologically, the subepithelial nature of the bulla is apparent with an intact epidermis or squamous epithelial layer forming the roof of the blister and is frequently associated with a heavy eosinophil inflammatory infiltrate. Immunohistochemistry shows typically linear deposits of IgG in the basement membrane (Fig. 15.12). The histological features of the four conditions above are shown in Fig. 15.13.

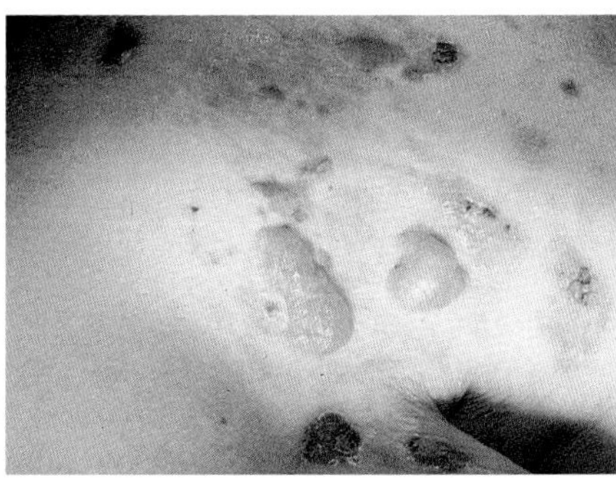
Fig. 15.10 Pemphigoid of the skin.

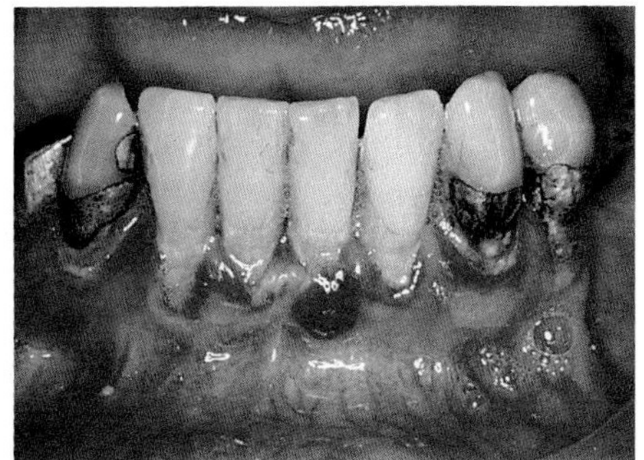
Fig. 15.11 Pemphigoid of the mouth.

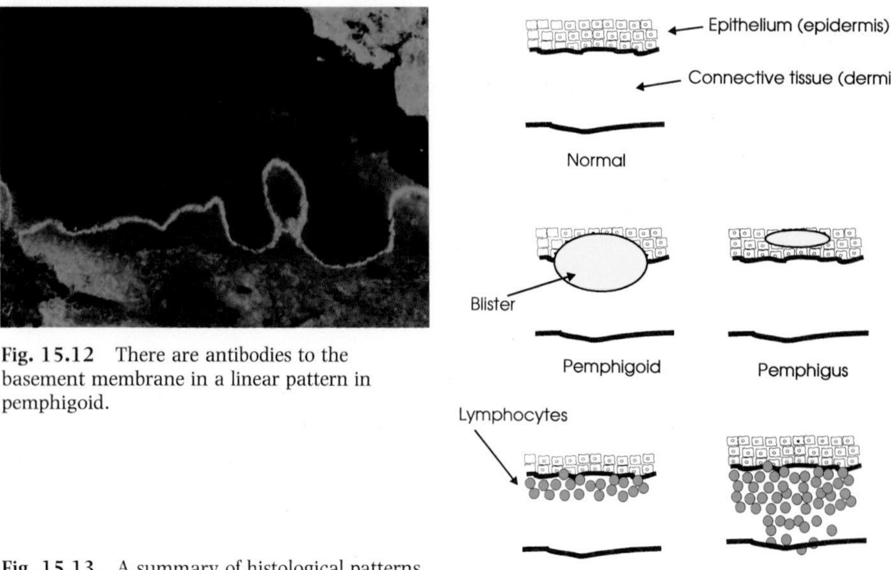

Fig. 15.12 There are antibodies to the basement membrane in a linear pattern in pemphigoid.

Fig. 15.13 A summary of histological patterns in skin disease.

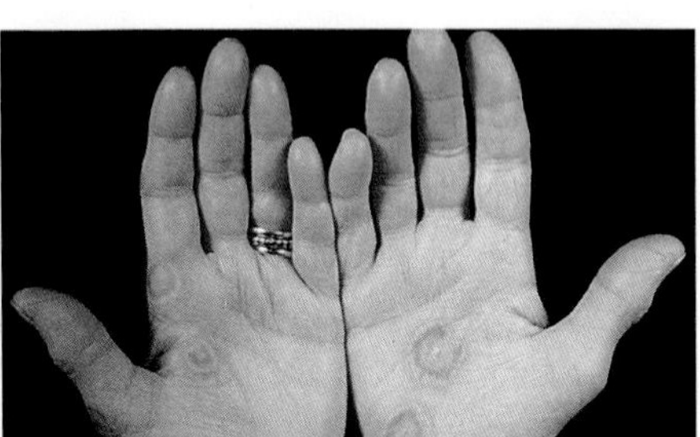

Fig. 15.14 Erythema multiforme of the skin.

Erythema multiforme

This is generally a skin rash of unknown cause but is occasionally associated with a viral or bacterial infection. Some drugs, particularly antibiotics such as sulphonamides may be associated with the condition. It is seen as large red areas of the skin, often oval in shape with a central pale area (Fig. 15.14). If the condition involves mucous membranes such as the mouth it may be severe, and is referred to as the Stevens–Johnson syndrome. The characteristic feature on histopathology is necrosis of individual epidermal cells. This may advance to form overt bulla. There is usually associated underlying inflammation. Striking oedema of underlying subepithelial connective tissue is frequently seen. Immunochemistry is negative or non-specific.

Dermatitis herpetiformis

This is an uncommon disease but is important as it is included in the differential diagnosis of blistering disorders. It generally occurs in middle-aged men. There is a marked itchy rash which is seen the outer surfaces of limbs and the lower trunk. Oral lesions may occur. The disease is strongly associated with coeliac disease which is a disorder which is associated with sensitivity to wheat-derived proteins such as gluten. On immunohistochemistry, granular deposits of IgA are seen in the basal membrane in either involved or uninvolved skin. Histologically there is a development of subepidermal bulla with small collections of acute inflammatory cells forming microabscesses.

Behçet syndrome

This is mentioned as it is a condition that shows presenting signs on the skin and in the mouth. It is a rare and unusual disease with a probable immunological origin, having an association with HLA type B5. It is characterized by orogenital ulcers of aphthous type, skin rash, and arthritis. There may also be conjunctivitis and inflammation of the uveal tract of the eye (the iris, ciliary body, and the choroid).

Sarcoidosis

This is a condition characterized by granulomas which involve various organ systems. It is well recognized in the skin. Histologically, there are well-formed epithelioid granulomas within the dermis. There is a similar condition which affects the mucous membranes such as the mouth and the term orofacial granulomatosis is often applied to sarcoid involving the mouth. This condition however may be part of a spectrum of disease including, for instance, Crohn's disease.

Scleroderma

This is an autoimmune disease of unknown cause in which there is striking fibrosis of the dermis; the other name for the disease is systemic sclerosis. The fibrosis can also involve internal organs such as the oesophagus and lungs. The scarring can severely restrict the opening of the mouth.

Epidermolysis bullosa

There is a group of very rare diseases characterized by an inborn abnormality of the basement membrane of the skin. Different varieties of the condition involve different layers of the basement membrane. The skin and oral mucosa show a fragile epithelium which develops blisters at the junction between the basement membrane and the epithelium.

OTHER SKIN DISORDERS

Psoriasis

This characteristically presents as a red raised skin rash with plaques associated with silver keratin scaly deposits. It is very common, involving up to 2 per cent of the population. It is of unknown cause the most marked feature is a marked increase in epithelial cell proliferation. In the skin it normally takes about 40–50 days for an epidermal cell to travel from the basal layer to the surface of the skin. In psoriasis this is strinkingly reduced to 7–10 days. On histology there is marked thickening of the epidermis with hyperkeratosis and abnormal keratinization with retention of nuclei in the corneal layer. This abnormal keratinization is called parakeratosis. There is associated acute inflammation involving the superficial parts of the epidermis.

Eczema

This is also known as dermatitis and is a very common condition. It may occur as an acute form where there is oedema of the epidermis with spongiosis. Small blisters may develop. There is frequently associated acute on chronic inflammation, particularly around blood vessels. Blood vessels are dilated causing the red rash. The inflammation is frequently very superficial. Chronic ezcema is characterized by marked thickening of the epidermis known as acanthosis with associated thickening of the keratin corneal layer known as hyperkeratosis.

The term eczema generally refers to the clinical condition where there is an allergic process underlying the disorder. There is often allergy to substances exposed to the skin such as chemicals or drugs.

Acne

This is a common disorder of adolescence in which there is marked plugging of hair follicles with heavy associated acute inflammation. There is often rupture of small cysts developing from these follicles causing scarring. It appears to be related to androgen exposure with abnormal response of the hair follicles.

Viral infections

Viral warts caused by the human papilloma virus are very commonly seen in the skin, and also in the oral mucosa. Viral warts show striking epithelial proliferation that is being driven by the viral infection. There may be viral inclusions in the epithelial cells. Some viral infections, particularly herpes virus, cause striking destruction of epidermal cells with blister formation.

SKIN TUMOURS

Seborrhoeic keratosis

This is otherwise known as a senile keratosis or basal cell papilloma. It frequently occurs in old age and presents as a heavily pigmented polypoid lesion which appears to be superficially attached to the skin. Histologically, there is marked proliferation of cells which resemble basal cells. The lesion is typically exophytic and it appears to grow outwards with no dermal invasion.

Epidermoid cysts

These may occur in association with trauma where there is implantation of epidermis into the dermis due to, for instance, a penetrating injury. This epidermis continues to grow and frequently forms a keratin-filled cyst. It is lined purely by squamous epithelium which is keratinizing. Cysts may occur particularly on the face in association with abnormal fusion of developing parts of the fetus. These are known as dermoid cysts in that they include hair follicles and sweat glands. Cysts may occur from hair follicle structures and frequently occur on the scalp. These are known as pilar cysts.

Solar keratosis

This is associated with heavy sun exposure and are characterized by abnormal epidermal cell growth. There is abnormal keratinization with retention of nuclei into the corneal layers and nuclear atypia. There is often changes of the elastic tissue underlying the epidermis known as solar elastosis. They are seen in some exposed areas of elderly people. They have a pre-malignant tendency.

Viral lesions

As with squamous papillomas of the oral mucosa, tumour-like lesions of the skin induced by the human papilloma virus (HPV) occur. The most frequent are the common wart (verruca vulgaris) associated with HPV types 2 or 4, and the venereally transmitted condyloma acuminatum, associated with HPV types 6, 11, and 16.

Bowen's disease

This is essentially carcinoma-*in situ* of the skin. There is severe dysplasia of the epidermis but no invasion of basement membrane into the dermis.

Squamous cell carcinoma

As with the mouth, this is a common primary malignant tumour of the skin (Figs 15.15 and 15.16). The histological appearances are identical in the skin and the mouth; the tumour is usually well diferentiated and tumour cells show abundant keratinization. Squamous cell carcinoma of the skin occurs in similar age and sex groups to oral cancer—particularly elderly men. This type of skin cancer is associated with sun exposure.

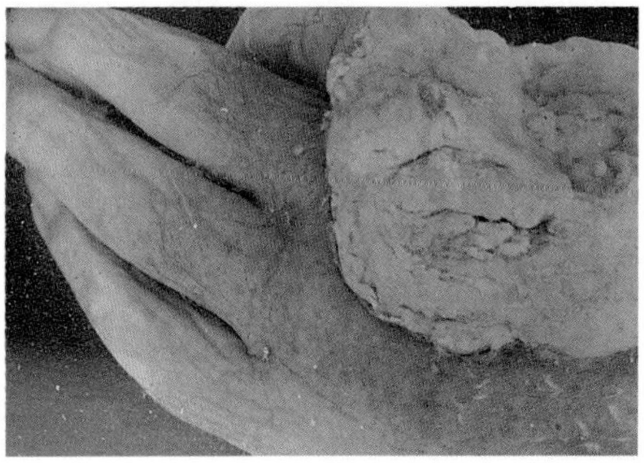

Fig. 15.15 Squamous cell carcinoma of the skin of the hand.

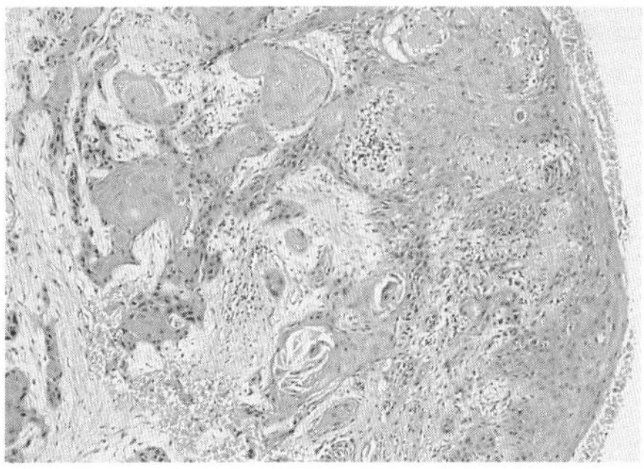

Basal cell carcinoma

This is a frequent tumour of sun exposed areas in elderly people. It characteristically occurs on the face, and although being slow-growing may be very destructive, hence the other term for this lesion is rodent ulcer. They very rarely metastasize unless they get very large. They present as a raised white lesion with a central crater (Fig. 15.17). Histologically, there is a malignant proliferation of epithelium which resembles primitive epidermis. There may be attempts at differentiation towards structures in the skin such as hair follicles or sweat glands.

Fig. 15.16 Invasive squamous cell carcinoma has similar features in both skin and oral mucosa.

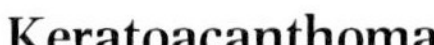

Keratoacanthoma

This is typically a rapidly growing lesion which occurs in the elderly and is biologically a self-limiting squamous cell carcinoma. It characteristically has a central crater filled with keratin and surrounded by atypical proliferating epithelium showing marked keratinization. The lesion is typically superficial. The feature that is distinct from squamous cell carcinoma is the rapid nature of its growth, occurring within weeks, and its resolution within only a few months. The overall architecture of the lesion is very distinctive.

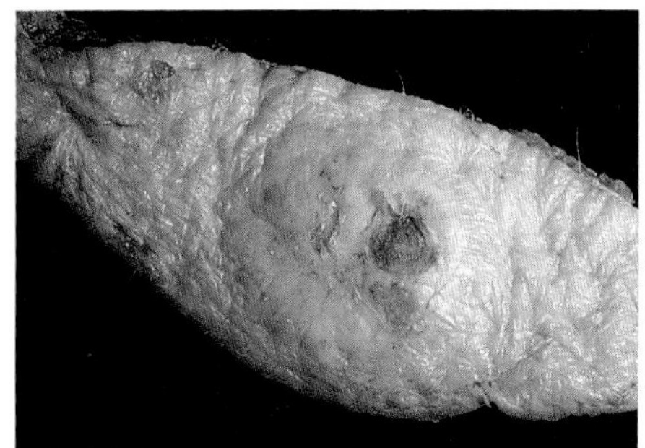

Fig. 15.17 A basal cell carcinoma of the skin.

Melanocytic naevus

These are commonly known as 'moles' and commonly appear as pigmented nodules which develop in early childhood and increase in number until early adult life. They then regress in old age. In the early phase, there is a proliferation of melanocytes at the dermal-epidermal junction (a 'junctional naevus'). In most established lesions there is a second population of melanocytes within the dermis (a 'compound naevus'). All the melanocytes eventually migrate into the dermis, forming an 'intradermal' naevus. In old age, these lesions regress, and eventually become fibrotic.

Malignant melanoma

This is a malignant proliferation of melanocytes which is associated with ultraviolet exposure. Heavy episodes of sun exposure in early childhood seems to be an important risk factor. There are four main types of melanoma listed in Table 15.2. A melanoma presents as a rapidly growing mole, with a history that does not fit into the pattern given for melanocytic naevi. They are irregular in shape and pigmentation, and may ulcerate (Fig. 15.18).

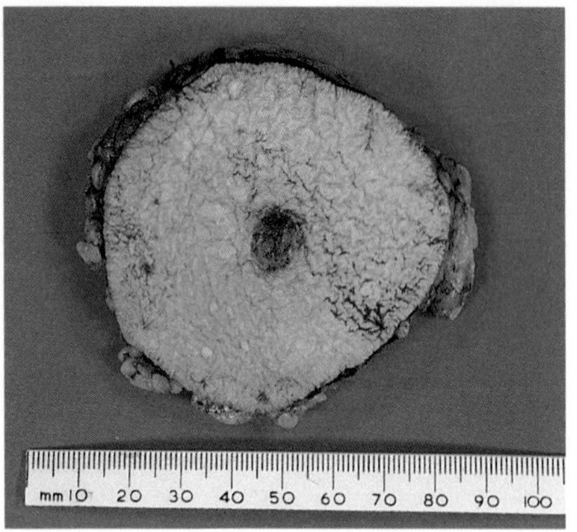

Fig. 15.18 A melanoma of the skin.

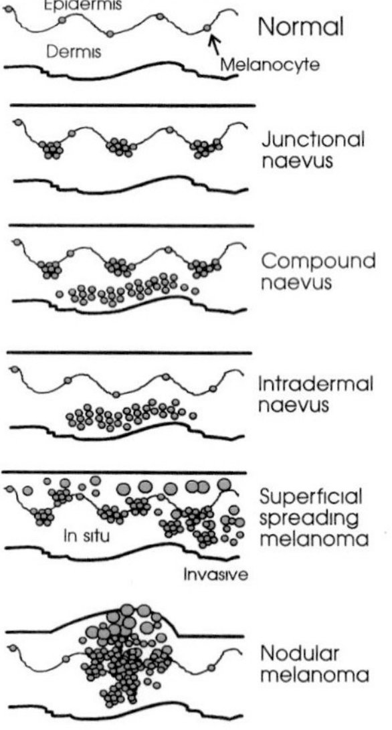

Fig. 15.19 A summary of melanocytic lesions.

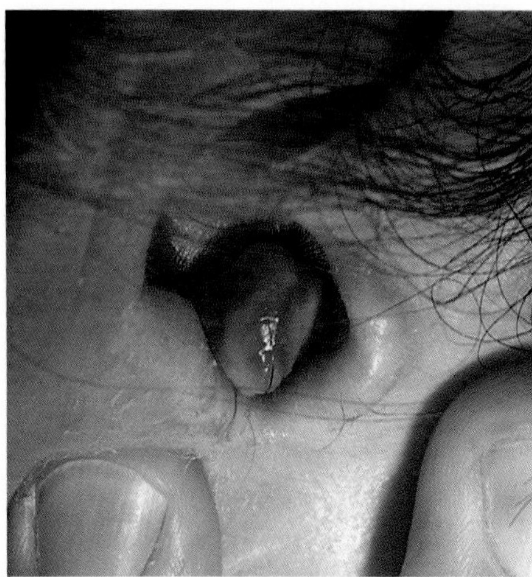

Fig. 15.20 A pyogenic granuloma arising in the ear.

Table 15.2 Types of malignant melanoma

1. Superficial spreading melanoma (a predominantly lateral growth phase)
2. Nodular melanoma (a predominantly 'vertical' growth phase)
3. Lentigo maligna
4. Acral melanoma (occurring on the periphery of the limbs)

Melanoma is an aggressive tumour; the prognosis relates to the thickness of the tumour. Tumours thinner than 0.75 mm have an excellent prognosis; those thicker than 0.75 mm have a poorer outlook. The structure of melanocytic lesions is summarized in Fig. 15.19. An important point is that melanoma occurs occasionally in sites other than the skin and oral mucosa, for example in the eye or oesophagus. The *in-situ* phase of a melanoma is referred to as 'melanocytic intraepithelial neoplasia'.

Pyogenic granuloma

This occurs both in the mouth and in the skin. It is really a benign capillary haemangioma which grows rapidly and may ulcerate (Fig. 15.20).

Dermatofibrona

This presents as a raised red dermal nodule. Histologically, it consists of a proliferation of cells which resemble histiocytes or fibroblasts.

Lymphoma

These are generally of T cell derivation. One type of T cell lymphoma is mycosis fungoides, a generally low-grade, only slowly progressive lymphoma. Secondary deposits of leukaemia may develop in the skin.

SUMMARY

Both the skin and the oral mucosa are lined by squamous epithelium and therefore have many diseases in common. *Skin diseases* that manifest in the mouth are:

–lichen planus
–systemic lupus erythematosus (SLE)
–pemphigus
–pemphigoid
–erythema multiforme (Stevens–Johnson syndrome)
–sarcoidosis

Other common skin diseases are:

–psoriasis
–eczema
–dermatitis herpetiformis (a bullous disorder)
–acne
–viral warts

Benign tumours of the skin

–seborrhoeic keratosis
–solar keratosis
–Bowen's disease (carcinoma *in situ*)
–melanocytic naevi

Malignant tumours

–squamous cell carcinoma (as in the mouth)
–basal cell carcinoma
–malignant melanoma
–lymphoma

16 Bone and joints

16 Bone and joints

BONE STRUCTURE

Bone is a much more dynamic structure than it may first appear, particularly with routine histology. It is effectively a composite of high tensile type I collagen forming the osteoid with high compressive strength calcium salts. In this sense it resembles reinforced concrete. The calcium is a complex of calcium and phosphate known as hydroxyapatite. On histology bone is composed of osteoid which is extensively calcified, containing regularly placed osteocytes within the bone substance. At the margins of the bone there is a population of osteoblasts capable of laying down osteoid. These are the equivalent of ameloblasts in tooth development, dentine being very similar to osteoid. There is also a second population of macrophage-like osteoclasts which are capable of digesting mineralized bone. Bone is therefore a dynamic tissue capable of adaptation to stress and injury. When osteoid is laid down, calcification soon follows, forming ossified bone. The osteoblasts and osteoclasts are in balance, bone continually being digested and then reformed.

Bone also provides a large buffer or reservoir of calcium. Calcium is under the control of two hormones, parathyroid hormone and vitamin D. Parathyroid hormone stimulates the resorption of calcium from bone and increases the reabsorption of calcium from the distal tubules of the kidney. Also, together with vitamin D, resorption of calcium from the intestine is increased.

Vitamin D is found in the diet as cholecalciferol. There is a drug, calciferol (vitamin D_2), which has the same action as vitamin D. Vitamin D becomes active after being metabolized by the liver to 25-hydroxycholecalciferol. Then the kidney metabolizes 25-hydroxycholecalciferol to 1,25-dihydroxycholecalciferol, the active form of vitamin D (D_3). This is why renal disease may interfere with calcium metabolism. Vitamin D_3 can also be formed in the skin by the action of ultraviolet light on 7-dehydroxycholesterol, a precursor.

Parathyroid hormone is secreted by the parathyroid glands. Calcitonin, which is produced by the C cells present within the thyroid, has an opposite effect to parathormone in that the hormone attempts to lower serum calcium; it also lowers serum phosphate. Calcitonin inhibits bone resorption and increases loss of phosphate and calcium by the kidneys.

METABOLIC BONE DISEASE

Hyperparathyroidism

Over-activity of the parathyroid glands can have a devastating effect on bone structure. The most common reason for hyperparathyroidism is a parathyroid adenoma which secretes excessive parathormone. This causes a dramatic increase in serum calcium due to increased breakdown of bone by osteoclasts. The hypercalcaemia of hyperparathyroidism is now usually picked up incidentally on routine biochemical testing, before serious bone lesions develop. The bone lesions may produce tumour-like destructive areas composed of large numbers of osteoclasts forming so-called giant-cell tumours. These may occur in the jaw, and a diagnosis of giant-cell tumour of the jaw always includes a differential diagnosis of hyperparathyroidism. Other causes of hypercalcaemia include excessive vitamin D intake, renal failure, sarcoidosis, destruction of bone by metastases, and parathormone-like activity by some malignant tumours, particularly squamous cell carcinoma of the lung and other organs.

The alteration of calcium metabolism in renal failure is due to a number of reasons, in particular, impaired conversion of vitamin D metabolites, disturbance in phosphate metabolism, and complications of prolonged haemodialysis, in particular osteomalacia.

Osteomalacia

This is when there is a disproportionate amount of osteoid for a given amount of mineralized bone. It occurs when there is impairment of calcification of new osteoid. It is seen as an increase in the amount of unmineralized osteoid in undecalcified bone sections. It is primarily due to a deficiency of vitamin D, and is the adult 'version' of rickets. This deficiency may be due to poor nutrition or malabsorption in the intestines, or renal disease. If there is vitamin D deficiency in children this causes rickets. This is characterized by a bending and distortion of bones in view of softening of the bones. Causes of intestinal malabsorption include loss of small bowel due to disease, or cystic fibrosis.

Biochemical investigation shows reduced serum calcium and raised serum phosphate, reduced urinary excretion of calcium, and a raised alkaline phosphatase, which is an enzyme secreted by osteoblasts.

Osteoporosis

This is a very common disease affecting predominantly elderly women. At least 25 per cent of elderly females are affected. Effectively, it is a softening of bone due to loss of osteoid and mineralized bone in equal proportions (Figs 16.1 and 16.2). It is, therefore, a normal ratio of osteoid to mineralized bone. There is a complete reduction in bone mass. It is characterized by striking softening of the bone and an increased incidence of fractures. It is really a general imbalance between the amount of bone resorption and the amount of bone formation. It has been shown that there is normally a continual loss of bone in adults from a relatively early age. It is particularly prevalent in post-menopausal women. As well as increased incidence of fractures, there may be slow deformity and distortion of the skeleton due to compression fractures, particularly of the vertebra. These can also present as pain.

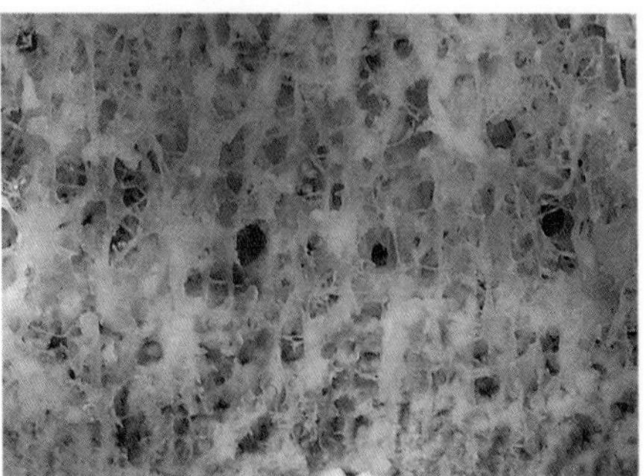

Fig. 16.1 The cut surface of osteoporotic bone as compared to normal in Fig. 16.2. Trabeculae are thinner and spaces in the bone larger.

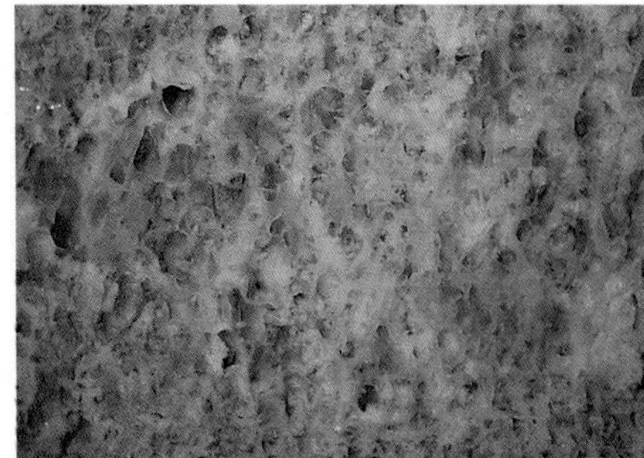

Fig. 16.2 Normal trabecular bone.

To the naked eye the bone appears more porous with trabeculae appearing much softer than normal. This can be seen particularly in the vertebral bodies and ribs. The neck of the femur is particularly prone to fracture. The cause of this reduction in bone mass is not known; there is evidence that dietary calcium supplements and oestrogens have preventative effects.

CONGENITAL DISORDERS

Some congenital conditions are described below.

Osteogenesis imperfecta

This is also known as 'brittle bone disease', and is a group of conditions where there is a genetic abnormality in the type I collagen which is the major component of osteoid. The bone is osteoporotic and very fragile with a tendency to fracture. Bones affected include the long bones and skull, although the jaw is not involved. Dentinogenesis imperfecta is a related condition of the teeth; dentine is very similar to osteoid.

Achondroplasia

This is an autosomal-dominant condition where there is a failure of normal enchondral ossification at the growth plates, with a reduction in the growth in length of long bones. The width of the bones in contrast is normal as there is no reduction in appositional growth on the sides of the bones. There is retarded growth of the skull base, with abnormal development of the maxilla leading to problems with occlusion of the teeth.

JOINT DISEASE

Osteoarthritis

This presents as pain in joints, particularly on movement and weight bearing. Osteoarthritis (also known as osteoarthrosis) particularly involves the large weight bearing joints, such as the knees, hip, and also some smaller joints such as the terminal joints of the fingers (the distal phalangeal joints). Up to a point osteoarthritis can be regarded as a 'wear and tear' phenomenon, although other mechanisms may well be involved in the development of the disease. Pathologically, the most striking feature is wearing and loss of the articular cartilage, with exposure of the underlying bone (Fig. 16.3). The underlying exposed bone may show cystic change and collapse. There is eventually severe destruction of the joint. The reduction in cartilage with effective loss of joint space can be seen on a plain X-ray. There may be protuberant growths of new bone around the affected joint. Osteoarthritis, also known as osteoarthrosis, occurs in a high proportion of the elderly, both men and women.

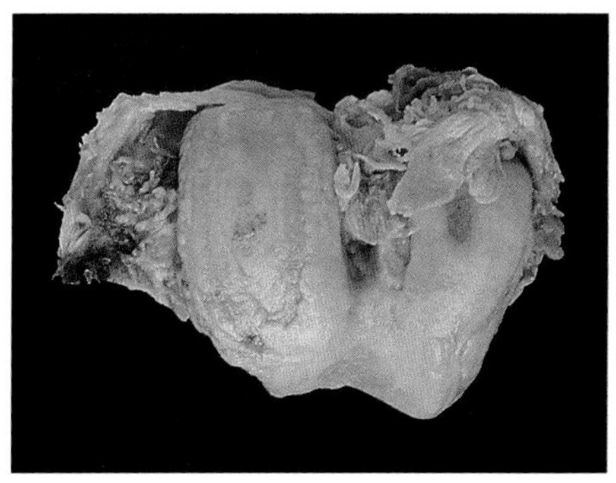

Fig. 16.3 A synovial knee joint showing osteoarthritis.

Rheumatoid arthritis

This is an example of a so-called autoimmune disease where there is an inappropriate immune reaction which particularly involves the joints, but may also occur in other organ systems. This is why the better name for this disease is rheumatoid disease, rather than rheumatoid arthritis, emphasizing the systemic

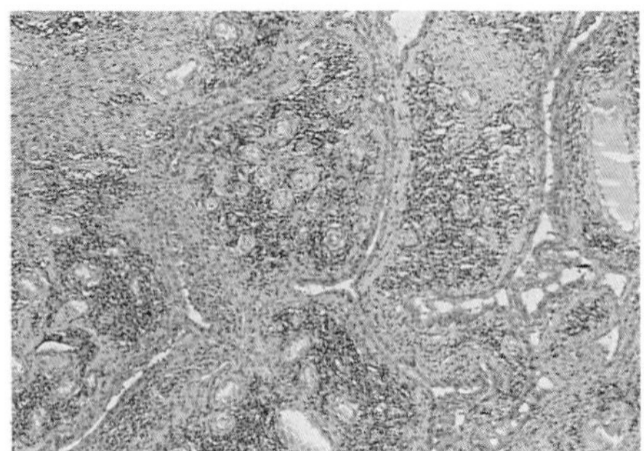

Fig. 16.4 Synovium from rheumatoid disease showing heavy chronic inflammation.

nature of the process. It is very common, affecting 1–3 per cent of the population, and occurs particularly in females. It is associated with certain HLA types, in particular DR4. Immunologically, 80 per cent of patients with rheumatoid disease show an immunoglobulin of IgM type directed against the patient's own IgG. This is known as the rheumatoid factor. Many of the immunological processes occurring in rheumatoid disease involve immune complex deposition, with complement activation. Lymphocytes and macrophages produce cytokines, such as interleukin-1 and tumour necrosis factor respectively, that are involved in the symptoms and joint destruction of rheumatoid disease. There is evidence that there is abnormal glycosylation of immunoglobulins in rheumatoid disease, allowing abnormal immunoglobulin binding. It has been suggested that Epstein–Barr virus or a parvovirus may initiate the process.

Because the arthritis is a common presenting and predominant symptom in rheumatoid disease this will be focused on.

The arthritis in rheumatoid disease is characterized by a very heavy chronic inflammatory infiltrate within the synovium and joint tissue (Fig. 16.4). The major cells seen are lymphocytes and plasma cells. Associated with this is destruction of the articular cartilage by an inflammatory mass composed of blood vessels and chronic inflammatory cells known as pannus. This chronic inflammatory infiltrate and destruction of cartilage causes very striking stiffness, pain, and swelling of joints. Joints that are predominantly involved are the hands, knees, and hip joints. In particular, the temporomandibular joints are frequently affected in up to 70 per cent of cases. Clinically, there is distortion of joints and frequent dislocation associated with distortion of associated supportive structures, such as tendons and ligaments.

The systemic nature of rheumatoid disease is supported by the association of other clinical diseases outside of the joints. In particular, these include autoimmune disease in other organs, such as the lungs, manifesting as fibrosing alveolitis. Immune complex-type vasculitis may develop in many sites, particularly in the skin. Patients may show anaemia or deposits of amyloid, representing a response to chronic disease. Patients may also develop a serious obliterative bronchiolitis in the lungs. Rheumatoid nodules may also develop in many sites, particularly the subcutis at sites of trauma, and within organs such as the lung. Sjögren's syndrome is also associated with rheumatoid arthritis, clinically seen as dry mouth and eyes due to reduced secretion of saliva and tears. On biopsy of the minor salivary glands, a lymphocytic infiltrate is frequently associated with rhematoid arthritis and Sjögen's disease. It is interesting that some manifestations of rheumatoid disease, particularly rheumatoid nodules, may precede the development of the overt disease.

Rheumatoid arthritis is a very important cause of severe disability in the elderly. Immunosuppressive treatment is frequently used. First line treatment includes anti-inflammatory drugs such as aspirin or non-steroidal anti-inflammatory agents. Other drugs that are used include immunosuppressives, such as steroids, and also empirical treatment, in particular gold. Patients with a positive rheumatoid factor (about 70 per cent of cases) have a more serious progression of disease as compared to rheumatoid factor-negative patients.

Ankylosing spondylitis

This apparent autoimmune disease is of interest because of its very close association with HLA B27 antigen. Almost 90 per cent of patients with ankylosing spondylitis are of this HLA type. Ankylosing spondylitis is a disease predominantly of males of young or middle age. Characteristically, it involves the vertebral column, although there is frequently an arthritis involving other joints. In contrast to rheumatoid arthritis it typically does not involve the hands. It is also closely associated with inflammatory bowel disease. The disease often starts in the pelvis, involving the sacro-iliac joints. There is an autoimmune chronic inflammatory process which involves ligaments and joints of the spine. There is frequently the development of joint fusion and new bone and the end result is immobility of the involved joints.

Reactive arthritis

Reiter's disease is a syndrome representing a variety of reactive arthritis which presents with arthritis, urethritis, and conjunctivitis. Lesions may also occur on the skin (palms, soles, penis) and oral mucosa.

Reactive arthritis is closely associated with urogenital or enteric infection by *Chlamydia trachomatis*, *Yersinia enterocolitica*, *Salmonella*, *Shigella*, and campylobacter. Up to 90 per cent of patients are HLA-B27 positive. The arthritis is sterile, and is probably triggered by an immune response in the joints to bacterial or chlamydial antigens.

Infective arthritis

Bacteria may infect joints. Well recognized bacteria that can cause a septic arthritis are shown in Table 16.1.

Table 16.1 Causes of infective arthritis

Staphylococcus aureus (80% of cases)
Staphylococcus albus
Streptococcus pyogenes (15–20% of cases)
Coliforms (15–20% of cases)
Salmonella (in sickle-cell anaemia)
Gonococcus (*Neisseria gonorrhoea*)
Haemophilus influenzae (particularly in children)
Tuberculosis

OSTEOMYELITIS

Osteomyelitis is acute or chronic inflammation of the bone usually due to bacterial infection. Most frequently, bacteria enter the bone substance via the bloodstream. However, there may be direct entry of bacteria to the bone if bone is exposed to the environment. For instance, bacteria may enter the ends of a bone fracture exposed to the air in a compound fracture. *Staphylococcus aureus* is a common cause of osteomyelitis in children. Tuberculosis is also a cause of osteomyelitis. In the development of osteomyelitis, bacteria frequently lodge in the area of bone towards the ends of long bones adjacent to the growth plate or epiphyseal plate. This area is known as the metaphysis, and is particularly vascular, probably explaining the vulnerability of this site to osteomyelitis. An acute inflammatory response develops with associated degeneration and necrosis of bone. This necrotic bone acts as a focus for continued infection and forms a so-called sequestrum. The adjacent periosteum shows reactive new bone formation forming an involucrum (Fig. 16.5). An overt abscess forms which may drain to the skin through a sinus opening. Effective antibiotic treatment and drainage of the abscess is essential to treat osteomyelitis.

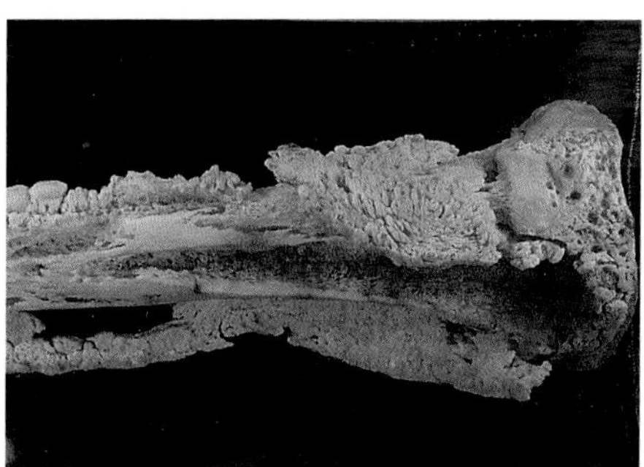

Fig. 16.5 Chronic osteomyelitis with marked new bone formation.

Osteomyelitis may involve the maxilla or mandible following tooth extraction, trauma, or a dental abscess. Previous radiotherapy may also induce osteomyelitis.

PAGET'S DISEASE

This is a disease which is characterized by a disordered proliferation and remodelling of bone which involves particularly the pelvis, spine, and tibia. The skull is also frequently involved. It has a very high incidence in some areas of the world, in particular the north-west of England. There appears to be no intrinsic abnormality of calcium metabolism, although the bone shows very marked osteoblastic activity. Histologically, there is evidence of continued bone absorption and bone formation in an irregular pattern. The actual architecture of the bone becomes disordered, bony trabeculae no longer connecting and although the bones may be thickened, they are softened and may easily deform. Bowing of the tibia, for instance, is a typical sign of Paget's disease. There may also be small fractures giving rise to bone pain, or overt fractures. Bone proliferation also causes narrowing of orifices through which nerves pass, particularly in the skull. Bone in Paget's disease passes through several stages with time. There is initially a phase of bone removal (osteolysis), followed by superimposed bone formation with distortion of the softened bone. A late phase then occurs in which the bone becomes re-formed, with a cessation of osteolysis.

The underlying cause is not known, although a viral aetiology has been suggested. Cranial nerve palsies are common in Paget's disease involving the skull. Osteosarcoma is a well-described complication of Paget's disease. The bone in Paget's disease is also extremely vascular and this probably explains the apparent heart failure that occurs in many Paget's patients.

With relevance to dentistry, Paget's disease may involve the mandible; it less frequently involves the maxilla. There may be distortion of the alveolar bone with displacement of the teeth.

BONE CYSTS

This is given a separate section because bone cysts may occur in the jaw and maxilla.

Solitary bone cyst

This lesion occurs in children and young adults in the mandible, frequently in relation to the premolar and molar teeth. The cysts appear empty on radiography, and are lined by connective tissue. This lesion may relate to trauma, although the definite cause is not known.

Aneurysmal bone cyst

This lesion may be traumatic in origin, or relate to another lesion and occurs in the mandible of young people. It is a very vascular lesion which presents as an enlarging bone mass.

BONE TUMOURS

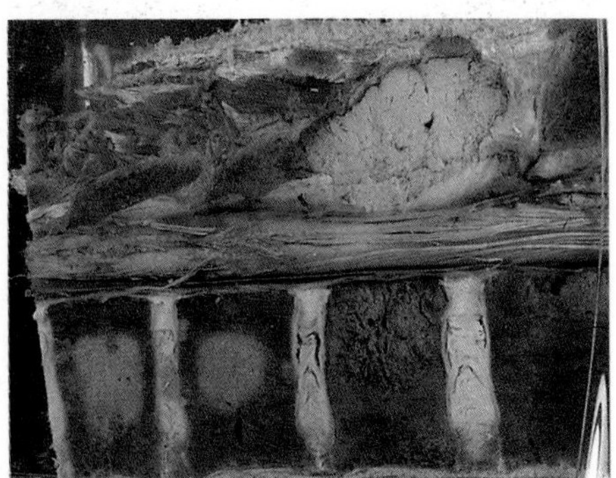

Fig. 16.6 Metastatic carcinoma in the vertebral colomn and spinal canal.

Metastatic carcinoma is the most common form of malignant bone tumour (Fig. 16.6). Common primary sites are the lung, breast, thyroid, prostate, and kidney. Primary tumours of bone are rare.

In general, the accurate diagnosis of a bone tumour is very much a clinico-pathological process. Before a diagnosis of a bone tumour is made, there is always a correlation made between the clinical findings, radiography, and available pathology. Very often the type of a bone tumour can be predicted by the site of the tumour and the age of the patient. Also there are many characteristic features of bone tumours on radiography. So, before a bone tumour is diagnosed, there must be an accurate clinical history, adequate radiographs, and relevant pathological material.

Benign tumours

Fibrous dysplasia (ossifying fibroma)

This is a locally aggressive fibrous lesion which involves ribs, the femur, tibia, skull, and frequently the jaws of children and young adults.

Giant-cell tumour

This is a tumour which has a dominant component of osteoclasts which involves long bones. This lesion is unusual in the jaw; there is a similar lesion of the jaw called a giant-cell reparative granuloma. The differential diagnosis always includes primary hyperparathyroidism giving rise to areas of excessive osteoclast activity.

Osteochondroma (bony exostosis)

This is one of the most common bone tumours and presents as a lump developing in the midpart of a long bone. It is composed of nodular cartilage overlying nodular proliferating bone. This usually occurs in young people.

Enchondroma

These are cartilagenous tumours that develop in middle-aged people and present as a diffuse swelling of a long bone. These tumours usually occur within the central part of a long bone, the medullary cavity. Histologically they are formed from mature cartilage.

Osteoid osteoma

This is a benign tumour which is a particularly structured lesion, with a central proliferating fibrovascular core with a surrounding rim of maturing bone. It commonly develops in long bones, particularly the tibia and femur. It is typically very painful.

Osteoma

This benign bony tumour composed of mature bone is relevant particularly in that it develops typically in the skull and nasal sinuses. It may occur in the mandible, or less commonly in the maxilla.

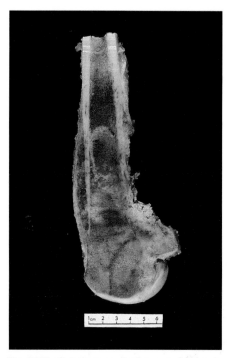

Fig. 16.7 Osteosarcoma in the upper humerus.

Malignant tumours

In view of the connective tissue nature of bone, most malignant tumours of bone are sarcomas.

Osteosarcoma

This is characterized by a tumour-forming malignant bone and typically affects young adults (Fig. 16.7). It most frequently develops in the lower femur, the upper tibia, or humerus. It occasionally occurs in the mandible. It is a very aggressive tumour which has a tendency to spread via the blood, particularly to the lungs.

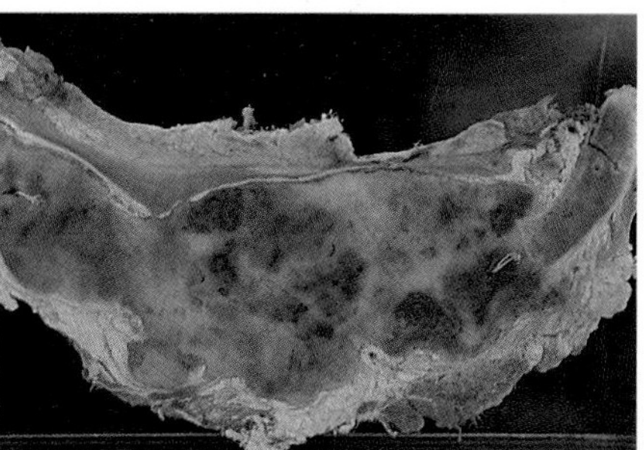

Fig. 16.8 Chondrosarcoma arising in the pelvis.

Chondrosarcoma

This is a tumour particularly of the elderly, and tends to arise in the midline, particularly in the pelvis, spine, and ribs (Fig. 16.8). It is rare in the jaws, but may occur in the maxilla and the back of the mandible.

Ewing's sarcoma

This is a very malignant tumour arising in the long bones of young people (10–30 years of age).

SUMMARY

- Bone is a composite of collagen and hydroxyapatite.
- Osteoblasts lay down bone.
- Osteoclasts resorb bone.
- Parathyroid hormone stimulates the resorption of calcium from bone and together with vitamin D increases serum calcium.
- Calcitonin acts to decrease serum calcium.

Metabolic bone disease

Hyperparathyroidism: this is over-activity of the parathyroid glands, either due to adenoma or hyperplasia. Presents with hypercalcaemia and resorption of bone.

Osteomalacia: this is decreased amount of mineralized bone with an increase of osteoid. It is primarily due to a deficiency of vitamin D. In children it presents as rickets. It may also occur with malabsorption.

Osteoporosis: this is reduction in bone mass causing bone to be soft and easily fracture. Typically occurs in elderly females. Is due to increased resorption of bone and reduced formation.

Congenital bone conditions

–osteogenesis imperfecta
–achondroplasia

Degenerative bone conditions

Osteoarthritis: this is a degenerative condition of bones characterized by reduction of cartilage within joints. It involves weight-bearing joints and probably relates to wear and tear with cartilage degradation.

Rheumatoid arthritis: a systemic autoimmune disease which shows particular manifestation within synovial joints but also involves other systems, particularly the lung and vascular system. It is of unknown cause—80 per cent of patients have a circulating antibody against IgG. Ankylosing spondylitis is a related autoimmune disease with arthritis involving the spinal joints.

Infective arthritis: this may also occur in association with systemic infection (reactive arthritis) or bacteria may directly involve joints and bone; septic arthritis or osteomyelitis develops respectively.

Paget's disease: this is of unknown cause which is characterized by very striking disordered proliferation and remodelling of bone involving particularly the pelvis, spine, and tibia. Also involves the skull. The bone shows disordered architecture and is weakened. Complications include nerve entrapment, osteosarcoma, and occasionally high volume heart failure.

Bone tumours

Benign bone tumours

–fibrous dysplasia
–giant-cell tumour
–osteochondroma
–enchondroma
–osteoid osteoma
–osteoma

Malignant tumours

–osteosarcoma
–chondrosarcoma
–Ewing's sarcoma

Metastases

Index